Pediatrics: Clinical Practice

Pediatrics: Clinical Practice

Editor: Vanessa Stevens

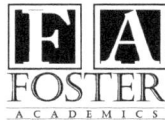

FA

FOSTER
ACADEMICS

www.fosteracademics.com

www.fosteracademics.com

FA FOSTER
ACADEMICS

Cataloging-in-Publication Data

Pediatrics : clinical practice / edited by Vanessa Stevens
    p. cm.
Includes bibliographical references and index.
ISBN 978-1-63242-776-2
1. Pediatrics. 2. Children--Diseases. 3. Children--Health and hygiene. I. Stevens, Vanessa.
RJ45 .P43 2019
618.92--dc23

Foster Academics,
118-35 Queens Blvd., Suite 400,
Forest Hills, NY 11375, USA

ISBN 978-1-63242-776-2 (Hardback)

Contents

Preface

The field of medicine associated with the care of infants, children, and adolescents is called pediatrics. An infant or neonate is significantly different from an adult in terms of physiology. During the developmental phase, genetic variance, congenital defects and developmental issues are of particular concern to pediatricians. Neonatology is a sub-field of pediatrics. It is concerned with the care of newborn infants. Neonatologists are the doctors who are specialist in this field. They usually deal with the cases of extremely ill or weak newborn infants. Some of the common medical conditions associated with neonatology include prematurity, sepsis, low birth weight, congenital malformations and birth asphyxia. Neonatal intensive care units (NICUs) are intensive care units especially designed for the care of ill and premature newborn infants. Incubators, blood pressure monitors, oxygen hoods and ventilators are some of the common equipments available in a neonatal intensive care unit. Different approaches, evaluations, methodologies and advanced studies on pediatrics have been included in this book. It brings forth some of the most innovative concepts and elucidates the unexplored aspects of pediatrics. Researchers, doctors, and students actively engaged in this field will find this book full of crucial and unexplored concepts.

The information contained in this book is the result of intensive hard work done by researchers in this field. All due efforts have been made to make this book serve as a complete guiding source for students and researchers. The topics in this book have been comprehensively explained to help readers understand the growing trends in the field.

I would like to thank the entire group of writers who made sincere efforts in this book and my family who supported me in my efforts of working on this book. I take this opportunity to thank all those who have been a guiding force throughout my life.

Editor

Child abuse and neglect in the Jaffna district of Sri Lanka – a study on knowledge attitude practices and behavior of health care professionals

M. G. Sathiadas (ID), Arunath Viswalingam and Karunya Vijayaratnam

Abstract

Background: Victims and perpetrators of child abuse do not typically self-report to child protection services, therefore responsibility of detection and reporting falls on the others. Knowledge on child protection is essential for the first contact person and such information is sparse in research literature originally coming from Sri Lanka. Anecdotally, several cases of child abuse have been missed out at the first contact level. Therefore we undertook this survey to assess the knowledge, attitudes towards child protection and the experiences of medical officers, nursing officers and social workers on child protection.

Method: This was a descriptive analytical study carried out in hospitals and the community during March–October 2016. An anonymous content validated self-administered questionnaire was used as the study instrument. Knowledge, Attitude, Practices and Behaviour were assessed via multiple choice questions and responses according to Likert score. Three anonymised case records were given as case vignettes to be studied by the participants and their responses were also recorded on the questionnaire.

Results: Among the 246 responders 156 (63.4%) were doctors. All groups of professionals identified the forms of child abuse correctly and the social indicators of child abuse was correctly identified in 152 (61.7%). Majority failed to identify the features of the perpetrator. Majority of the professionals showed a favourable response in attitude when dealing with child maltreatment. 153 (62%) had suspected child abuse in their career and 64% of them had reported it to the authority. Fifty two (21%) had attended a training workshop on child abuse and 65.8% of the responders were not satisfied with their knowledge. 229(93%) of them indicated that they wanted some form of education on child maltreatment. The Knowledge, Attitude and Behaviour towards child abuse were significantly good on people with experience in the field of Paediatrics and Judicial Medical work, when compared to those who did not have the experience in these two fields. (p value< 0.01).

Conclusion: Although the knowledge among health professionals regarding child abuse and care was satisfactory, further areas need reinforcement. The attitude was more positive, the behavior and practices on child maltreatment needed reinforcement via workshops and continuing medical education.

* Correspondence: docsathiadas@hotmail.com
Department of Paediatrics, University of Jaffna, PO Box: 57, Adiyapatham
Raod, Jaffna, Sri Lanka

Background

Child Maltreatment or Abuse has been a worldwide problem and continues to be a major crisis in our current society as well. Child maltreatment is defined by the World Health Organisation (WHO) as abuse and neglect that occurs to children under 18 years of age. It includes all types of physical, sexual abuse, neglect and negligence of the child, emotional ill treatment and exploitation for commercial and non-commercial reasons. This can lead to problems in child's health, survival and dignity of the child especially in responsibility, trust and power [1]. The National Society for the Prevention of Cruelty to Children also describes the types of abuse similarly to the WHO [2].

The physical signs of abuse may include unexplained bruising, marks or injuries on any part of the body, multiple bruises which are unexplained, cigarette burn marks, broken bones and scalds, with upward splash marks [2]. Changes in behaviour can also indicate physical abuse. The symptoms can be child's fear anticipating the parents being approached for an explanation by the autorities, aggressive behaviour or severe temper tantrums, flinching when touched, depression and withdrawn behaviour [2].

Visible evidences are seen in physical abuse whereas these are absent in emotional abuse or neglect but can leave deep, long lasting scars in their minds. When abused children get help early, their chances of recovery and healing from it is greater [3].

Most common forms of child abuse have been recorded in South Asian region and in addition to them, conscription of children during armed conflict, which is a new form of child abuse, has also been recorded especially in Sri Lanka and Nepal [4]. The 2006 UN Study on Violence against Children, estimated that in South Asia, between 41 and 88 million children witness violence at home every year. Evidence also indicates that half of the world's child brides live in South Asia, where 46% of women aged 20–24 are first married or in union before they reach the age of 18 and that around 44 million children are engaged in child labour across the region. Sexual abuse and exploitation, as well as child trafficking and corporal punishment raise additional concerns in the region. No data are provided on sexual abuse and exploitation, despite the importance of these phenomena in the region. Abuse is often not reported and is shrouded in secrecy; hence the regional data is scarce [5].

The reports on child abuse, neglect and exploitation are increasing in Sri Lanka as well. According to the figures tabled in the Sri Lankan Parliament in April 2013, there are about 15,000 legal trials pending Nationwide and more than 4,000 (27%) involve some form of violence towards a child. Around 1500 cases per year are reported for issues related to children. The same report says there were 1,750 cases of child rape, 5,475 cases of child molestation and 1,194 cases of child abuse in 2012 [6]. The number reported is much less than the actual incidence, because large number of children do not report abuse [6].

Another major reason for underreporting of child maltreatment in this region is due to the sociocultural impact it makes as most of the abuse victims are alienated and hence do not get reported. Primary caretakers from Asian countries were less likely to report the abuse to authorities when compared to the other caretakers [7, 8]. Most of the primary caretakers from Asia disbelieved child abuse, hence the children do not self-report to the carer. Discussing family problems to anyone outside the family can be considered shameful. The cultural pressures makes the victim to internalise the conflict and they are least supported. They express more suicidal impulses rather than anger and hostility [8].

Diagnosis and management of child abuse is a challenge and has to be done through a multidisciplinary approach involving medical and legal professionals. Therefore, precise knowledge on the subject of child maltreatment is essential among these professionals [9].

Events of child abuse and neglect are commonly not detected as first responders in child care fail to identify injuries, conditions, or behaviours. In the absence of timely intervention, an abused child has a 10% risk of having fatal injuries [10]. A study done in Central Gujarat India suggests that medical and dental residents are not prepared in detecting and managing children with issues related to protection [11]. A significant gap was seen in recognising and responding effectively. Mandated training on detecting and management of child abuse and neglect, to all medical and allied professionals will improve reporting of suspected child abuse [12].

It is known that victims and perpetrators of child abuse do not usually self-report to child protection services [5] Medical officers, being the first responders in most cases, are in an ideal position to report abuse. Hence, it is very important for medical officers to be familiar on medico-legal aspects of child abuse.

Therefore, the objective of this study was to describe the knowledge, attitudes and experiences of medical officers, nursing officers and social workers regarding child abuse in the Jaffna District of Sri Lanka, and to assess the associations with socio demographic factors, experience in the field of Paediatrics and Judicial Medicine towards child abuse.

Methods

Study design

This was a descriptive analytical study which was carried out in hospitals and community in the Jaffna District of Sri Lanka from March to October 2016.

Setting

The Jaffna District, Sri Lanka is situated in the North of Sri Lanka and has one tertiary care centre and three general hospitals. The tertiary care centre has specialists care and receives referrals from all the general hospitals. All these hospitals together, cater for the entire population of 610,640. [13] and would see approximately 200,000 per annum at the outpatient and emergency departments. Children seen for child abuse at the peripheral units also get referred to the tertiary unit for specialised care.

Participants

Simple random sampling was done among the doctors, nurses in all 4 hospitals and social workers from the community. This included, all the medical and dental officers (includes Consultants, Senior Registrars, Registrars, Senior House Officers (SHO), Resident House Officer (RHO), Intern Medical Officers (IMO)) and Nursing Officers working in different hospitals. Social workers are personals who work mainly in the community and play a role in identifying child abuse and neglect in the field.

Sample size was calculated using the Daniel [14] formula and the p was 13% according to Starling et al. [15]. Level of confidence was 95% with z being 1.96 and the non-response rate was 20%. This gave a total sample size of 208, enough to obtain a 95% confidence interval that the results could be generalised to a wider population [15].

As there was definite sampling frame, a simple random sampling was done. Eligible sample of participants were informed and a written informed consent was obtained. Ethical approval was obtained from Faculty of Medicine, University of Jaffna, Sri Lanka. (J/ERC/16/72/NDR/0143).

Data collection and analysis

An anonymous pre-tested and standardised self-administered questionnaire was used as the study instrument. The questionnaire included questions to assess the socio-demographic factors of medical, nursing and social workers. The 24-item questions were in the native language comprising of multiple choice or true false format based on the literature, to assess the knowledge, and a 10 item questions to assess the attitude. A field test was conducted with 10 experts in the field of child abuse to measure the content validity. Content Validity Ratio (CVR) was calculated using Lawshe's formula $CVR = (N_e - N/2)/(N/2)$, in which the N_e is the number of panellists indicating "essential" and N is the total number of panellists [16]. The CVR for the whole questionnaire was 0.80. The questionnaire was modified as per the expert suggestions, and the modified version was used as the study tool.

Three case vignettes were prepared from anonymised case records. The cases were physical abuse, sexual abuse and neglect based on delay in seeking medical help. These case histories were given in paper format and confidence in the story was assessed on a 5 point scale (1 being not confidant and 5 being very confident) and reporting and taking action on the individual cases was assessed by "yes"/ "no" responses. Cronbach alpha was used to assess the reliability of the scores.

To assess the knowledge, questions regarding types of child abuse, identifying features of abuse and characteristics of the perpetrator were considered. Questions were analysed by responses to each of the question separately and were expressed as percentage. Chi-square test for significance of difference among proportions was calculated.

To assess the attitude of the participants regarding child abuse and neglect, each respondent was asked 10-item questions.. Responses were recorded as "strongly agree" or "disagree", or "somewhat agree" or "disagree", or "don't know"/ "can't say". Depending on whether it was a proper attitude or not, scores from 1 to 4 were allotted. A score of '0' was given for "don't know"/ "can't say". Six items had negative statements and they were allocated the reverse scores. A total 40 was then divided into sub scores which were defined as 0–9 Very Poor, 10–18 considered as there are many issues which need changing, 19–27 as more positive attitudes and 28–40 as having a good overall attitude. Analysis of variance for significance of difference among means was calculated and Cronbach alpha was used to assess the reliability of the scores.

To assess the experiences of participants, five questions in the questionnaire were provided and the responses were expressed as percentage. Each respondent was asked if s/he undertook any particular action in the previous year that would help towards having better practices.

The data was described using frequencies and percentages. P value of < 0.05 was considered as statistically significant. Data was coded and entered in SPSS version 20.

Results

A Total of 273 were selected for the survey and number of responders was 246(90.1%). Among the responders, 156 (63.4%) were medical officers, 59 (24%) were nursing officers and others were social workers. Mean age of the subjects was 34.70 ± 7.924 yrs. Male female ratio was 1:1.29. Most of them (149–60.6%) were married, 108 (43.7%) had experience less than 5 years in their respective fields and 107 (43.5%) had children of their own. The characteristics of the responders along with their experiences in the profession are provided in Table 1. Among those in the medical profession 33(21.2%) were intern medical officers, who were the first contact in most of the cases when a patient is admitted, 19(12.2%) were consultants and 104(66.7%) belonged to the middle grade, whose experience varied from 1.5–15 years.

Table 1 Characteristics of the responders and their experience

Feature		Medical officers (N = 156)	Nursing officers (N = 59)	Social and probation (N = 31)
Age (years)	26–30	73(46.8%)	26(44.1%)	2(6.4%)
	31–35	36(23.1%)	11(18.6%)	11(35.5%)
	36–40	21(13.5%)	4(6.8%)	10(32.3%)
	> 40	26(16.7%)	18(30.5%)	8(25.8%)
Gender	Male	77 (49.4%)	18 (30.5%)	12 (38.7%)
	Female	79(50.6%)	41(69.5%)	19(61.3%)
Experience (years)	0–4.9	76(48.7%)	22(37.3%)	10(32.3%)
	5–9.9	36(23.1%)	16(27.1%)	10(32.3%)
	> 10	44(28.2%)	21(35.6%)	11(35.5%)
Marital Status	Single	67(42.9%)	23(39%)	7(22.6%)
	Married	89(57.1%)	36(61%)	24(77.4%)
Having children	Yes	62(39.7%)	26(44.1%)	19(61.3%)
	No	94(60.3%)	33(55.9%)	12(438.7%)
Experience in paediatrics and judicial work	Yes	69(44.2%)	21(35.6%)	0(0%)
	No	87(55.8%)	38(64.4%)	0(0%)

Knowledge of the responders

All groups of professionals were able to identify the forms of child abuse correctly and there was no significant difference between the groups, except on seeking timely medical advice. Frequency of identifying the types of child abuse is provided in Table 2.

The knowledge of the social indicators of child abuse was correctly identified by 152 (61.7%). The knowledge on the features of the perpetrators was satisfactory in 74%($n = 182$). The knowledge of the perpetrator being known to the family was identified in 75%($n = 187$), perpetrator being abused as a child in 62%($n = 153$) and having a psychiatry background in 61%($n = 152$). There was no significant difference between the groups in the identifying features of the perpetrators. (p value > 0.5).

Knowledge of the physical indicators was satisfactory in all groups of health workers. (Table 3).

The three case vignettes were mainly of child physical abuse, sexual abuse and seeking delayed medical help (Neglect). All categories of people identified the type of abuse correctly. Cronbach alpha was 0.81 in confidence in reporting, suggesting good internal consistency. The mean scores for confidence in reporting were 2.7, 3.1 and 1.4 for

cases of physical, sexual abuse and neglect respectively. The differences in the mean scores also had a significant difference between the groups. (P value < 0.001) The decision to report to the authority was 90% ($n = 222$) in the case of physical abuse, 97% ($n = 240$) in sexual abuse and 65% ($n = 160$) in the case of neglect. The decision to report was significant between the groups in dealing with the case of neglect (*p value < 0.001*) but not in physical and sexual abuse. (*p values > 0.5*) Experience in the field of paediatrics and judicial work did not have a significant association in identification and reporting of the cases given in the case vignettes.

The source of knowledge was mainly through the university education system (54.1%) followed by reading the literature (52.8%) and following Continuing Medical Education (CME) programme on child abuse (41.1%).

Attitude of the responders

Mean attitude scores were 20.16 ± 3.3, 20.25 ± 4.04, 23.84 ± 5.3 for doctors, nurses and social-workers respectively. (F = 12.55 $p = 0.000$) Even though the majority of the professionals showed a more positive attitude, there are many issues that need changing. (Table 4) Majority

Table 2 Frequency of identifying type of abuse

Type of child abuse or neglect	Medical officers (N = 156)	Nursing officers (N = 59)	Social workers (N = 31)	X^2 (p value)
Failure to seek needed medical treatment	148(94.9%)	39(69.6%)	30(96.8%)	36.58 (p = 0.000)
Neglect of child education	147(94.2%)	53(89.8%)	31(100%)	3.751 ($p = 0.153$)
Beating causing injury	139(89.1%)	55(93.2%)	31(100%)	4.240 ($p = 0.120$)
Non-injurious spanking	110(70.5%)	39(66.1%)	16(51.6%)	4.216 ($p = 0.121$)
Verbal humiliation	139(89.1%)	54(91.5%)	31(100%)	3.792 ($p = 0.150$)
Sexual abuse	148(94.8%)	57(96.6%)	31(100%)	1.835 ($p = 0.400$)

Table 3 Knowledge of the physical indicators

Question	True	False	Not responded
Bruising over bony prominence is an indication of abuse	142(57.7%)	98[a](39.8%)	06(2.4%)
Burns are associated with abuse	148[a](60.1%)	90(36.5%)	08(3.25%)
Bite marks on the shoulder be investigated for child abuse	107[a](43.49%)	79(32.1%)	60(24.3%)
Child expresses fear of going home after a period in the hospital	213[a](86.5%)	31(12.6%)	02(0.8%)
A history that is vague and defers each time tells it is a possible indicator of abuse	172[a](69.9%)	72(29.2%)	02(0.8%)
Torn frenulum indicates child sexual abuse	76(30.9%)	68[a](27.6%)	102(41.4%)
Sexualised behaviour in the child may be due to sexual abuse	146[a](59.5%)	97(39.4%)	03(1.2%)

[a]correct answer

(76.4%) were confident in reporting child abuse and 24% said they would defer reporting until firm evidence was present. 60.5% were confident in giving evidence in a court of law and 45% were not familiar with the legal issues. Only 24.3% were satisfied with the local child protection services (Table 5).

Practices and behaviour

Majority of the professionals (62%) suspected child abuse in children and only 64% had reported child abuse to the authorities previously. All the cases suspected were not reported to the authorities and the main reasons provided being: Lack of adequate history and evidence (56,6.1%), uncertainty of the diagnosis (55, 22.3%), possible harmful effects on the child's family (31, 12.6%), lack of knowledge of the referral procedure (25, 10.1%), aggressive and angry parents (15, 6.1%), possible effect on my professional career (13, 5.28%) and fear and anxiety of the court proceedings (11, 4.47%).

All the professionals indicated that education on child protection is essential but only 52(21%) had attended training workshops on child abuse. Different practices adopted by the professionals are provided in Table 6.

Analysis of the data showed knowledge regarding child abuse (p 0.001), knowledge of the characteristics of the perpetrator (p 0.04), attitude of more positivity towards Child abuse and neglect (*p* value 0.01), behaviour of detecting and reporting of child abuse and neglect (p 0.001) and the awareness of the law of child protection had a significant differences with the experience of the person and the speciality of paediatrics and judicial medical work. The

inexperienced felt that the doctor was responsible for the stigma that occurred to these children (p 0.001).

The participants have indicated that the preferred methods of updating the knowledge on child abuse and neglect were to undertake continuing education and workshops on child abuse (70.3%) followed by information booklets (48%) and online self-study (28.5%).

Discussion

Our study aimed at identifying the knowledge and practices of professionals, first in contact with the children who have been abused and neglected. Our study indicated satisfactory overall knowledge and it correlated well with the experience and speciality of the responders. Awareness and Basic knowledge on child abuse and neglect are the important prerequisite for reporting suspected cases of child abuse. The ability to detect and diagnose when an abused child presents, is also vital to the care of the child. When compared to studies done in Gujarat and Karnataka in India, our study indicates overall knowledge is satisfactory [11, 17].

The knowledge regarding indicators of abuse was unsatisfactory as only 68(27.6%) answered all seven responses correctly. The torn oral fraenum was identified as a form of abuse earlier but in current literature it has been disproved [18]. In this study the torn fraenum was identified as a form of abuse by 76% of the responders. This study indicates that there may be a deficiency of updated knowledge about changes to these concepts. Thomas et al. [19] have explained that this lack of

Table 4 Attitude scores in health professionals

	Medical officers (N = 156)	Nursing officers (N = 59)	Social workers (N = 31)	Total	Statistical analysis
Mean attitude score	20.16 ± 3.3	20.2 ± 4.0	23.84 ± 5		F (2,243) = 12.55 $p = 0.000$[a]
Issues need changing (10–18)	51(32.7%)	17(28.8%)	8(25.8%)	76(30.9%)	X²(4,N = 246) = 30.3 $p = 0.001$[b]
More positive attitudes (19–27)	101(64.7%)	41(69.5%)	15(48.4%)	157(63%)	
Good feeling overall (28–36)	4(2.6%)	1(1.7%)	8(25.8%)	13(5.3%)	

[a]Analysis of variance for significance of difference among means
[b]Chi-square test for significance of difference among proportions
Crohnbach alpha 0.74

Table 5 Attitude towards child abuse

Attitudes	Positive Responses			ANOVA
	Medical officers (N = 156)	Nursing officers (N = 59)	Social workers (N = 31)	
Professional is responsible for the stigma that occurs to the family[b]	74(30.1%)	27(11.0%)	11(4.5%)	F(2,243) = 4.933 (p = 0.008)
Confidence in reporting child abuse[a]	112(45.5%)	50(20.3%)	26(10.6%)	F(2,243) = 1.443 (p = 0.238)
Confident in giving evidence in a court of law[a]	93(37.8%)	33(13.4%)	23(9.3%)	F(2,243) = 1.443 (p = 0.136)
Not familiar with the legal issues[b]	77(31.3%)	27(11.0%)	7(2.8%)	F(2,243) = 6.220 (p = 0.002)
Reported only if persistence of abuse[b]	19(7.7%)	6(2.4%)	3(1.2%)	F(2,243) = 1.548 (p = 0.215)
Defer reporting if no firm evidence[b]	43(17.5%)	10(4.1%)	6(2.4%)	F(2,243) = 7.344 (p = 0.001)
Satisfaction with the local child protection services[a]	27(11.0%)	20(8.1%)	13(5.3%)	F(2,243) = 3.580 (p = 0.029)
The child should be removed from home and familiar surroundings[b]	19(7.7%)	30(12.2%)	8(3.3%)	F(2,243) = 16.422 (p = 0.000)
Change the school is advised in abused children[b]	44(17.9%)	33(13.4%)	11(4.5%)	F(2,243) = 6.803 (p = 0.001)

[a]Positive attitude
[b]Negative attitude

updated knowledge may arise from the failure of reinforcement in the clinical setting of knowledge gained in the undergraduate classroom.

The knowledge among the medical doctors and nurses was higher when compared to the social workers about various types of abuse and physical indicators. Even though it was statistically not significant, the community social workers should have adequate knowledge of child abuse for early detection, which would prevent detrimental effects [20].

The perpetrators of Child Sexual Abuse (CSA) are usually known to the family and may have been also abused as child. This fact should be understood clearly by all healthcare professionals to prevent future perpetrators from initiating abuse [21]. In our study 23% (57) did not know the characteristic features of the perpetrators. Hence further training is needed in this aspect.

The responses to the case vignettes highlight the current knowledge and course of action. Case vignettes on physical and sexual abuse the responders were

Table 6 Practices and behaviour of the professionals in child protection

	Medical officers (N = 156)	Nursing officers (N = 59)	Social workers (N = 31)	X^2 (p value)
Suspect CAN	96(61.5%)	28(47.4%)	28(90.3%)	15.827 (p = 0.001)
Report CAN	74(47.4%)	23(39.0%)	27(87%)	20.324 (p = 0.001)
Aware of process of reporting	114(73.1%)	38(64.4%)	28(90.3%)	6.955 (p = 0.031)
Awareness of Sri Lankan laws	92(60.0%)	22(37.3%)	23(74.2%)	13.080 (p = 0.001)
Importance of child abuse education	156(100%)	58(98%)	31(100%)	4.743 (p = 0.315)
Attended training on CAN	13(8.3%)	16(27.1%)	23(74.2%)	68.956 (p = 0.001)
Self-satisfaction of knowledge	45(28.8%)	21(35.6%)	18(58.1%)	9.890 (p = 0.007)
Wish to improve the knowledge	150(96.2%)	54(91.5%)	25(80.6%)	9.964 (p = 0.010)

confident and the course of action of reporting was 90. 2% in physical abuse and 97.5% in sexual abuse. Van Haeringen et al. [9] stated that only 69% of the health professionals reported the highest level of suspected physical abuse where as our study indicated the opposite. Case vignette of a delay in seeking medical help and neglect had the minimum score with minimum number (65%) reporting it to the authorities.

The keenness to improve the knowledge has been shown by all the professionals by indicating their interest to improve their knowledge base and interest in attending a continuing medical programme and workshops on Child abuse. The interest to be trained is a good initiative to detect child abuse and possibilities towards future introduction of screening for child abuse and neglect at emergency and outpatient settings [22].

The attitude towards more positive and good were seen in 69% of the responders and this is similar (65.5%) to a study done in Karnataka by Kirankumar et al. [17]. Attitudes towards reporting child abuse are another aspect that was studied. A suspected case of child abuse and neglect has to be reported to the authorities without delay but this can be traumatic to the parents, carers and the health care professionals. Since the stigma involved in abuse is profound in this part of the world where reporting can be a serious issue. Our study also indicated that the responders had suspected but not reported due to various reasons. This may have been due to lack of adequate history and evidence, uncertainty of the diagnosis, possible harmful effects on the child's family, lack of knowledge of the referral procedure, aggressive and angry behaviour of parents, possible effect on the profession and fear and anxiety toward possible court proceedings. Similar fears were also noted in the study done by Deshapande et al. in Gujarat [11].

A study done by Jones et al. [23] on child abuse reporting experience, found that even at the highest levels of suspicion, only 73% of injuries were reported to child protective services and many factors hindered the reporting. This includes the clinician's level of closeness with the family, some issues in the history and the expectations of the child protection services. In our study the health professionals indicated they were either not satisfied with the services or were not aware of the availability of the services. Training and continuing medical education along with a support system to overcome the fears can alleviate this problem. In addition, strengthening the child protection services and making health providers aware of the existence of the services, can improve child abuse being detected and reported early.

Behaviour and practices by the health care professionals towards child abuse also plays a major role in identifying cases of abuse. The need to improve the knowledge is clearly stated in our study which indicates

the professionals are committed to learn and improve the services rendered. Our study found several gaps especially in the reporting system and the awareness of the existing law. All felt the importance of the issue as 99. 5% indicated that education regarding child abuse was important. Even though they felt the importance, only 21.1% had attended a workshop or CME on child abuse and neglect. This was also identified in the study by Reiniger et al [12]. Modern methods of CME like on-line courses may be more appropriate in this fast moving modern world.

Self-awareness of the level of knowledge on child abuse and neglect is important for further improvements in knowledge. Our study states that 65.8% of the responders were not satisfied with their knowledge and 93% of them indicated they wanted some form of CME on abuse. It is reported that physicians in rural regions of Austria possessed basic knowledge on child abuse but were not aware of the referral system [24]. To improve diagnosis, reporting, strengthening the interaction with experts and to reduce fears in handling child abuse victim, better training is needed.

In regards to the practices of child abuse, some responders had misbeliefs, mainly in the aspect of removing the child from home (63%) after the incident irrespective of the situation that it took place. They also indicated to remove the child from the school as the family may face social isolation (35.7%). This practice can be detrimental to the child. Significant and lifelong adverse effects on the child's mental health and development are seen in all forms of abuse. Support is needed not only medically, but also in psychosocial aspect, for the speedy recovery of the child. A child's experience of maltreatment may cause great stress and disruption in the family and making them feel guilty about what has already occurred in the home. There is a chance that other members in the family too may have been affected. Health professionals also feel the stigma in the family and society and thereby inappropriate decisions like moving the child away from home and school has been suggested as a way of management.

Experience in the field of paediatrics and Judicial medical work indicated that the knowledge, attitude and behaviour towards child abuse and neglect were good when compared to the professionals in other specialities. As the experienced person is not the first contact person, it is mandatory to train the first responder on child abuse [8].

This study has few strengths and limitations. The random sampling technique has minimised the selection bias. The questionnaire was self-administered hence the issues that arise from face to face were overcome. The questionnaire was tested for content validity, but we were not able to perform the Pearson's product moment correlation coefficient as the field experts were contacted only once, and the time tested second administration was not performed due to practical difficulties and unavailability of the experts. Even though this is a descriptive analytical study, a qualitative study or a mixed method study could have assessed the attitude and practices of child abuse better. This study can be generalised to the South Asian region as it involves a large number of responders both from the clinical and community level who belong to the same socio-cultural background.

Conclusion

The results reveal that the knowledge, attitude and behaviour of the different health care professionals are satisfactory with few deficiencies, mainly in the areas of identifying the perpetrator and the decision they will take in the case of neglect. All the groups felt their knowledge was satisfactory and wanted to further their knowledge through various continuing medical programmes. The experience and professionals involved in child care and judicial work had a statistically significant good knowledge, attitude and behaviour regarding child abuse.

There were barriers in reporting despite a legal requirement; hence support of the child protection services and the effectiveness of these services need to be evaluated. The gap between detecting and reporting can be overcome by improving the knowledge base.

Understanding and clinical competencies in detecting child abuse are crucial knowledge and skills that are required to evaluate the effectiveness of curricula and the programmes involved in CME, in preparing future healthcare professionals to identify, manage and prevent child abuse. A regular check on the outcome of the education has to be assessed and improvements must be made according to latest evidences. Professional education programmes must sensitise all health care professionals of the occurrences and instruct them on how and when to report a suspected case of child abuse and neglect.

Abbreviations
CME: Continuing medical education; CSA: Child sexual abuse; IMO: Intern medical officer; RHO: Resident house officer; SHO: Senior house officer; WHO: World Health Organisation

Acknowledgements
The authors thank all the responders who participated in the study.

Funding
Self-funded by the researchers.

Authors' contributions
MGS - Designed and developed the protocol, monitored data collection, reviewed and revised the manuscript and approved the final document, AV - Data collection, analysis and approved the final manuscript and KV - Data collection, manuscript preparation and approved the final manuscript.

Competing interests
The authors declare that they have no competing interests.

References
1. WHO fact sheet on child abuse 2017. http://www.who.int/en/news-room/fact-sheets/detail/child-maltreatment. Accessed 15 Aug 2017.
2. National Society for the Prevention of Cruelty to Children (NSPCC), Child Protection Fact Sheet, definitions and signs of abuse April 2009; https://www.ncl.ac.uk/studentambassadors/assets/documents/NSPCCDefinitionsandsignsofchildabuse.pdf. Accessed 12 July 2017.
3. Kudagammana S. Defining and comprehending child abuse at present times. An appraisal. Sri Lanka J Forensic Med Sci Law. 2011;1(2):28–32. https://doi.org/10.4038/sljfmsl.v1i2.2726.
4. De Silva H. Children needing protection – experience from South Asia. Arch Dis Child. 2007;92:931–4. https://doi.org/10.1136/adc.2006.101196.
5. UNICEF report on violence against children in South Asia. https://books.google.lk/books?id=hwdQDQAAQBAJ&pg=PA313&lpg=PA313&dq=UNICEF+report+on+violence+against+children+in+South+Asia.+https://www.unicef.org/+rosa/protection_7735.htm.&source=bl&ots=XOe2ZOq0F4&sig=_6YD4NfzC6mwbM9LstuKcaqi9S8&hl=en&sa=X&ved=0ahUKEwiZlrjj9eraAhVEPo8KHc7AAUAQ6AEILzAC#v=onepage&q=UNICEF%20report%20on%20violence%20against%20children%20in%20South%20Asia.%20https%3A%2F%2Fwww.unicef.org%2Frosa%2Fprotection_7735.htm.&f=false. Accessed 26 Mar 2018.
6. UNICEF 2013 report on violence against children, https://www.unicef.org/srilanka/VAC(3).pdf. Accessed 20 June 2017.
7. Browne A, Finkelhor D. Impact of child sexual abuse: a review of the research. Psychol Bull. 1996;99:66–77.
8. Rao K, DiClemente RJ, Ponton LE. Child sexual abuse of Asians compared with other populations. J Am Acad Child Adolesc Psychiatry. 1992;31(5):880–6.
9. Van Haeringen AR, Dadds M, Armstron KL. The child abuse lottery-will the doctor suspect and report? Physician attitudes towards and reporting of suspected child abuse and neglect. Child Abuse Negl. 1998;22(3):159–69.
10. Kinght B, Saukko P. Knight's forensic pathology. 3rd ed: Edward Arnold publishers; 2004. ISBN: 978 0 340 76044 4, ch22 fatal child abuse, pp 462-479
11. Deshapande A, Macwan C, Poonach KS, Bargale S, Dhillon S, Porwal P. Knowledge and attitude in regards to physical child abuse amongst medical and dental residents of Central Gujarat: a cross-sectional survey. Journal of Indian Society of pedodontics and preventive dentistry. 2015; 33(3):177–82.
12. Reiniger A, Robinson E, McHugh M. Mandated training of professionals: a means for improving reporting of suspected child abuse. Child Abuse Negl. 1995;19(1):63–9.
13. http://www.jaffna.dist.gov.lk/index.php?option=com_content&view=article&id=145&Itemid=244&lang=en. Accessed 3 Apr 2018.
14. Daniel WW. Biostatistics: a Foundation for Analysis in the health sciences. 7th ed. New York: John Wiley & Sons; 1999.
15. Starling S, Heisler K, Paulson J, Youmans E. Child abuse training and knowledge: a National Survey of emergency medicine, family medicine, and pediatric residents and program directors. Pediatrics. 2009;123(4):e595–602.
16. Lawshe CH. A quantitative approach to content validity. Pers Psychol. 1975; 28:563–75.
17. Kirankumar SV, Noorani H, Shivprakash PK, Sinha S. Medical professional perception, attitude, knowledge and experience about child abuse and neglect in Bangalkot district of North Karnataka: a survey report. J. Indian Soc. Pedod. Prev. Dent. 2011;29(3):193–7.
18. Maguire S, Hunter B, Hunter L, Sibert JR, Mann M, Kemp AM, for the Welsh Child Protection Systematic Review Group. Diagnosing abuse: a systematic review of torn frenum and other intra-oral injuries. Arch Dis Child. 2007;92: 1113–7. https://doi.org/10.1136/adc.2006.113001.
19. Thomas H, Straffon L, Inglehart MR. Child abuse and neglect: dental and dental hygiene students educational experiences and knowledge. J Dent Educ. 2006;70:558–65.
20. Dias A, Sales L, Hessen DJ, Kleber RJ. Child maltreatment and psychological symptoms in a Portuguese adult community sample: the harmful effects of emotional abuse. Eur. Child Adolesc. Psychiatry. 2015;24(7):767–78.
21. McGee H, O'Higgins M, Garavan R, Conroy R. Rape and child sexual abuse. J. Interpers. Violence. 2011;26(17):3580–93. https://doi.org/10.1177/0886260511403762.
22. Louwers ECFM, Korfage IJ, Affourtit MJ, et al. Detection of child abuse in emergency departments: a multi-Centre study. Arch Dis Child. 2011;96:422–5.
23. Rise J, Flaherty EG, Binns HJ, Price LL, Slora E, Abney D, Harris DL, Christoffel KK, Sege RD. Clinicians' description of factors influencing their reporting of suspected child abuse: report of the child abuse reporting experience study research group. Pediatrics. 2008;122(2):259–66. https://doi.org/10.1542/peds.2007-2312.

2

Effectiveness of Cognitive Orientation to daily Occupational Performance over and above functional hand splints for children with cerebral palsy or brain injury

Michelle Jackman[1,2*], Iona Novak[1,3], Natasha Lannin[4], Elspeth Froude[5], Laura Miller[6] and Claire Galea[3]

Abstract

Background: Functional hand splinting is a common therapeutic intervention for children with neurological conditions. The aim of this study was to investigate the effectiveness of the Cognitive Orientation to daily Occupational Performance (CO-OP) approach over and above conventional functional hand splinting, and in combination with splinting, for children with cerebral palsy or brain injury.

Methods: A multisite, assessor-blinded, parallel, randomized controlled trial was conducted in Australia. Participants ($n = 45$) were randomly allocated to one of three groups; (1) splint only ($n = 15$); (2) CO-OP only ($n = 15$); (3) CO-OP + splint ($n = 15$). Inclusion: age 4–15 years; diagnosis of cerebral palsy or brain injury; Manual Ability Classification System I–IV; hand function goals; sufficient language, cognitive and behavioral ability. Primary outcome measures were the Canadian Occupational Performance Measure (COPM) and Goal Attainment Scale (GAS). Treatment duration for all groups was 2 weeks. CO-OP was provided in a group format, 1 h per day for 10 consecutive weekdays, with parents actively involved in the group. Hand splints were wrist cock-up splints that were worn during task practice. Three individual goals were set and all participants were encouraged to complete a daily home program of practicing goals for 1 h. Analyses were conducted on an intention to treat basis.

Results: The COPM showed that all three groups improved from baseline to immediately post-treatment. GAS showed a statistically significant difference immediately post-intervention between the splint only and CO-OP only groups $p = 0.034$), and the splint only and CO-OP + splint group ($p = 0.047$) favoring CO-OP after controlling for baseline.

Conclusions: The CO-OP Approach™ appeared to enhance goal achievement over and above a functional hand splint alone. There was no added benefit of using hand splints in conjunction with CO-OP, compared to CO-OP alone. Hand splints were not well tolerated in this population. Practice of functional goals, through CO-OP or practice at home, leads to goal achievement for children with cerebral palsy or brain injury.

Keywords: Upper limb, Task-specific training, Motor training, Cognition, Orthoses, Goal-directed, Occupational therapy

* Correspondence: Michelle.jackman@hnehealth.nsw.gov.au
[1]School of Child and Adolescent Medicine, The University of Sydney, Sydney, Australia
[2]Occupational Therapy Department, John Hunter Children's Hospital, Newcastle, Australia
Full list of author information is available at the end of the article

Background

Cerebral palsy (CP) and brain injury (BI) can significantly impair a child's ability to use their hands [1]. Therapeutic modalities to improve hand function have progressed significantly over the past 20 years, and there is now a substantial body of evidence to support task-specific upper limb (UL) training interventions in this population [2, 3]. In clinical practice, usual care includes functional hand splinting to promote functional hand use. We wanted to know, whether or not, "Cognitive Orientation to Occupational Performance (CO-OP)", a new task-specific intervention for the cerebral palsy and brain injury populations, had any clinical benefits over and above functional hand splinting. There also remains limited empirical evidence regarding whether combining UL therapies has any additive effect [2, 3]. We therefore sought to measure the combined effect.

Functional splints are worn when performing an activity, with the aim of supporting one or more joints to maximize the function of the UL during a task. Within the International Classification of Functioning, Disability and Health (ICF) [4], functional splints are a 'body function and structure' and 'environmental' intervention which aims to support changes in activities by changing the position of the hand. Functional splints are made from various materials, including, but not limited to, neoprene, Lycra™, thermoplastic or tape. Common examples of functional hand splints are a wrist cock-up splint to assist with cutlery use during meal times, a supination splint to assist with catching a ball or a thumb abduction splint to assist with pencil grasp during handwriting [5]. There are a small number of randomized trials investigating functional hand splints [6–10], although there are wide variations in the type of splints investigated, quality of evidence and reliability of outcome measures used in these studies [11]. Functional splints, like many interventions used with children with CP and BI, are often used in combination with other interventions including task-specific training.

Task-specific training is a term used to describe a group of interventions that involve active use of the UL [3]. In the pediatric neurological population, there is high level evidence to support the use of task-specific training, including approaches such as constraint-induced movement therapy (CIMT) and bimanual training [2, 3, 12]. The Cognitive Orientation to daily Occupational Performance (CO-OP) [13] is another task-specific training option. The CO-OP Approach™ combines both motor learning theories with cognitive approaches [14], and shares many of the key ingredients of task-specific training [15] with the important and unique feature of individual child-led problem-solving and strategy choice. In CO-OP, children set their own therapy goals and are guided to discover and develop their own cognitive strategies for successfully carrying out the goal, through the use of the global problem-solving strategy "goal-plan-do-check" [14]. Children are guided to discover their own successful strategies for carrying out a task, instead of the therapist selecting a successful strategy from task analysis and training task performance, which is the convention in other forms of task-specific training. Once a successful strategy has been discovered by the child, children are encouraged to practice the task consistently, as is done in other task-specific UL approaches, in order to bring about the neuroplastic changes in function that underpin motor learning [16]. CO-OP is conventionally carried out over 12 weekly individual therapy sessions, as per the inventor's recommendations. The CO-OP Approach™ has been piloted in children with CP and BI [13, 17, 18] although there exists limited high level evidence in this population.

The theoretical underpinnings of splinting and CO-OP are very different. When considered in light of the ICF, CO-OP is directly focused on addressing 'activities', through cognitive and training strategies, whilst splinting is focused on addressing the 'impairment' with the aim of improving function. It is therefore important to explore which of these interventions is most effective, and whether or not there is benefit to combining such interventions. There are currently three different theories that seek to explain the relationship between functional splints and task-specific training. One theory is that a functional splint will allow the user to carry out a task more effectively immediately, with a carry-over effect once the skill is learnt and the splint removed. Another theory is that a functional splint will in fact inadvertently hinder active movement of the limb during task practice, which is vital in the motor learning process. Finally, the "orthotic effect" theory, where the splint is considered to have a neutral effect on motor learning and improved function. The splint improves function when donned, but does not facilitate learning, nor does it inhibit learning. All three theories are currently untested.

The aim of this randomized controlled trial (RCT) was to investigate whether the CO-OP Approach™ led to greater achievement of goals for children with CP or BI over and above conventional splinting alone or when used in combination. The hypotheses for this trial were (1) Children with CP or BI who received CO-OP combined with a splint will achieve comparable improvements in goal achievement and hand function when compared to children who receive CO-OP alone, (2) Children with CP or BI who participate in CO-OP alone will achieve clinically significant changes in goal achievement when compared to children who receive a splint alone.

Our study rationale was that historically therapists sought to induce functional goal achievement using 'impairment' interventions (e.g. splinting), whereas newer paradigms preferentially recommend 'activities' interventions (e.g. CO-OP or task-specific training). Our hypotheses sought to examine the relative effectiveness of these two different paradigms within the same study.

Method

Design and sample size

We conducted a single-blinded RCT that was registered with the Australian New Zealand Clinical Trials Register (ACTRN12613000690752). Detailed study procedures have been previously published [19]. Sample size power calculations were estimated from a previously published 3-group RCT using the same population and outcome measures [20]. We sought an effect size of 0.9, which required 15 participants per each of the three groups, to produce an 80% probability of detecting a 2-point clinically significant change on the 10 point Canadian Occupational Performance Measure [21] (COPM) scale. Statistical significance was set at $p < 0.05$.

Participants

Children were eligible to participate if they met the following inclusion criteria: (a) Age 4 to 15 years, (b) Diagnosis of CP or BI (minimum 12 months post-injury), (c) Manual Ability Classification System (MACS) I–IV, (d) Impaired hand function as a result of the neurological condition, (e) Child-set goals focused on improving hand function, (f) Sufficient language, cognitive and behavioral skills to set goal topics using the COPM, interact with therapist and participate within a group context (according to CO-OP guidelines), (g) Parents able to commit to a 2 week block of therapy. Exclusion criteria: (a) Impaired hand function resulting from secondary condition (e.g. fracture), (b) Significant intellectual or language impairment (CO-OP guidelines), or (c) Known allergy to splinting materials.

Procedures

Ethical approval was granted from participating organizations and the University of Notre Dame, Australia. Participants were recruited to this multicenter study through tertiary children's hospitals and community agencies across three states of Australia from 2013 to 2016. Potential participants were initially screened via email and phone contact. Those deemed likely to be eligible were invited to attend an eligibility assessment. Prior to full baseline assessment, study procedures were fully explained and written consent obtained from the carers of all participants. Participants were randomized immediately following baseline assessment. The randomization sequence was generated using a computer random number generator, with concealment of group undertaken using sequentially numbered and sealed opaque envelopes, stored and opened by an independent offsite officer. To assign group allocation, the principal researcher telephoned the independent

officer, who opened the envelope and advised on the assigned group. Blinding of subjects and therapists was not possible due to the nature of the treatment. Masked assessment was carried out at baseline, immediately following the 2 weeks of treatment (primary endpoint) and 8 weeks following completion of treatment by a qualified occupational therapist masked to group allocation. Participants were not provided with previous COPM scores at re-assessment. Data entry was conducted by an independent person masked to group allocation.

Intervention

Participants were randomly allocated to one of three treatment groups: (1) functional hand splint only, (2) CO-OP only, or (3) CO-OP + a functional hand splint. The total duration of the treatment for all groups was 2 weeks. Each participant's individual goals, identified on the COPM, were the focus of therapy. All participants were encouraged to complete 1 h of daily home practice of goals, recorded in a logbook. Detailed information regarding the interventions are available in the study protocol [19].

Functional hand splinting

All the functional hand splints were a wrist cock-up splint fabricated in either thermoplastic or neoprene with a static insert on the volar surface to support the wrist and block wrist flexion. The prescriber aimed to position the wrist in approximately 20–30° of wrist extension as per splinting conventions, however if this negatively impacted on the individual's ability to actively extend their fingers and/or functionally grasp, the splint was fabricated in their maximum possible wrist extension with full finger extension. An additional support at the thumb or for supination was included, depending on the child's hand function and individual goals. To improve wearing tolerance, child and family preference of material were considered. Participants allocated to splint groups were instructed to wear the splint during goal practice (1 h each day), although practice with and without the splint was recorded. Participants in the splint only group were instructed to practice goals at home and did not undertake any face-to-face intervention with a therapist.

Cognitive Orientation to daily Occupational Performance (CO-OP)

A total of 10 sessions were carried out over 10 consecutive weekdays, for approximately 1 h per session, within the clinic environment. This study aimed to adhere to the critical components of CO-OP, and CO-OP fidelity checklists [22] were utilized to ensure that CO-OP was being provided and not some other task training. The study aimed to provide CO-OP training to participants within a small group (3–4 children). Due to recruitment numbers and randomization sequence factors, the groups varied in the number of participants (range 2–5) depending on recruitment rates at that site. This meant some participants needed to receive individual CO-OP intervention ($n = 6$) because they were a "group of one". Parents were active participants within the sessions.

Functional hand splinting + CO-OP

Participants randomized to the CO-OP + splint group undertook CO-OP, whilst being prescribed with a hand splint, as described above. Children were expected to wear their splint at all times during practice of goals, both within the CO-OP group and during home practice. Logbooks recorded time spent with the splint on and off during goal practice. In line with ethical considerations, if a child did not assent to wearing the splint their wishes were respected. Researcher and parent notes were taken regarding reasons the child chose to discontinue wearing the splint.

Outcome measures

All outcome measures collected are reported in this paper. Outcome measures were collected at baseline, immediately following the 2 weeks of intervention, and primary outcome measures only were collected at 8 weeks post intervention (follow up).

Primary outcome measures

Primary outcome measures were the COPM [21] and Goal Attainment Scale (GAS) [23], with the study powered to detect a change on the COPM. The COPM is the ICF activities level recommended tool of choice when using CO-OP, according to the developer of CO-OP's recommendations [14]. COPM is a standardized goal setting and outcome measurement tool commonly used in pediatric rehabilitation practice and research [21, 24] and is validated for both child report and parent proxy report. The COPM enables the participant to rate their performance, as well as satisfaction on a scale of 1–10 for each individual goal. As per the COPM administration manual, children who were able to understand the concept of rating the COPM scored themselves. Whereas if the child had difficulty understanding the numeracy concepts of scoring, parents completed the COPM proxy-scoring, which is known to be valid, reliable and responsive in young children with cerebral palsy [25]. For example, children with intellectual disability or children younger than 8 years old. Whoever rated the COPM at baseline assessment also rated at follow up assessment. COPM raw scores (range 0–10) were used to determine change.

The GAS is a standardized measure of goal achievement that measures change in an individuals goals [23], according to a five point scale, in which – 2 is the current level of function, 0 is the expected level of function and + 2 far

exceeds the expected level of function following the treatment. GAS scores were not weighted. Data analysis utilized GAS T-scores (range 22–78).

Secondary outcome measures

Secondary outcome measures included the Box and Block Test [26] (BBT) and wrist range of motion (ROM), which are ICF body structures level measures that reflect the therapeutic intent of splinting. The BBT is an assessment of grasp and release, in which the participant transfers individual blocks from one side of a box, over a partition to the other side, over a 60s period [26]. The score is the total number of blocks moved (range 0–150). A number of studies have utilized the BBT for children with CP [27–29], although reliability and validity in this population is unclear. Strong test-retest and interrater reliability has been shown in typically developing children [26, 30].

Wrist ROM comprised of passive wrist ROM (with fingers flexed), Volkmann's angle [31] (with fingers extended) and active wrist ROM (with fingers flexed). An external wrist ROM device was utilized to standardize ROM measurements in an effort to improve interrater reliability. Joint angle was measured using a digital inclinometer, with change measured in whole numbers of degrees (range 0–180).

Statistical analysis

Participant characteristics were analyzed using descriptive statistics. A one-way ANCOVA controlling for COPM performance at baseline was also conducted to ensure no significant baseline differences between all three groups. All data were assessed for normality using Shapiro-Wilks and visual inspection of boxplots. All analyses were conducted on an intention to treat basis, as per the study protocol. Statistical significance was set at $p < 0.05$ (two-tailed). Two-way mixed ANOVA with repeated measures were undertaken to account for expected correlation within participant scores over the three time points. ANCOVA controlling for baseline score were conducted when only two time points were used. Where there was contamination between the treatment groups, i.e. participants deviated from the treatment protocol, post-hoc secondary analyses on primary outcomes were run using the same analysis methodology as intention to treat. All data were analyzed using SPSS (V.24) and STATA (STATA, Version 14, StataCOrp, College Station, TX, USA). Findings are reported according to the CONSORT statement [32].

Results

A total of 45 children (22 females and 23 males) were randomized to the three intervention groups. Participant flow is shown in Fig. 1.

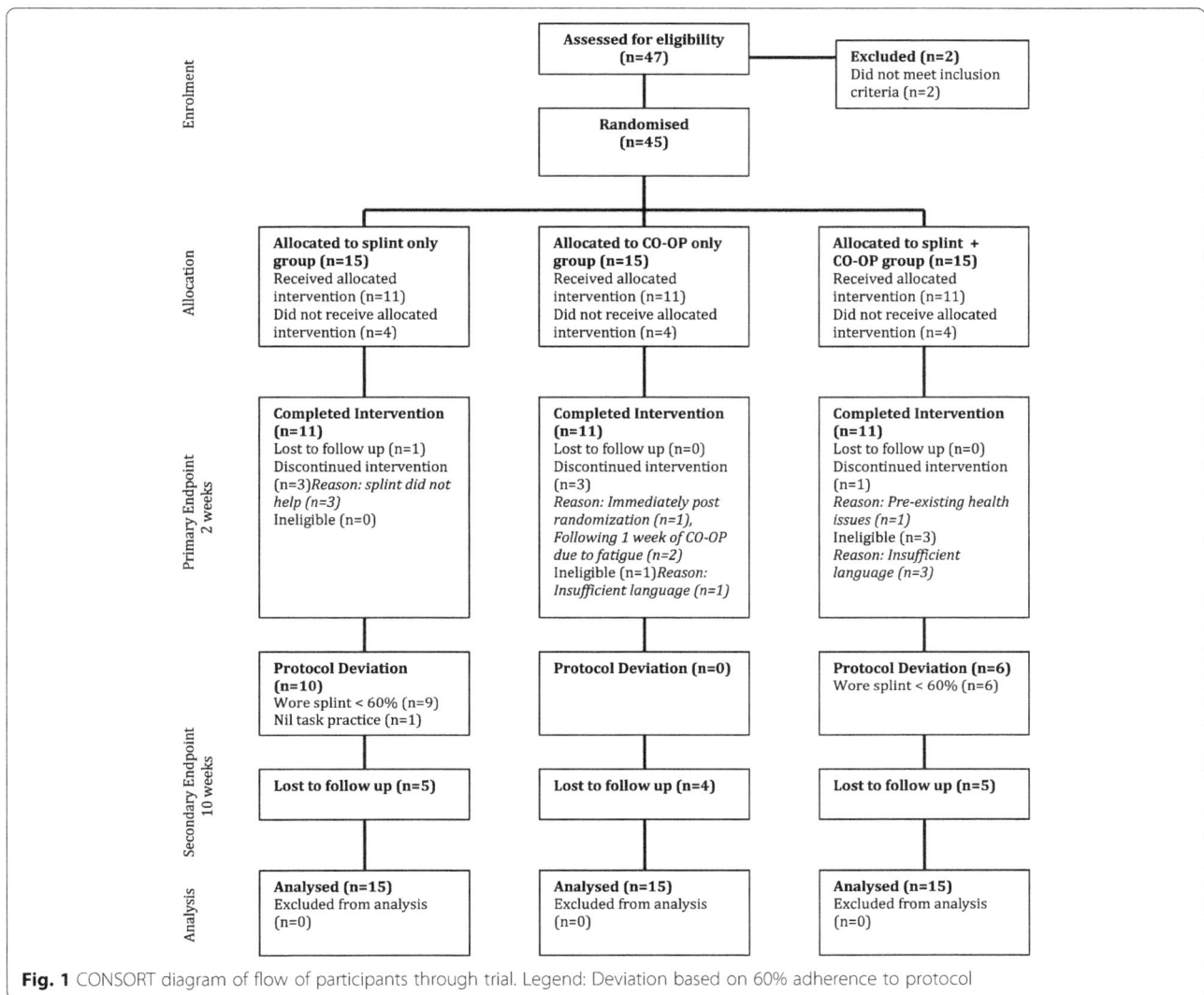

Fig. 1 CONSORT diagram of flow of participants through trial. Legend: Deviation based on 60% adherence to protocol

Participants ranged from 4.1 to 15.2 years, MACS I–IV and GMFCS I–V. Participant baseline characteristics are shown in Table 1. Overall, 33 of the 45 participants completed the intervention (Splint only group n = 11[73%], CO-OP only group n = 11[73%], CO-OP + splint group n = 11[73%]). The only variable different between the groups at baseline was unilateral impairment topography. Analyses were conducted using the MACS classification, which is known to be more objective and stable.

Primary outcomes
COPM
All groups improved on both COPM performance and COPM satisfaction scores from baseline to immediately post-intervention (Table 2). There were no statistically significant differences between the three groups immediately following the intervention (after controlling for baseline)

or 8 weeks post-intervention (repeated measures) on COPM Performance or COPM Satisfaction, as shown in Table 3. Between-group intervention contamination occurred, as children abandoned their splints, preferring to carry out goal practice splint free (refer to dose of practice section).

Of the 45 participants who were enrolled into the study, 26 participants were able to score the COPM independently. Nineteen participants were unable to independently score the COPM. Of these 19, three children scored the COPM with assistance from a parent and in the other 16 cases the parents scored the COPM for the child. The reason for a parent needing to score the COPM was primarily age (n = 10 participants were under 6 years of age). Children over 6 years of age were given the opportunity to determine their own scores on the COPM, however the assessing

Table 1 Baseline characteristics of participants

Participant Information	Whole Sample $n = 45$	Group 1 (Splint only) $n = 15$	Group 2 (CO-OP only) $n = 15$	Group 3 (CO-OP + Splint) $n = 15$
Age (mean (SD))	8.4 (2.7)	8.3 (2.8)	8.1 (2.3)	8.8 (3.1)
Gender				
Male (n, %)	23 (51)	8 (53)	8 (53)	7 (47)
Female (n, %)	22 (49)	7 (47)	7 (47)	8 (53)
Diagnosis				
Cerebral Palsy (n, %)	40 (89)	13 (87)	15 (100)	12 (80)
Brain injury (N, %)	5 (11)	2 (13)	0	3 (20)
Limbs affected				
Unilateral (n, %)	32 (71)	14 (93)	11 (73)	7 (47)[a]
Bilateral (n, %)	13 (29)	1 (7)	4 (27)	8 (53)
Motor Type				
Spastic (n, %)	28 (62)	9 (60)	11 (73)	8 (53)
Dystonic (n, %)	5 (11)	2 (13)	0	3 (20)
Mixed (n, %)	11 (24)	4 (27)	3 (20)	4 (27)
Ataxic (n, %)	1 (2)	0	1 (7)	0
MACS				
I (n, %)	5 (11)	3 (20)	1 (7)	1 (7)
II (n, %)	28 (62)	10 (67)	10 (67)	8 (53)
III (n, %)	9 (20)	2 (13)	3 (20)	4 (27)
IV (n, %)	3 (7)	0	1 (7)	2 (13)
GMFCS				
I (n, %)	24 (53)	9 (60)	8 (53)	7 (47)
II (n, %)	10 (22)	4 (27)	4 (27)	2 (13)
III (n, %)	4 (9)	1 (7)	0	3 (20)
IV (n, %)	6 (13)	1 (7)	3 (20)	2 (13)
V (n, %)	1 (2)	0	0	1 (7)
House				
1 (n, %)	20 (44)	6 (40)	7 (47)	7 (47)
2 (n, %)	4 (9)	2 (13)	0	2 (13)
3 (n, %)	14 (31)	4 (27)	7 (47)	3 (20)
4 (n, %)	3 (7)	1 (7)	0	2 (13)
No contracture	4 (9)	2 (13)	1 (7)	1 (7)
COPM score, mean (SD)				
COPM-P	2.75 (1.34)	2.78 (1.32)	2.16 (0.98)	3.32 (1.48)
COPM-S	3.38 (1.47)	3.37 (1.43)	3.07 (1.38)	3.69 (1.62)

Legend: *MACS* Manual Ability Classification System, *GMFCS* Gross Motor Function Classification System, *House* House thumb classification, *COPM-P* Canadian Occupational Performance Measure Performance Score, *COPM-S* Canadian Occupational Performance Measure Satisfaction Score; [a] Statistically different at baseline

therapist, in conjunction with the parent, made a decision regarding the participant's ability to rate the COPM independently. Reasons for children over the age of six requiring parental assistance included cognitive delay ($n = 5$), attention deficit ($n = 2$) and language delay ($n = 2$) (Additional file 1: Table S1).

GAS

For GAS scores, there was a statistically significant difference between the splint only and the CO-OP only groups ($p = 0.034$) as well as the splint only and CO-OP + splint ($p = 0.047$) immediately post-treatment, in favor of the CO-OP group. Analyses indicated a type II error

Table 2 Results at baseline, immediately following treatment (2 weeks), and at follow up (10 weeks)

Outcome measure	Outcome Score		
	Splint only	CO-OP only	CO-OP + Splint
COPM-Per Mean(SD)			
Baseline	2.78 (1.32)	2.16 (0.98)	3.32 (1.48)
Immediate	5.43 (2.12)	5.89 (2.37)	6.11 (2.43)
Follow up	5.41 (2.00)	5.36 (2.21)	6.33 (2.05)
COPM–Sat Mean(SD)			
Baseline	3.37 (1.43)	3.06 (1.38)	3.69 (1.62)
Immediate	5.78 (2.20)	6.47 (2.26)	6.34 (2.32)
Follow up	5.88 (2.19)	6.51 (2.21)	6.33 (2.19)
GAS, Mean (SD)			
Baseline	22.79 (0.67)	22.61 (0.0)	22.79 (0.67)
Immediate	39.24 (9.95)	50.91 (14.14)	50.41 (18.89)
Follow up	39.24 (15.26)	49.02 (14.53)	49.92 (17.18)
BBT, Mean (SD)			
Baseline	12.1 (10.2)	12.4 (10.6)	11.5 (11.0)
Immediate	12.1 (10.7)	14.5 (11.9)	12.6 (11.8)
Wrist Extension PROM, degrees (Mean, SD)			
Baseline	53.4 (25.2)	60.8 (21.1)	60 (29.5)
Immediate	59.6 (21.4)	64 (21)	63.5 (24.5)
Wrist Extension AROM, degrees (Mean, SD)			
Baseline	19.9 (42.4)	23.4 (35.1)	37.1 (37.4)
Immediate	30.1 (35.1)	28.6 (32.2)	40.5 (31)
Volkmann's angle, degrees (Mean, SD)			
Baseline	36.9 (38.1)	43.2 (34.8)	37.7 (47.3)
Immediate	40.7 (38.2)	37.9 (50.1)	32.7 (54.3)

Legend: *COPM-Per* Canadian Occupational Performance Measure – Performance, *COPM-Sat* Canadian Occupational Performance Measure – Satisfaction, *GAS* Goal Attainment Scale, *BBT* Box and blocks test, *PROM* Passive range of motion, *AROM* Active range of motion. *P* value significance set at $p < 0.05$

for GAS data, suggesting that the study was underpowered. GAS data, as shown in Table 2 suggested a trend towards greater improvements in the CO-OP only and CO-OP + splint groups compared to the splint only group.

Secondary outcomes – BBT and ROM

There was a statistically significant within group difference between splint only and CO-OP only (p = 0.047) immediately post-treatment in favor of CO-OP only. There were no other statistically significant between group differences after controlling for baseline (Table 3).

Dose of practice

Information regarding dosage of task practice and splint wear is detailed in Table 4. At study commencement, all three groups were instructed to practice tasks at home at the exact same dosage, and the two splint groups (Groups 1 & 3) were instructed to wear the splints during the home practice for the same dosage. However, not all participants adhered to the prescribed dosage for splint-wearing or task practice at home. For both the CO-OP groups (Groups 2 & 3), CO-OP was provided face-to-face, in addition to the home practice with or without splint wearing depending on group allocation. The mean (SD) dose of the home-based task practice for each group in minutes, self-selected by participants, was: Splint only = 353 (186); CO-OP only = 856 (438); CO-OP + Splint = 893 (450). In the splint only group, participants adhered to the prescribed splint wearing on average 47.1% of the expected prescribed minutes, and in the CO-OP + splint group, participants adhered to the prescribed splint wearing on average 47.3% of the expected prescribed minutes. One participant in the CO-OP + splint group withdrew due to ill health arising from a pre-existing medical condition, which is a known confounder in childhood disability trials.

At completion of the study, children and parents were asked "If given the choice would you have worn the splint during practice of goals?", to which 64% (16/25) responded no. Reasons given by children and parents included: the splint restricted movement, making it difficult to grasp and release; the splint made practice of goals more difficult; and the splint was poorly tolerated by the child.

Per protocol post hoc secondary analyses were run and no additional statistically significant between group differences were identified with dropouts removed (Additional file 1: Table S2).

Discussion

In this three group, pragmatic RCT, all groups showed statistically significant within-group improvements following 2 weeks of treatment. Between-groups, goal attainment was greater for those who received CO-OP, compared to a functional hand splint and practicing goals at home. Combined use of CO-OP and splinting had no additive effect over CO-OP alone. Splints were not well tolerated by our participants, and participants deviated from the protocol by practicing goals without the splint on. The dose of task practice required to achieve significant improvements in this study was much lower than suggested minimum UL task-specific training dosage [3]. CO-OP, as well as task-specific practice of goals at home, may be effective interventions that lead to goal achievement when collaborative client-centered goals are set, a short, intense block of therapy is prescribed and the treatment is focused on active practice of the child's chosen goals.

We investigated whether CO-OP added any benefits over and above a functional hand splint alone and when

Table 3 Intention to treat (ITT) Results and between group ANCOVA analyses immediately following treatment (2 weeks), and repeated measures at follow up (10 weeks). Analyses used are specified within table

Outcome Measure	Group	Estimated Mean	Estimated 95% CI	P value
Repeated measures analysis (3 Time points) n = 45				
COPM PER	Splint	4.54	3.72–5.36	p = 0.052
	COOP	4.47	3.65–5.29	
	CO-OP + Splint	5.25	4.43–6.07	
COPM SAT	Splint	5.02	4.15–5.88	p = 0.756
	COOP	5.35	4.48–6.21	
	CO-OP + Splint	5.45	4.59–6.32	
GAS	Splint	33.76	28.75–38.76	p = 0.072
	COOP	40.85	35.84–45.86	
	CO-OP + Splint	41.04	36.03–46.05	
ANCOVA (Controlling for baseline 2 time points pre and immediately following intervention)				
COPM PER	Splint	5.41	4.24–6.59	Splint – COOP p = 0.371
	COOP	6.17	4.95–7.40	Splint – CO-OP + splint p = 0.618
	CO-OP + Splint	5.83	4.62–7.05	COOP – CO-OP + Splint p = 0.702
COPM SAT	Splint	5.79	4.70–6.89	Splint – COOP p = 0.268
	COOP	6.66	5.55–7.76	Splint – CO-OP + Splint p = 0.647
	CO-OP + Splint	6.15	5.04–7.25	COOP – CO-OP + Splint p = 0.518
GAS	Splint	39.12	32.23–46.91	Splint – COOP p = 0.034
	COOP	51.16	43.32–59.00	Splint – CO-OP + Splint p = 0.047
	CO-OP + Splint	50.29	42.50–58.08	COOP – CO-OP + Splint p = 0.875
BBT	Splint	11.97	10.55–13.40	Splint – COOP p = 0.047
	COOP	14.02	12.60–15.45	Splint – CO-OP + Splint p = 0.250
	CO-OP + Splint	13.14	11.71–14.57	COOP – CO-OP + Splint p = 0.382
PROM[a]	Splint	62.00	52.21–71.59	Splint – COOP p = 0.893
	COOP	60.94	50.57–71.32	Splint – CO-OP + Splint p = 0.932
	CO-OP + Splint	62.48	52.84–72.13	COOP – CO-OP + Splint p = 0.827
WROM[a]	Splint	34.35	22.93–45.76	Splint – COOP p = 0.482
	COOP	28.50	16.29–40.70	Splint – CO-OP + Splint p = 0.661
	CO-OP + Splint	30.64	18.29–42.99	COOP – CO-OP + Splint p = 0.804
Volkmann's angle[a]	Splint	42.25	21.90–62.60	Splint – COOP p = 0.461
	COOP	31.25	9.36–53.14	Splint – CO-OP + Splint p = 0.550
	CO-OP + Splint	33.69	13.32–54.01	COOP – CO-OP + Splint p = 0.871

Legend: *COPM-Per* Canadian Occupational Performance Measure – Performance, *COPM-Sat* Canadian Occupational Performance Measure – Satisfaction, *GAS* Goal Attainment Scale, *BBT* Box and blocks test, *PROM* Passive range of motion, *AROM* Active range of motion. P value significance set at $p < 0.05$
[a]PROM, WROM and Volkmann's angle –ANCOVA results should be interpreted with caution model fit poor

used in combination. Children provided with CO-OP in addition to splint demonstrated no greater improvement in goal achievement than children who completed CO-OP alone. In contrast to our findings, Elliott and colleagues [7] found that children who received a splint plus goal-directed training improved more on GAS scores than children who completed goal-directed training alone. Further research may be needed, however given the poor tolerance of splints in our study it may

be ethically challenging to justify a larger trial of this nature.

CO-OP was shown to lead to goal achievement, therefore may be another beneficial task-specific training option for children with CP or BI. Task-specific UL training approaches, that involve active practice of a task, rather than addressing underlying impairments, are now widely recognized as best practice in this population [33]. CO-OP may be utilized with children who are

Table 4 Dosage of intervention (time in minutes)

DOSE	Splint only ($n = 11$)	CO-OP only ($n = 13$)	CO-OP + Splint ($n = 13$)
Total dosage of task practice, minutes			
Mean (SD)	353(186)	856 (438)	893 (450)
Range	40–600	300–1680	240–1860
Dosage of CO-OP, minutes			
Mean (SD)	N/A	485 (111)	466 (139)
Range		300–600	180–600
Dosage of task practice at home, minutes			
Mean (SD)	330 (188)	372 (382)	427 (398)
Range	40–600	0–1080	60–1320
Time splint worn, minutes			
Mean (SD)	174 (157)	N/A	459 (421)
Range	0–450		30–1440
% time splint worn during task practice			
Mean %	47.1%	N/A	47.3%
Range %	0–100%		3.6–100%

N/A Not applicable

able to set their own goals, have the communication and cognitive skills to problem-solve and are motivated to persist with practice of goals. CO-OP can be used with children with unilateral or bilateral impairment, with a range of functional abilities. In other populations, CO-OP has been shown to have the additional benefit of transfer of problem-solving skills to future goals and functional skills [34]. We did not investigate transfer of skills, although a study of CO-OP for children with BI suggested transfer may not be achieved [18], warranting further investigation. As CO-OP is a promising intervention in this population, there is a need to provide CO-OP training to therapists in an effort to translate this new evidence into clinical practice.

Splints were not well tolerated by children in our study and this in itself is an important finding. Dislike of splint wearing and self-selected abandonment has been observed in other clinical populations [35–37]. Participants in the splint group, who were expected to practice their goals daily with their hand splint on, generally chose not to wear their splint, but instead to practice their goals without the splint on. The majority of children who were provided with a splint chose to wear it less than 50% of the time during goal practice, despite instructions to wear the splint 100% of the time. It appears that if participants did not find the splint useful, it was discarded and they continued to practice goals without the splint. Intervention contamination between-groups therefore occurred, and the splint only group were completing goal-directed, task-specific training at home. In doing so, these participants were able to achieve their goals, suggesting children may have discerned what was working, and

thus were motivated to practice using the effective goal-direct task-specific training strategy. Daily, targeted practice of goals within the home may be another effective task-specific training option, consistent with previously reported benefits of home programs [20]. The lack of difference between the groups was therefore not surprising given the number of children in the splint only group that did not adhere to the protocol, and instead carried out task-specific training in a home program format, which has similarities with the CO-OP approach. Previous head-to-head trials of different types of task specific training for children with cerebral palsy (e.g. Constraint Induced Movement Therapy versus Bimanual Training), have showed no differences in outcomes between types of task-specific training interventions [2, 3]. It is interesting that the children performing home programs achieved similar outcomes on the COPM, because home programs provide a low-cost alternative with no travel requirements for parents. Previous splinting studies have reported poor tolerance of external garments by children [38] and static splints by adults [35–37], however there have also been studies that have reported no issues with splint tolerance [7, 8, 38].

Dose, or total amount of practice has been identified as an essential consideration in task-specific training [32]. Previous studies have suggested a minimum of 40 h of practice may be required to achieve significant improvements in UL function [3]. In our study, the dose of practice was much less than this suggested minimum dosage, consistent with previous CO-OP studies in the developmental coordination disorder population [14, 33]. The splint only group improved with an average of approximately 6 h of self-selected goal practice at home and the CO-OP groups improved with approximately 14 h of practice over a 2 week period (10 h face-to-face plus 4 h at home) (Table 3). Possible explanations for these positive results from lower dose intervention include: (a) the interventions in this study focused solely on practice of the three goals as chosen by each individual child, whereas in other cerebral palsy and brain injury studies [3, 12], participants may practice many tasks that target improved upper limb function. It is possible that a smaller dose of practice, such as the 6–14 h achieved in our study, is enough to successfully achieve three individual goals, whereas a larger dose, for example 40 h, is required in order to not only achieve goals, but also to improve hand function as measured on the Assisting Hand Assessment (AHA) and Quality of Upper Extremity Skills Test (QUEST) [3]; (b) CO-OP is more effective than other task specific approaches at low doses in the cerebral palsy population, because CO-OP teaches a global problem solving strategy that the child can use to solve problems at home when the therapist is not present [13]. The only previous study of CO-OP in the cerebral palsy population found that CO-OP led to greater generalization, supporting this proposition [13]; (c) In regard to outcome measures, the COPM and GAS, which measure changes in 'activities and participation' were of interest in this study, in keeping with the ICF focus in pediatric rehabilitation and newer theories of motor learning. In our study the primary outcome measures were the COPM and GAS, whereas previous task-specific training studies have utilized assessments such as the AHA or QUEST in combination with goal achievement outcomes. The COPM and GAS are known to be highly responsive to detecting small individualized gains. The differences between the COPM and GAS outcomes are not clear, however one theory is that the COPM is more subjective than the GAS. It has previously been suggested that participants are likely to perceive whichever therapy they receive as effective, and this may be reflected in COPM outcomes. The GAS may be more objective, and therefore may be more likely to reflect actual improvements in goal achievement, rather than perceived improvement. Moreover, although the BBT provided a basic measure of hand function, it is understandable that children did not improve on the BBT as a result of CO-OP as they did not practice grasping and releasing blocks as part of their treatment. Participants practiced their own goals and therefore we wanted to measure if those goals had been achieved; and (d) Undertaking CO-OP with a therapist face-to-face where motivation and the "just right challenge" for learning is implemented, as opposed to prescribing a splint with self-directed practice at home, perhaps is more likely to lead to a greater dose of training and therefore a better outcome.

Future directions

The results of our study further support the benefits of task-specific training approaches in various forms for children with CP or BI. Further research comparing CO-OP or task-specific home programs to proven task-specific training approaches, such as CIMT or bimanual training is warranted, particularly as dose requirements appear lower enabling cost effective services. Further research is needed regarding the types of children with CP or BI who may respond best to the CO-OP Approach™. A larger sample would enable sub-group analyses by etiology and type of cerebral palsy and brain injury, which would provide valuable information to clinicians about responders. Education regarding CO-OP is needed for therapist working with children with cerebral palsy and brain injury in order to translate this new evidence into practice in this population. Future studies should plan to recruit a much larger sample size, based on a power calculation using this new pilot data.

Limitations

This was a pragmatic trial that had small numbers and included a very broad population in regard to age, diagnosis and motor abilities, this is a study limitation. There are several other limitations to this pilot study, and the results must be interpreted cautiously. First, there were a large number of withdrawals in each group, and a number of participants who deviated from the study protocol (Fig. 1). It is possible that children who may benefit from CO-OP differ from those who may benefit from functional hand splints. Pre-trial participant treatment preferences may have biased recruitment and adherence. Poor splint wearing adherence, affected the statistical power for both the between-group analysis and dose response analysis. Second, it is difficult to prescribe one splint that is suitable for three goals, each of which may require a different hand position. It is possible that poor design of the splint led to poorer hand function, although measures were in place to limit this possibility. Block randomization would have been beneficial in order to facilitate homogeneous CO-OP groups. Third, the comparison of CO-OP in center-based group format, to individualized splint-wearing at home, introduces another confounder that may explain the study results. Fourth, the use of a self-reported goal-based measure as a primary end-point rather than an objective hard end-point measure, may have influenced the results. Fifth, the combined use of child self-reporting and parent proxy-reporting of the primary end-point measure (COPM) may have influenced the results. Sixth, contamination of trial groups led to small sample sizes for regression analysis. Cautious interpretation of the results is therefore recommended.

Conclusion

Task-specific training continues to be best practice in supporting goal achievement for children with CP or BI, with CO-OP being a new form of task-specific training useful in these populations. CO-OP or task-specific training at home may be intervention options that require a lower dose to achieve individual goals, although CO-OP because of its structured problem-solving approach is likely to be more effective than child-led home practice alone. Combined use of CO-OP and functional hand splints did not lead to any additional benefits over CO-OP alone, and splints were not well tolerated by our participants. Therapy can be maximized through child-chosen goals, setting short, intensive timeframes and treatment including active practice of goals.

Abbreviations
AHA: Assisting hand assessment; BBT: Box and Blocks Test; BI: Brain injury; CIMT: Constraint-induced movement therapy; CO-OP: Cognitive Orientation to daily Occupational Performance; COPM: Canadian Occupational Performance Measure; CP: Cerebral palsy; GAS: Goal attainment scale; GMFCS: Gross motor function classification system; ICF: International Classification of Functional, Disability and Health; MACS: Manual abilities classification system; QUEST: Quality of Upper Extremity Skills Test; RCT: Randomised controlled trial; ROM: Range of motion; UL: Upper limb

Acknowledgements
Sincere thanks to the children and dedicated families who participated in this research. Thankyou also to Noni Payling, Amanda Orr, Dr. Brian Hoare, Megan Thorley, Amanda Cauchi, Sarah Wilkes-Gillan, Carly Stewart, Kate Morris and Jane Berry.

Funding
This study was supported by a National Health and Medical Research Council postgraduate scholarship (MJ 1074570). The funding body, NHMRC, did not contribute to the design of this trial or the content or preparation of this manuscript in any way.

Authors' contributions
MJ, IN and NL conceptualized and designed the study. MJ, IN, EF and LM were involved in the acquisition of data. CG, MJ, IN and NL analysed and interpreted the data. MJ drafted the manuscript. IN, NL and CG critically revised the manuscript. All authors reviewed and approved the final manuscript.

Competing interests
The authors declare that they have no competing interests.

Author details
[1]School of Child and Adolescent Medicine, The University of Sydney, Sydney, Australia. [2]Occupational Therapy Department, John Hunter Children's Hospital, Newcastle, Australia. [3]Cerebral Palsy Alliance Research Institute, The University of Sydney, Sydney, Australia. [4]Alfred Health, La Trobe University, Melbourne, Australia. [5]School of Health Science, Australian Catholic University, Sydney, Australia. [6]School of Health Science, Australian Catholic University, Brisbane, Australia.

References
1. Arner M, Eliasson AC, Nicklasson S, Sommerstein K, Hägglund G. Hand function in cerebral palsy. Report of 367 children in a population-based longitudinal health care program. J Hand Surg. 2008;33:1337–47.
2. Novak I, McIntyre S, Morgan C, Campbell L, Dark L, Morton N, Stumbles E, Wilson S-A, Goldsmith S. A systematic review of interventions for children with cerebral palsy: state of the evidence. Dev Med Child Neurol. 2013;55:885–910.
3. Sakzewski L, Ziviani J, Boyd RN. Efficacy of upper limb therapies for unilateral cerebral palsy: a meta-analysis. Pediatrics. 2014;133:e175–204.
4. Rosenbaum P, Stewart D. The World Health Organization international classification of functioning, disability, and health: a model to guide clinical thinking, practice and research in the field of cerebral palsy. Semin Pediatr Neurol. 2004;11:5–10.
5. Lannin Natasha A, Novak I. In: Curtin M, Molineaux M, Supyk J, editors. Orthotics for Occupational Outcomes. 6th ed. London: Elsevier; 2010. p. 507–26.
6. Elliott C, Reid S, Hamer P, Alderson J, Elliott B. Lycra(®) arm splints improve movement fluency in children with cerebral palsy. Gait Posture. 2011;33: 214–9.
7. Elliott CM, Reid SL, Alderson JA, Elliott BC. Lycra arm splints in conjunction with goal-directed training can improve movement in children with cerebral palsy. In: NeuroRehabilitation; 2011. p. 47–54.
8. Keklicek H, Uygur F. Effects of hand taping on upper extremity function in children with cerebral palsy. In: Neurorehabilitation and neural repair, vol. 26; 2012. p. Np7–np8.
9. Kara OK, Uysal SA, Turker D, Karayazgan S, Gunel MK, Baltaci G. The effects of Kinesio taping on body functions and activity in unilateral spastic cerebral palsy: a single-blind randomized controlled trial [with consumer summary]. Dev Med Child Neurol. 2015;57:81–8.
10. Azzam AM. Efficacy of enhancement forearm supination on improvement of finger dexterity in hemiplegic cerebral palsy children. Indian J Physiother Occup Ther. 2012;6:5–8.
11. Jackman M, Novak I, Lannin Natasha A. Hand splinting for children with cerebral palsy and brain injury: a systematic review with meta analysis. In: Australian Occupational Therapy Conference, vol. 62. Melbourne: Australian Occupational Therapy Journal; 2015. p. 142.
12. Hoare Brian J, Wasiak J, Imms C, Carey L. Constraint-induced movement therapy in the treatment of the upper limb in children with hemiplegic cerebral palsy. In: Cochrane Database of Systematic Reviews: Wiley; 2007. www.cochranelibrary.com.
13. Cameron D, Craig T, Edwards B, Missiuna C, Schwellnus H, Polatajko HJ. Cognitive orientation to daily occupational performance (CO-OP): a new approach for children with cerebral palsy. Phys Occup Ther Pediatr. 2016;37 (2): 1–16.
14. Polatajko HJ, Mandich A. Enabling Occupation in Children: The Cognitive Approach to Occupational Performance (CO-OP) Approach. Ottawa: COAT Publications ACE; 2004.
15. Wright V. Practical applicaiton of motor learning approaches in PT/OT - are we using motor learning strategies to their fullest extent in our sessions? In: Australasian Academy of Cerebral Palsy and Developmental Medicine. Adelaide; 2016.
16. Gauthier LV, Taub E, Perkins C, Ortmann M, Mark VW, Uswatte G. Remodeling the brain: plastic structural brain changes produced by different motor therapies after stroke. Stroke. 2008;39:1520–5.
17. Mandich AA, Polatajko HJ, Zilberbrant A. A cognitive perspective on intervention. In: Eliasson AC, Burtner P, editors. Improving Hand Function in Children with Cerebral Palsy. London: Wiley; 2008.
18. Missiuna C, DeMatteo C, Hanna S, Mandich A, Law M, Mahoney W, Scott L. Exploring the use of cognitive intervention for children with acquired brain injury. Phys Occup Ther Pediatr. 2010;30:205–19.
19. Jackman M, Novak I, Lannin N. Effectiveness of functional hand splinting and the cognitive orientation to occupational performance (CO-OP) approach in children with cerebral palsy and brain injury: two randomised controlled trial protocols. BMC Neurol. 2014;14:144.
20. Novak I, Cusick A, Lannin N. Occupational therapy home programs for cerebral palsy: double-blind, randomized, controlled trial. Pediatrics. 2009; 124:e606–14.
21. Law M, Baptiste S, Carswell A, McColl M, Polatajko HJ, Pollock N. COPM Canadian Occupational Performance Measure. 4th ed. Ottawa: CAOT Publications ACE; 2005.
22. McEwan, Polatajko, Wolf, Baum. CO-OP Fidelity Checklist. Revised 2015 edition. CO-OP Academy Executive; 2015. http://co-opacademy.ca/wp-content/uploads/2018/04/CO-OP-Fidelity-Checklist-Apr-4-2018.pdf. Accessed 13 July 2018.
23. Kiresuk TJ, Smith A, Cardillo JE. Goal attainment scaling: Applications, theory, and measurement. Hillsdale, England: Lawrence Erlbaum Associates, Inc; 1994.
24. Cusick A, McIntyre S, Novak I, Lannin N, Lowe K. A comparison of goal attainment scaling and the Canadian occupational performance measure for paediatric rehabilitation research. Pediatr Rehabil. 2006;9(2):149–57.

25. Cusick A, Lannin NA, Lowe K. Adapting the Canadian occupational performance measure for use in a paediatric clinical trial. Disabil Rehabil. 2007;29:761–6.

26. Mathiowetz V, Federman S, Wiemer D. Box and blocks test for manual dexterity: norms for 6–19 year olds. Can J Occup Ther. 1985;52:241–5.

27. Öhrvall A-M, Krumlinde-Sundholm L, Eliasson A-C. Exploration of the relationship between the manual ability classification system and hand-function measures of capacity and performance. Disabil Rehabil. 2013;35: 913–8. 916

28. Geerdink Y, Aarts P, Geurts AC. Motor learning curve and long-term effectiveness of modified constraint-induced movement therapy in children with unilateral cerebral palsy: a randomized controlled trial. Res Dev Disabil. 2013;34:923–31.

29. Sakzewski L, Miller L, Ziviani J, Abbott DF, Rose S, Macdonell RAL, Boyd RN. Randomized comparison trial of density and context of upper limb intensive group versus individualized occupational therapy for children with unilateral cerebral palsy. Dev Med Child Neurol. 2015;57(6): 539–547.

30. Jongbloed-Pereboom MG, Nijhuis-van der Sanden MW, Steenbergen B. Norm scores of the box and block test for children ages 3–10 years. Am J Occup Ther. 2013;67:312–8. 317

31. Bassini L, Patel M. Pediatric Hand Therapy. In: Cooper C, editor. Fundamentals of Hand Therapy: Clinical Reasoning and Treatment Guidelines for Common Diagnoses of the Upper Extremity. St Louis: Mosby Elsevier; 2007.

32. Schulz KF, Altman DG, Moher D. CONSORT 2010 statement: updated guidelines for reporting parallel group randomised trials. BMC Med. 2010;8(1):18.

33. Sakzewski L, Gordon A, Eliasson A-C. The state of the evidence for intensive upper limb therapy approaches for children with unilateral cerebral palsy. J Child Neurol. 2014;29:1077–90.

34. Polatajko HJ, Mandich AD, Miller LT, Macnab JJ. Cognitive orientation to daily occupational performance (CO-OP): part II – the evidence. Phys Occup Ther Pediatr. 2000;20:83–106.

35. Cebesoy O, Kose KC, Kuru I, Altinel L, Gul R, Demirtas M. Use of a splint following open carpal tunnel release: a comparative study. Adv Ther. 2007;24:478–84.

36. Safaz İ, TÜRk H, YaŞAr E, Alaca R, Tok F, TuĞCu İ. Use and abandonment rates of assistive devices/orthoses in patients with stroke. Gulhane Med J. 2015;57:142–4.

37. Lannin NA, Horsley SA, Herbert R, McCluskey A, Cusick A. Splinting the hand in the functional position after brain impairment: a randomized, controlled trial. Arch Phys Med Rehabil. 2003;84:297–302.

38. Nicholson JH, Morton RE, Attfield S, Rennie D. Assessment of upper-limb function and movement in children with cerebral palsy wearing lycra garments. Dev Med Child Neurol. 2001;43:384–91.

3

The antipyretic efficacy and safety of propacetamol compared with dexibuprofen in febrile

Seung Jun Choi[1,2], Sena Moon[3], Ui Yoon Choi[3], Yoon Hong Chun[3], Jung Hyun Lee[3], Jung Woo Rhim[3], Jin Lee[4], Hwang Min Kim[5] and Dae Chul Jeong[3,6]* (iD)

Abstract

Background: We aimed to compare the antipyretic efficacy, safety, and tolerability between oral dexibuprofen and intravenous propacetamol in children with upper respiratory tract infection (URTI) presenting with fever.

Methods: Patients aging from 6 months to 14 years admitted for URTI with axillary body temperature ≥ 38.0 °C were enrolled and randomized into the study or control group. Patients in the study group were intravenously infused with propacetamol and subsequently oral placebo medication was administered. Patients in the control group were intravenously infused with 100 mL of 0.9% sodium chloride solution without propacetamol and then oral dexibuprofen was administered. We checked the body temperature of all patients at 0.5 h (hr), 1 h, 1.5 h, 2 h, 3 h, 4 h, and 6 h after oral placebo or dexibuprofen had been applied.

Results: A total of 263 patients (125 in the study group) were finally enrolled. The body temperatures of patients in the study group were significantly lower until 2 h after administration (37.73 ± 0.58 vs 38.36 ± 0.69 °C ($p < 0.001$), 37.37 ± 0.53 vs 37.88 ± 0.69 °C ($p < 0.001$), 37.27 ± 0.60 vs 37.62 ± 0.66 °C ($p < 0.001$), 37.25 ± 0.62 vs 37.40 ± 0.60 °C ($p = 0.0452$), at 0.5 h, 1 h, 1.5 h, and 2 h, respectively). The two groups showed no significant differences in terms of the range of body temperature decrease, the Area Under the Curve of body temperature change for antipyretic administration-and-time relationship, the maximum value of body temperature decrease during the 6 h test period, the number of patients whose body temperature normalized (< 37.0 °C), the mean time when first normalization of body temperature, and the development of adverse events including gastrointestinal problem, elevated liver enzyme, and thrombocytopenia.

Conclusions: Intravenous propacetamol may be a safe and effective choice for pediatric URTI patients presenting with fever who are not able to take oral medications or need faster fever control.

Keywords: Children, Dexibuprofen, Fever, Propacetamol, Upper respiratory tract infection

* Correspondence: jdcped@hanmail.net
[3]Department of Pediatrics, College of Medicine, The Catholic University of Korea, 222, Banpodaero, Seocho-gu, Seoul 06591, Republic of Korea
[6]Vaccine Bio-research Institute, College of Medicine, The Catholic University of Korea, Seoul, Republic of Korea
Full list of author information is available at the end of the article

Background

Fever is a common symptom in numerous pediatric diseases including infection and works as a positive response that aids in immune function [1–4]. However, fever confers discomfort, may lead to increased body water loss and dehydration, and may delay overall recovery due to decreased activity and appetite. In such circumstances, antipyretics are used in the pediatric population to alleviate secondary effects of fever like dehydration. Acetaminophen and nonsteroidal anti-inflammatory drugs (NSAIDs) including ibuprofen are commonly used. However, since these drugs are administered via oral route, uses are limited, not being able to be provided for those who cannot take oral medications.

Propacetamol is a prodrug of paracetamol (acetaminophen); 0.5 g of paracetamol can be obtained through plasma esterase-involved hydrolyzation of 1 g of propacetamol [5, 6]. In adult patients, intravenous propacetamol is indicated for fever and acute pain relief. A limited number of previous studies have presented the antipyretic efficacy of intravenous propacetamol in children [7–10]. Furthermore, there have not been previous comparison studies over oral antipyretics and intravenous propacetamol.

Here, we aimed to evaluate and verify the non-inferiority of intravenous propacetamol compared to dexibuprofen in terms of antipyretic efficacy and safety for fever reduction in pediatric upper respiratory tract infection (URTI) patients.

Methods

Study design and procedures

This study was a multicenter, randomized, double-blind, comparative, phase 3 clinical trial that was designed to test the antipyretic efficacy of propacetamol (Yungjin Pharm. Co. Ltd., Seoul, Republic of Korea) compared with dexibuprofen (Hanmi Pharm. Co. Ltd., Seoul, Republic of Korea). Subjects from hospitals of The Catholic University of Korea were evaluated for appropriateness for enrollment and were randomized to either the study or control group. The sample size was calculated according to the assumptions stated in the following steps. The level of significance was 0.05, and the power of test was set as 80%. The mean change in body temperature at 6 h after a single dose of 5 mg/kg of dexibuprofen was 0.8 °C with a standard deviation of 1.0 °C. The equivalence margin was − 0.35 with a drop-out rate of 20%.

Study group subjects were administered propacetamol when fever (defined as axillary temperature ≥ 38 °C) developed at a dose of 15 mg/kg in patients weighing < 10 kg and 30 mg/kg in patients weighing ≥10 kg. The dosage of propacetamol was determined according to the previous study [7] which had elucidated the antipyretic effect of intravenous propacetamol, which was administered to children aging from 3 to 12 years at a dose of 30 mg/kg.

Because younger and smaller children were included in our study, the dosage of propacetamol for children weighing < 10 kg was determined based on another reference [11]; the propacetamol was mixed with 100 mL of 0.9% sodium chloride solution and given as an intravenous infusion over 30 min. Oral placebo was subsequently administered. The control group subjects were administered intravenous infusion with 100 mL of 0.9% sodium chloride solution without propacetamol for 30 min followed by a single 6 mg/kg dose of oral dexibuprofen. If the subject vomited within 15 min of placebo or dexibuprofen administration, another dose of previously administered oral agent was administered. Body temperature was checked at 0.5 h (hr), 1 h, 1.5 h, 2 h, 3 h, 4 h, and 6 h after placebo or dexibuprofen administration. No further antipyretics and no antibiotics were administered within 6 h of placebo or dexibuprofen administration unless judged necessary by the attending pediatrician.

The study was conducted in accordance with the ethical principles of the Declaration of Helsinki. Written informed consent was obtained from parents or legal guardians and from the child, if possible. The clinical studies were approved by the Korean Food and Drug Administration. The protocol was approved by the Institutional Research Board (IRB) of each institution. Once a patient qualifying the inclusion criteria was enrolled, this patient was prospectively registered in the IRB registry and was then grouped at the ratio of one-to-one into A or B group consecutively by block randomization. The IRB numbers of the participating hospitals are as follows: KC13MDMT0120 at Seoul St. Mary's Hospital; VC13MDMT0024 at St. Vincent's Hospital; KMC2015–009 at Hanjin General Hospital; DC14MDMT0006 at Daejeon St. Mary's Hospital; PS13MDMT0015 at St. Paul's Hospital; OC13MDMT0025 at Incheon St. Mary's Hospital; and CR115093 at Yonsei Christian Hospital.

Inclusion and exclusion criteria

Patients ranging in age from 6 months to 14 years admitted for URTI and presenting with fever (defined as body temperature of the axillar fossa ≥38.0 °C) at the time of admission were included. URTI was diagnosed based on disease history and physical examination carried out by the attending pediatricians. Patients were excluded under the following circumstances: the patient had been administered antipyretics within 4 h prior to admission, a history of febrile crisis within the past 6 months, the presence of severe hematological abnormality, currently receiving treated for or was treated within the past 6 months for nephrologic, hepatologic, pulmonary, endocrine, hematologic, or cardiologic illnesses, neurologic or central nervous system abnormality, diabetes currently not under control, suspected lower respiratory tract infection, severe hemolytic anemia, under maintenance therapy for bronchial asthma, asthma, urticarial, or allergic reaction history when using aspirin or NSAIDs, physical or psychological status deemed inappropriate for a clinical trial, participation in another clinical trial involving other drug(s) within the past 4 weeks, and failure to receive informed consent from the patient or parent.

Efficacy assessments

The primary efficacy variable was the difference in body temperature reduction at 4 h after antipyretic administration between the study and control groups. The secondary efficacy variables were range of body temperature reduction at 4 h after antipyretic administration, the Area Under the Curve (AUC) of body temperature change until 6 h after antipyretic administration-and-time relationship, the maximum value of body temperature reduction within the 6 h after antipyretic administration, the number of patients whose body temperature normalized (< 37.0 °C) at 6 h after antipyretic administration, and the time point when body temperature first reached < 37.0 °C.

Safety assessments

Before the administration of antipyretics and at the second visit (3 days after the initial administration), physical examination and laboratory tests with complete blood cell count, blood chemistry analysis, and urinalysis were done. Adverse events were monitored throughout the whole study period and any occurrences were charted.

Statistical analysis

Test power was set at 80%, and significance level was set at $p < 0.05$. With an expected drop-out rate of 20%, the sample size was calculated to be 161 subjects in each group.

For characteristics analysis, t-tests were used for continuous variables, and Chi-square or Fisher's exact test were used for categorical variables. For assessing primary efficacy – which is the difference in body temperature reduction at 4 h after antipyretic administration between the study and control groups – propacetamol was considered at least as effective as dexibuprofen if the lower boundary of the 95% confidence interval (CI) for the difference in body temperature reduction (dexibuprofen minus propacetamol) was zero or greater at the equivalence margin of 0.35 °C. Secondary efficacy variables were tested using t-tests, except for the number of patients whose body temperature normalized (< 37.0 °C) at 6 h after antipyretic administration, and the incidence of adverse events during the study period was tested with Chi-square or Fisher's exact test.

Results

Three hundred eleven subjects were enrolled during the study period and were randomly assigned to either group

(157 in the study group and 154 in the control group). Among them, 23 in the study group and 8 in the control group were excluded due to wanting to drop-out during the study period (12 in the study group and 4 in the control group), withdrawing informed consent (6 in the study group and vs 1 in the control group), receiving prohibited medication during the study period (5 in the study group and vs 3 in the control group). One hundred thirty four subjects in the study group and 146 subjects in the control underwent per protocol analysis, and 17 more subjects were excluded for various reasons (administration of drugs prohibited for concomitant use, withdrawal of parental consent, violation of the time point of body temperature measurement, etc.). The subjects ultimately qualified to be enrolled in our study were selected, and finally 125 subjects in the study group and 138 subjects in the control group were enrolled (Fig. 1). Of the 125 study group subjects, 17 (13.6%) weighed < 10 kg and received 15 mg/kg of propacetamol, and 108 (86.4%) weighed ≥ 10 kg and received 30 mg/kg of propacetamol. The demographics and basic characteristics were not significantly different between the two groups (Table 1).

Efficacy results

The lower boundary of the primary efficacy variable (the difference of body temperature reduction at 4 h after antipyretic administration: dexibuprofen minus propacetamol) was – 0.34, which was within the equivalence margin of 0.35 (Table 2).

The area under the curve (AUC) of body temperature change at 6 h after antipyretic administration-and-time relationship did not significantly differ between the two groups. None of the secondary efficacy variables were statistically different between the test and control groups (Table 3).

Body temperatures at 0.5 h, 1 h, 1.5 h, and 2 h after antipyretic administration were significantly lower in the study group (37.73 ± 0.58 °C versus 38.36 ± 0.69 °C, 37.37 ± 0.53 °C versus 37.88 ± 0.69 °C, 37.27 ± 0.60 °C versus 37.62 ± 0.66 °C, and 37.25 ± 0.62 °C versus 37.40 ± 0.60 °C [study vs control group]), while the temperatures at 3, 4, and 6 h after medication administration did not significantly differ. Body temperature < 38 °C was achieved within 0.5 h after administration of propacetamol, while it took approximately 1 h to achieve body temperature < 38 °C after administration of dexibuprofen. For both types of antipyretics, body temperature achieved the lowest value at 2 h after administration (Fig. 2).

Safety results

A total of 84 adverse events in 64/263 patients were reported. Adverse events included vomiting, diarrhea, abdominal pain, constipation, rash, elevated liver enzyme, and thrombocytopenia. Laboratory adverse events were

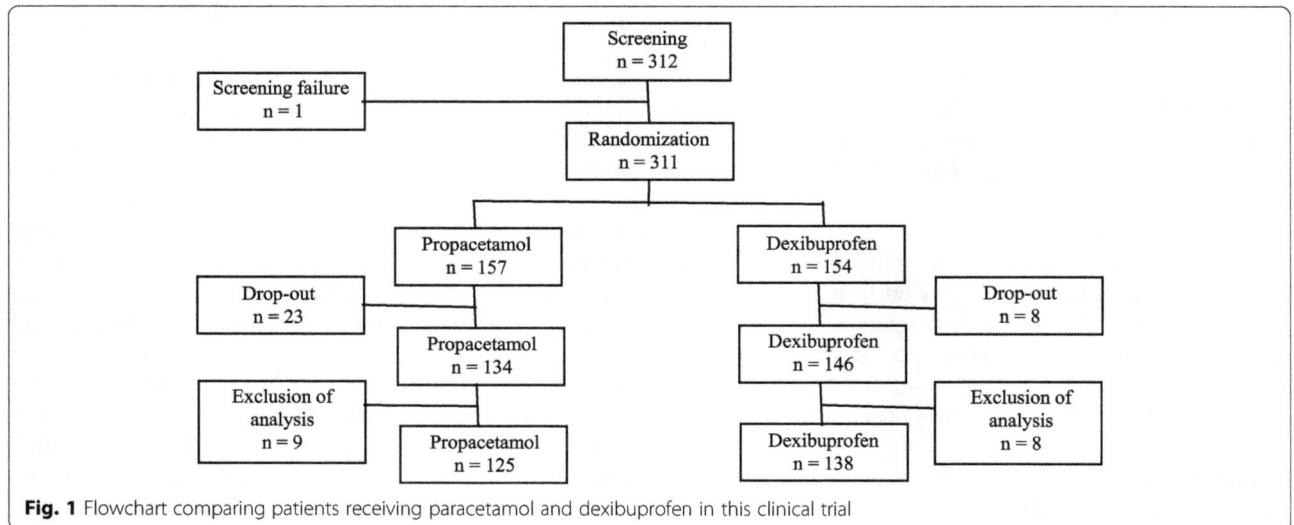

Fig. 1 Flowchart comparing patients receiving paracetamol and dexibuprofen in this clinical trial

developed in 21 patients in the study group versus 36 in the control group. AST elevation was found in 8 patients in the study group versus 14 in the control group. ALT elevation was found in 5 patients in the study group versus 9 in the control group. Thrombocytopenia was found in 8 patients in the study group versus 13 in the control group. These laboratory adverse events were assessed as unlikely to be related or unrelated with the type of antipyretics administered. There was no statistically significant difference in adverse event levels between the study group and control group (Table 4). There was no case of study interruption or antipyretic dosage change due to adverse events. There were no serious adverse events in which the patient(s) had been exposed to a danger to life,

required a longer hospital stay, or had acquired permanent or major sequalae.

Discussion

Based on our study results, the antipyretic effect of intravenous propacetamol compared to dexibuprofen used in pediatric URTI patients presenting with fever was similar. In addition, concerning safety issues, intravenous propacetamol was tolerable based on our data analysis.

Dexibuprofen and acetaminophen are the two most widely used antipyretic drugs in the pediatric population. The former is an enantiomer of racemic ibuprofen, an effective and tolerable antipyretic and analgesic drug for pediatric use [12–14], and an equal effect at a lower

Table 1 Demographic and clinical characteristics of the study groups

Characteristics	Study groups (n = 125)	Control group (n = 138)	p-value
Gender, male (%)	63 (50.4)	70 (50.7)	0.957
Age (years)	3.0 [0–14.0]	3.0 [0–13.0]	0.730
0.5–1 year (%)	35 (28.0)	41 (29.7)	0.700
2–5 years (%)	65 (52.0)	68 (49.3)	
6–10 years (%)	20 (16.0)	26 (18.8)	
11–14 years (%)	5 (4.0)	3 (2.2)	
Weight (kg)	13.9 [7.4–88.0]	15.0 [7.5–51.0]	0.515
Baseline temperature (°C)	38.6 ± 0.5	38.7 ± 0.5	0.159
Laboratory test results (at admission)			
White blood cell count ($\times 10^3$/μL)	9.7 [2.7–28.3]	9.6 [1.9–27.7]	0.555
Neutrophil (%)	60.0 [7.7–91.0]	63.7 [16.9–95.0]	0.208
Lymphocyte (%)	29.1 [4.0–86.8]	24.8 [2.0–73.2]	0.134
Platelet ($\times 10^3$/μL)	246.0 [102.0–583.0]	251.0 [91.0–504.0]	0.824
C-reactive protein (mg/μL)	1.68 [0.1–105.1]	2.33 [0.1–139.1]	0.486

Results are presented as median [range] or as mean ± standard deviation or as a percentage (%)

Table 2 Difference in axillary body temperature reduction at 4 h after antipyretic administration: dexibuprofen minus propacetamol

Efficacy variable	mean ± standard deviation	95% confidence interval	equivalence margin
Dexibuprofen minus propacetamol	−0.13 ± 0.11	(− 0.34, 0.03)	0.35

dose than ibuprofen has been shown in previous studies [15–17], some including pediatric upper respiratory tract infection (URTI) patients presenting with fever [18, 19]. Acetaminophen is another popular choice of pediatric antipyretic drug, which is generally administered via oral route. However, a rectal route may be used in cases when the oral route is not tolerable, such as when the patient is vomiting, in respiratory distress, or has decreased mental status. In such a case, its bioavailability is substantially reduced (54% lower than that for the oral route), making it difficult to quantify the targeted drug concentration [20]. In such circumstances, intravenous antipyretic like propacetamol (a prodrug of acetaminophen as previously mentioned) would be a preferred choice.

In addition, if prompt alleviation of fever is warranted in severe pyrexia, intravenous antipyretics may be indicated [21]. In our study, the body temperature during the first 2 h after intravenous propacetamol administration was significantly lower than that after dexibuprofen administration. While intravenous drug concentrations reach maximum levels within 40 min when propacetamol is intravenously administered [22], it takes more than 2 h for dexibuprofen to reach its maximum concentration after oral administration [15]. This difference may have influenced our results concerning the superior antipyretic effect of intravenous propacetamol within the first 2 h after administration. Such rapid antipyretic effect of propacetamol may be promising in preventing recurrent febrile seizures, because approximately half of the recurrent seizure events are encountered in the first 2 h after a second fever episode [23]. Beyond 3 h after antipyretics administration, the BT change between the two groups did not differ significantly. This may be associated with the half-life of each antipyretic drug (1.8–3.5 h for dexibuprofen and 2.1–4.8 h for propacetamol) [24, 25]. Once the plasma concentration of the drug is reduced, the

antipyretic effect would be diminished and thus lead to sequential rise in BT, minimizing the significant difference of BT between the two groups in the later hours after antipyretic administration.

Furthermore, propacetamol has another advantage over NSAIDs in that it interferes less with platelet functions. In previous literature, propacetamol was shown to be related with reversible platelet dysfunction but at a lesser extent compared to ketorolac [26]. Further, in more recent reports, paracetamol – the hydrolyzed product of propacetamol – has been studied for its efficacy and safety in preterm infants for treatment of patent ductus arteriosus, and has shown less adverse effects concerning platelet function [27]. Therefore, propacetamol may be safely used in patients with hemorrhage risks or underlying hematologic diseases. Also, the safety profile of propacetamol is known to be superior to that of NSAIDs for use in patients with a history of peptic ulcers or asthma [28].

Meanwhile, the recommended dosage of acetaminophen varies depending on the age or weight of the patient. For example, Fusco et al. [29] administered 7.5 mg/kg, 10 mg/kg, and 15 mg/kg of acetaminophen to children < 3 months, ≥ 3 months and < 24 months, ≥ 24 months old, respectively. In our study, we administered 15 mg/kg of propacetamol (7.5 mg/kg of acetaminophen) in patients weighing < 10 kg and 30 ml/kg of propacetamol (15 mg/kg of acetaminophen) in patients weighing ≥10 kg. Complying with this set criteria, the actual dosage administered was equal to or less than previously known dosages (provided that a child reaches 10 kg at 12 months of age), but the antipyretic effect was satisfactory and the safety profiles were acceptable.

The adverse effect(s) of a drug is also an issue to take a cautious notice in. Pain at the injection site is a typical adverse event of intravenous propacetamol administration, which was shown to reach 10.0% in a previous publication

Table 3 Efficacy analysis

Efficacy variable	Study group ($n = 125$)	Control group ($n = 138$)	p-value
AUC of BT change at 6 h after administration-and-time relationship	5.98 ± 3.87	5.78 ± 4.01	0.683
BT reduction at 4 h after administration (°C)	0.97 ± 0.90	1.16 ± 0.92	0.09
Maximum value of BT reduction during the 6 h after administration (°C)	1.63 ± 0.66	1.64 ± 0.70	0.855
Number of patients whose BT normalized (< 37.0 °C) at 6 h after administration, n (%)	26 (20.8)	23 (16.7)	0.390
Time point when BT first reached < 37.0 °C, hour	1.73 ± 1.29	2.13 ± 1.06	0.064

Results are presented as mean ± standard deviation or as a percentage (%)
BT Body Temperature
AUC Area Under the Curve

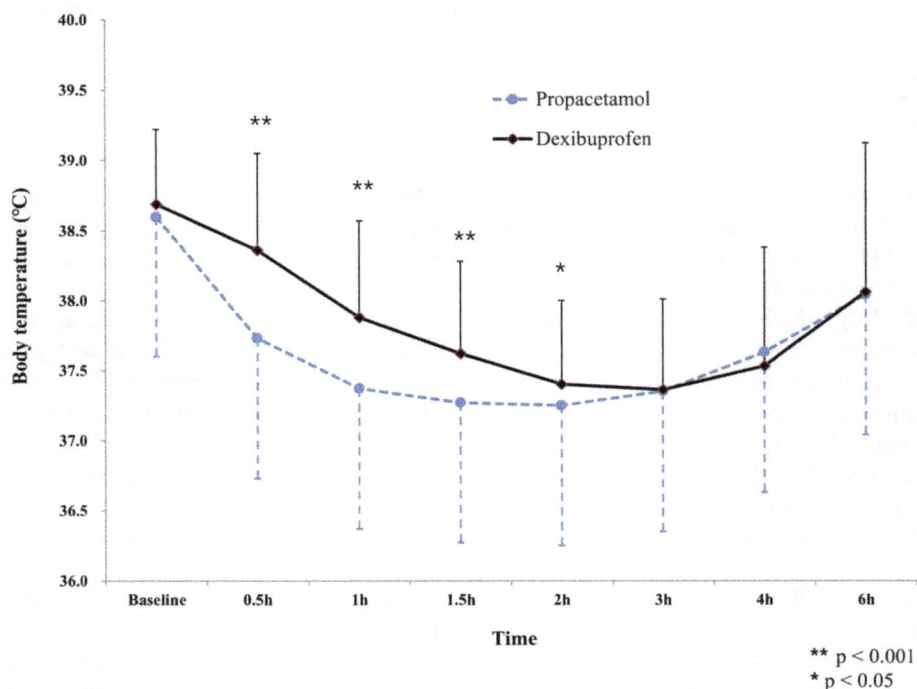

Fig. 2 Changes of mean temperature (°C) after the administration h: hour

by Walson et al. [7]. However, Walson and colleagues showed that pain at the injection site was 9.5% even in the placebo group. Such pain can be alleviated by slow infusion of the drug [5]. In this study, we diluted propacetamol in 100 ml of 0.9% sodium chloride solution and slowly intravenously infused the drug for 30 min, and pain at the injection site was not reported.

This study is limited in that intention-to-treat analysis was not done, which necessitates complements in future researches. Also, future studies are warranted to evaluate the antipyretic efficacy and safety of intravenous propacetamol involving more various disease entities. Furthermore, supplemental researches over the combination or alternation therapy of propacetamol and other po antipyretic (i.e, NSAIDs) are required.

Conclusion

We were able to verify the antipyretic efficacy and safety of intravenous propacetamol in febrile pediatric URTI patients. Intravenous propacetamol may be used effectively in patients for whom oral antipyretics cannot be administered or a prompt antipyretic is warranted.

Table 4 Number of children with adverse events

	Study group (n = 125)	Control group (n = 138)	p-value
Vomiting	1 (0.8)	4 (2.9)	0.373
Diarrhea	3 (2.4)	7 (5.1)	0.340
Abdominal pain	0 (0)	1 (0.7)	–
Constipation	1 (0.8)	0 (0)	–
Rash	5 (4.0)	5 (3.6)	–
Elevated liver enzyme level			
AST	8 (6.4)	14 (10.1)	0.373
ALT	5 (4.0)	9 (6.5)	0.420
Thrombocytopenia	8 (6.4)	13 (9.4)	0.495

Results are presented as a percentage (%)
AST aspartate aminotransferase
ALT alanine aminotransferase

Abbreviations
NSAIDs: Nonsteroidal anti-inflammatory drugs; URTI: Upper respiratory tract infection

Funding
This study was financially supported by Yungjin Pharm. Co. Ltd., Seoul, Republic of Korea (research grant number: YJ9–301).

Authors' contributions
SJC designed the study, carried out statistical analyses, interpreted data, and wrote the draft and final version of the manuscript. SNM, UYC, YHC, JHL, JWR, JL, and HMK collected data. SNM critically revised the manuscript. DCJ supervised the whole process, critically revised the manuscript, and approved the final version. All authors read and approved the final manuscript.

Competing interests

The authors declare that they have no competing interests.

Author details

[1]Department of Pediatrics, Asan Medical Center Children's Hospital, University of Ulsan College of Medicine, Seoul, Republic of Korea. [2]Graduate School of Medicine, The Catholic University of Korea, College of Medicine, Seoul, Republic of Korea. [3]Department of Pediatrics, College of Medicine, The Catholic University of Korea, 222, Banpodaero, Seocho-gu, Seoul 06591, Republic of Korea. [4]Department of Pediatrics, Hanjin General Hospital, Seoul, Republic of Korea. [5]Department of Pediatrics, Yonsei Christian Hospital, Wonju, Republic of Korea. [6]Vaccine Bio-research Institute, College of Medicine, The Catholic University of Korea, Seoul, Republic of Korea.

References

1. Kohl KS, Marcy SM, Blum M, Jones MC, Dagan R, Hansen J, Nalin D, Rothstein E, The Brighton Collaboration Fever Working Group. Fever after immunization: current concepts and improved future scientific understanding. Clin Infect Dis. 2004;39:389–94.
2. Crocetti M, Moghbeli N, Serwint J. Fever phobia revisited: have parental misconceptions about fever changed in 20 years. Pediatrics. 2001;107(6):1241–6.
3. Evans SS, Repasky EA, Fisher DT. Fever and the thermal regulation of immunity: the immune system feels the heat. Nat Rev Immunol. 2015;15(6):335–49.
4. Hasday JD, Garrison A. Antipyretic therapy in patients with sepsis. Clin Infect Dis. 2000;31(suppl 5):S234–41.
5. Depre M, van Hecken A, Verbesselt R, Tjandra-Maga TB, Gerin M, de Schepper PJ. Tolerance and pharmacokinetics of propacetamol, a paracetamol formulation for intravenous use. Fundam Clin Pharmacol. 1992;6:259–62.
6. Autret E, Dutertre JP, Breteau M, Jonville AP, Furet Y, Laugier J. Pharmacokinetics of paracetamol in the neonate and infant after administration of propacetamol chlorhydrate. Dev Pharmacol Ther. 1993;20:129–34.
7. Walson PD, Jones J, Chesney R, Rodarte A. Antipyretic efficacy and tolerability of a single intravenous dose of the acetaminophen prodrug propacetamol in children: a randomized, double-blind, placebo-controlled trial. Clin Ther. 2006;28:762–9.
8. Granry JC, Rod B, Boccard E, Hermann P, Gendron A, Saint-Maurice C. Pharmacokinetics and antipyretic effects on an injectable prodrug of paracetamol (propacetamol) in children. Paediatr Anaesth. 1992;2:291–5.
9. Reymond D, Birrer P, Lüthy AR, Rimensberger PC, Beck MN. Antipyretic effect of parenteral paracetamol (propacetamol) in pediatric oncologic patients: a randomized trial. Pediatr Hematol Oncol. 1997;14:51–7.
10. Duhamel JF, Le G, Dalphin ML, Payen-Champenois C. Antipyretic efficacy and safety of a single intravenous administration of 15 mg/kg paracetamol versus 30 mg/kg propacetamol in children with acute fever due to infection. Int J Clin Pharmacol Ther. 2007;45:221–9.
11. Duggan ST, Scott LJ. Intravenous paracetamol (acetaminophen). Drugs. 2009;69:101–13.
12. Walson PD, Galletta G, Chomilo F, Braden NJ, Sawyer LA, Scheinbaum ML. Comparison of multidose ibuprofen and acetaminophen therapy in febrile children. Am J Dis Child. 1992;146:626–32.
13. Autret E, Breart G, Jonville AP, Courcier S, Lassale C, Goehrs JM. Comparative efficacy and tolerance of ibuprofen syrup and acetaminophen syrup in children with pyrexia associated with infectious diseases and treated with antibiotics. Eur J Clin Pharmacol. 1994;46:197–201.
14. Amdekar YK, Desai RZ. Antipyretic activity of ibuprofen and paracetamol in children with pyrexia. Br J Clin Pract. 1985;39:140–3.
15. Kaehler ST, Phleps W, Hesse E. Dexibuprofen: pharmacology, therapeutic uses and safety. Inflammopharmacology. 2003;11:371–83.
16. Singer F, Mayrhofer F, Klein G, Hawel R, Kollenz CJ. Evaluation of the efficacy and dose-response relationship of dexibuprofen [S(+)-ibuprofen] in patients with osteoarthritis of the hip and comparison with racemic ibuprofen using the WOMAC osteoarthritis index. Int J Clin Pharmacol Ther. 2000;38:15–24.
17. Dionne RA, McCullagh L. Enhanced analgesia and suppression of plasma beta-endorphin by the S(+)-isomer of ibuprofen. Clin Pharmacol Ther. 1998;63:694–701.
18. Kim CK, Callaway Z, Choung JT, Yu JH, Shim KS, Kwon EM, Koh YY. Dexibuprofen for fever in children with upper respiratory tract infection. Pediatr Int. 2013;55:443–9.
19. Yoon JS, Jeong DC, Oh JW, Lee KY, Lee HS, Koh YY, Kim JT, Kang JH, Lee JS. The effects and safety of dexibuprofen compared with ibuprofen in febrile children caused by upper respiratory tract infection. Br J Clin Pharmacol. 2008;66:854–60.
20. Anderson BJ, Holford NH, Woollard GA, Kanagasundaram S, Mahadevan M. Perioperative pharmacodynamics of acetaminophen analgesia in children. Anesthesiology. 1999;90:411–21.
21. Babl FE, Theophilos T, Palmer GM. Is there a role for intravenous acetaminophen in pediatric emergency departments? Pediatr Emerg Care. 2011;27:496–9.
22. Holmer Pettersson P, Owall A, Jakobsson J. Early bioavailability of paracetamol after oral or intravenous administration. Acta Anaesthesiol Scand. 2004;48:867–70.
23. van Stuijvenberg M, Steyerberg EW, Derksen-Lubsen G, Moll HA. Temperature, age, and recurrence of febrile seizure. Arch Pediatr Adolesc Med. 1998;152:1170–5.
24. Zhang X, Liu X, Gong T, Sun X, Zhang Z-R. In vitro and in vivo investigation of dexibuprofen derivatives for CNS delivery. Acta Pharmacol Sin. 2012;33(2):279–88.
25. Allegaert K, Van der Marel CD, Debeer A, Pluim MAL, Van Lingen RA, Vanhole C, Tibboel D, Devlieger H. Pharmacokinetics of single dose intravenous propacetamol in neonates: effect of gestational age. Arch Dis Child Fetal Neonatal Ed. 2004;89(1):F25–8.
26. Niemi TT, Backman JT, Syrjälä MT, Viinikka LU, Rosenberg PH. Platelet dysfunction after intravenous ketorolac or propacetamol. Acta Anaesthesiol Scand. 2000;44:69–74.
27. El-Mashad AE, El-Mahdy H, El Amrousy D, Elgendy M. Comparative study of the efficacy and safety of paracetamol, ibuprofen, and indomethacin in closure of patent ductus arteriosus in preterm neonates. Eur J Pediatr. 2017;176:233–40.
28. Hyllested M, Jones S, Pedersen JL, Kehlet H. Comparative effect of paracetamol, NSAIDs or their combination in postoperative pain management: a qualitative review. Br J Anaesth. 2002;88:199–214.
29. Fusco NM, Parbuoni K, Morgan JA. Drug utilization, dosing, and costs after implementation of intravenous acetaminophen guidelines for pediatric patients. J Pediatr Pharmacol Ther. 2014;19:35–41.

4

Illness recognition and appropriate care seeking for newborn complications in rural Oromia and Amhara regional states of Ethiopia

Y. Amare[1]* (ID), S. Paul[2] and L. M. Sibley[3]

Abstract

Background: Ethiopia has made significant progress in reducing child mortality but newborn mortality has stagnated at around 29 deaths per 1000 births. The Maternal Health in Ethiopia Partnership (MaNHEP) was a 3.5-year implementation project aimed at developing a community-oriented model of maternal and newborn health in rural Ethiopia and to position it for scale up. In 2014, we conducted a case study of the project focusing on recognition of and timely biomedical care seeking for maternal and newborn complications. In this paper, we detail the main findings from one component of the case study – the narrative interviews on newborn complications.

Methods: The study area, comprised of six districts in which MaNHEP had been implemented, was located in the two most populous federal regions of Ethiopia, Oromia and Amhara. The final purposive sample consisted of 16 cases in which the newborn survived to 28 days of life, and 13 cases in which the newborn died within 28 days of life, for a total sample size of 29 cases. Narrative interview were conducted with the main caregiver and several witnesses to the event. Analysis of the data included thematic content analysis and the determination of care seeking pathways and levels and timeliness of biomedical care seeking.

Results: Mothers and other witnesses do recognize certain symptoms of newborn illness which they often mentioned in clusters. The majority considered the symptoms to be serious and in some case hopeless. Perceived causes were mostly natural. Forty-one percent of care seekers sought timely biomedical care in the neonatal period. Surprisingly, perceived severity did not necessarily trigger care seeking. Facilitators of biomedical care seeking included accessibility of health facilities and counseling by health workers, whereas barriers included perceived vulnerability of newborns, post-partum restrictions on movements, hopelessness, wait-and-see atttitudes, poor communication and physical inaccessibility of health facilities.

Conclusions: Symptom recognition and care seeking patterns indicate the need to strengthen focused locally relevant health messages which target mothers, fathers and other community members, to further enhance access to health care and to improve referral and quality of care.

Keywords: Newborn complications, Symptom recognition, Care seeking, Illness narratives

* Correspondence: yaredamare@yahoo.com
[1]Consultancy for Social Development, P.O. Box – 70196, Addis Ababa, Ethiopia

Background

Globally, 2.6 million newborns died in 2016. In Ethiopia, as in much of the developing world, the death rate among children under 5 years of age has declined at a higher rate than among newborns which has remained around 29 deaths per 1000 live births in 2016. [1] Consequently, 48% of deaths in children under 5 in Ethiopia occur in the neonatal period. [2] The most important causes of newborn death globally are pre-term birth complications (36%), intra-partum related events (24%), sepsis or meningitis (16%) and congenital abnormalities (11%). [2] Low levels of facility delivery, poor newborn care practices and limited care seeking for complications are underlying factors behind high rates of newborn morbidity and care seeking.

The Maternal Health in Ethiopia Partnership (MaNHEP) was a 3.5-year implementation project funded by the Bill & Melinda Gates Foundation to develop a community-oriented model of maternal and newborn health in rural Ethiopia and to position it for scale up. [3] Emory University implemented MaNHEP, in collaboration with John Snow Research and Training Inc., University Research Co. LLC, and Addis Ababa University. In 2014, Emory conducted a case study of the project focusing on recognition of and biomedical care seeking for maternal and newborn complications. The Ethiopia case study, was one of six country studies that included India, Indonesia, Nigeria, Tanzania and Uganda. All case studies were framed by the Delay Model. [4] In an earlier 2016 publication, we focused on findings pertaining to illness recognition and care seeking for maternal complications. [5] In this paper, we detail the main findings on illness recognition and care seeking for newborn complications and their implications for policy, programming and research.

Methods

Study site

As described in our recent publication focusing on illness recognition and care seeking for maternal complications [5], the study was conducted in the two most populous federal regions of Ethiopia, Oromia and Amhara (Fig. 1). [1] The districts were largely rural and included Degem, Kuyu and Warra Jarso in Oromia Region and North Achefer, South Achefer and Mecha in Amhara Region (estimated population 350,000). Each district has an urban center and around six health centers each of which oversee five or six health posts. From each district, one health center and two health posts were randomly selected. Cases of newborn complications occurring within the previous 6 months were identified and sampled from the catchment areas of these facilities, as described below. A case was defined as a mother, her newborn and the witnesses to the newborn's illness event.

Sampling and data collection

This section presents a summary of sampling and data collection procedures. For further details on sampling, the interview guide, reporting and maintainance of data

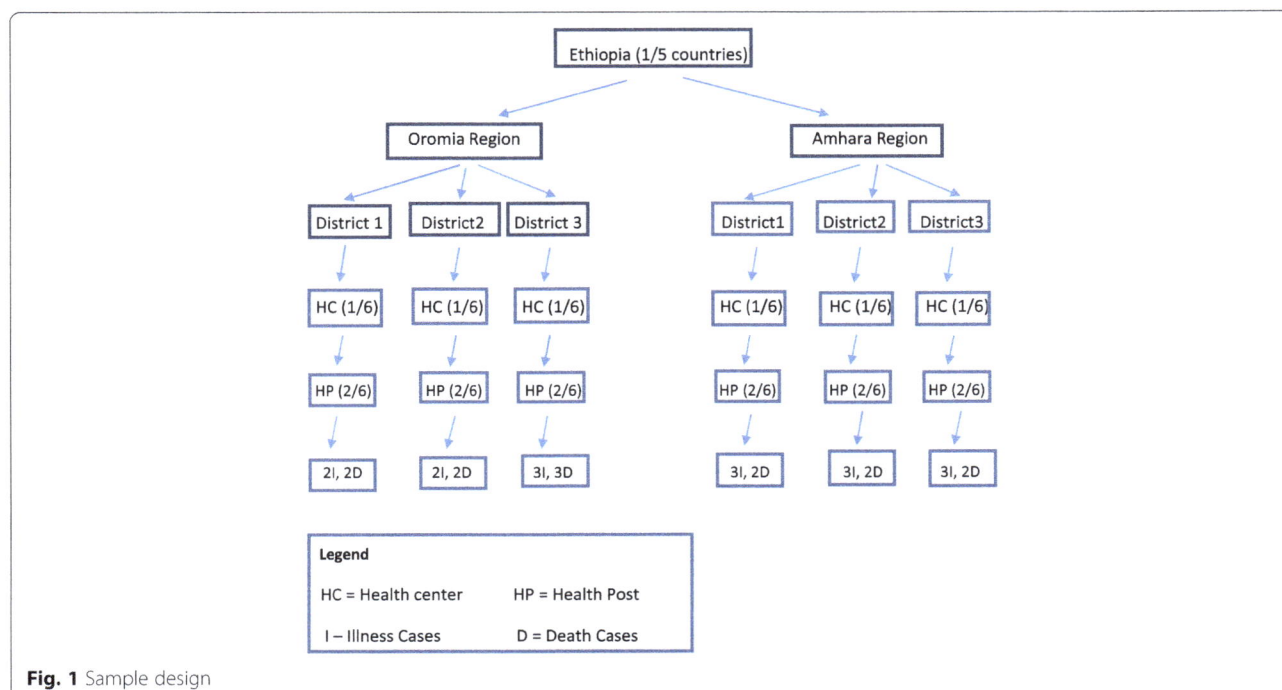

Fig. 1 Sample design

quality, see our previous publication on recognition and care seeking for maternal complications [5].

In the six districts, the study aimed to involve 30 cases: for each of the six districts, 3 mothers who perceived that their newborn became ill during the first month of life and was alive at 28 days of life, 2 mothers whose newborn became ill and died within 28 days of life and several witnesses to each event . Representation of diverse views and availability of cases were considerations in sampling. The inclusion criteria for these mothers were: female, age 18–49 years, gave birth in the previous 6 months, residence in the MaNHEP project area, perceived her newborn became ill within the first month of life and willing and able to participate. The final sample consisted of 16 cases in which the newborn survived to 28 days of life, and 13 cases in which the newborn died within 28 days of life, for a total sample size of 29 cases (Fig. 1).

After obtaining verbal informed consent using standard disclosure procedures, the study team used illness narrative interviews to collect data. The illness narrative is a qualitative rendering of an illness event by those who experienced the illness, along with those who were witnesses to the event. [6]

The narrative interviews were conducted with a primary caregiver, usually the mother of the newborn, and several witnesses to the illness event, who varied in number from one-to-three additional persons including her husband, mother-in-law, mother, sibling or neighbor. Although the interviews prioritized the primary caregiver who was usually the mother, other witnesses participated to a greater or lesser extent depending on personality and their role in the management of the illness episode. Thus, it turned out that the main or only respondent(s) in 13 of the 29 interviews was the mother; the mother and her husband in seven interviews; the mother and another person such as her mother-in-law or mother in five interviews; and persons other than the mother in four interviews.

Shortly after the interviews were conducted, "expanded field notes" on them were developed from memory, field notes, and audiotape recordings.

Analysis

. Coding procedures are detailed in our previous publication on illness recognition and care seeking for maternal complication. [5] A codebook, based on the illness narrative guide content and containing code definitions and inclusion and The analysis involved thematic content analysis using NVivo 10 based on the Delay Model [4]; re-coding of care-seeking pathways into: biomedical and non-biomedical or late biomedical categories; and univariate analysis to identify respondent characteristics and thematic code frequencies. Further details on these

analyses are available in an earlier publication on care seeking for compications of pregnancy and child birth. [7] We also conducted a multiple correspondence analysis (MCA) to detect underlying structures in the illness recognition data. MCA is an exploratory qualitative data analysis technique. Perceived symptoms and causes (please refer below to the list of symptoms and causes) were treated as nominal variables with multiple levels, and the correlations among them were projected in a 2-dimensional visual "map." Proximity between different levels of these variables and between groups of individuals associated with the levels in the map were examined for clusters or patterns of symptoms and causes in relation to outcomes. A clustering of symptoms and causes suggests illness recognition on the part of respondents. Grouping individuals by an external outcome variable allow one to examine whether clusters of symptoms and causes are associated with differential outcomes-e.g. babies survived or did not survive the first 28 days of life. MCA was performed using the statistical software R [8].

Ethical approval

Before initiating the study, ethical review of and approval for the study was obtained from Emory University Institutional Review board and the Oromia and Amhara Regional State Health Bureaus.

Results
Sample characteristics

Of the 29 cases, a majority of mothers were between 19 and 29 years of age (55%) and had never attended school (62%). A majority of mothers (62%) also had given birth in a health facility. Mothers from Oromia attended more years of school than their Amhara counterparts (80% versus 43%). Of the cases, 13 cases involved newborns that had died. Of the newborns that had died, nearly all died within the first week of life (11 died day 1–3, 1 died between 4 and 7 days, and 1 died between 7 and 28 days). There were no notable differences in maternal age or education between the the group of newborns who died and those who survived. On the other hand, more babies born at home died than babies born in a health facility (eight out of the nine babies versus five of eighteen babies, respectively). The two babies who were born on the way to a health facility both survived.

Delay 1
Perceived symptoms and their severity

Mothers and witnesses to the illness event mentioned a number of symptoms in their newborns. In order of frequency, many mothers mentioned inability to breastfeed (72%), followed by vomiting (41%), fever (38%), coughing, sneezing and/or stuffy nose (38%), continuous crying and weak or difficult breathing (31% each) and cold body (24%). Symptoms mentioned by between 10 and 20% of mothers included swollen uvula, weak or no crying, weakness and diarrhea. Lastly, symptoms mentioned by less than 10% of mothers included inability to pass urine or stool, change in stool color and weight loss, as well as hiccups, frothing from the mouth, bleeding from the nose and mouth, moaning, rash, swollen umbilical cord, and swelling on the back of the head and neck.

Symptoms were often mentioned in clusters. For example, eight Amhara mothers and witnesses among the total of 29 mothers noticed that the baby was unable to breastfeed, vomited and/or had a fever, high temperature on the back of the neck, in addition to a red swollen uvula. Three mothers and witnesses observed that their baby had a cough, congested nose or difficult breathing in conjunction with inability to breastfeed, fever or vomiting. Others mentioned continuous crying, inability to breastfeed, vomiting and diarrhea, along with fever and increasing weakness.

> "He refused to suck my breast and when he did suck on it, he vomited soon afterwards. He cried a lot and he was sweating and had high fever. There was a sound inside his stomach when he was crying."(Mother, Oromia).

Of the 13 babies who died, several mothers and witnesses reported that their baby cried continuously after birth, was unable to breastfeed, lost weight and had a fever. Another mother noticed that her baby felt very cold and was silent until she died, whereas a father and his mother observed that their twin babies were coughing and had a congestion, difficulty breathing and were cold. Finally, one mother and the two grandmothers realized that their twin babies were born too soon, observing that they were very small and thin, weak and/or making moaning sounds.

Seventeen of the twenty-nine mothers and witnesses believed that their newborn's illness symptoms were serious; whereas in four cases, they thought the symptoms indicated the babies' condition was hopeless. One woman, whose newborn experienced two separate illness episodes, perceived the initial illness to be serious, but the second illness episode as not serious.

> "Yes, I was worried that the baby had fever and spent the whole night crying. I was worried that he may die. A baby cries and stops but my baby cried continuously. He also did not breastfeed and had vomiting and diarrhea." (Mother, Amhara).

> "When they [twins] came out from the womb, they were born with many problems. Even if the elder one was crying, they were coughing since birth and their

body was as cold as iron. So I did not think they would start breastfeeding." (Grandmother, Oromia).

Some mothers and witnesses also reported changing perceptions of severity as symptoms presented. In three out of the 29 cases, they thought that the symptoms were not serious or that the baby would get better. Four families believed that the symptoms were not serious, but then serious when these symptoms persisted or other symptoms appeared.

> As one mother poignantly described, "I did not think that the baby was going to die. It was in the evening around nine that she was born and started to have difficulty breathing and sucking the breast. I was thinking that she may start sucking the breast next morning but she did not and her breathing problem persisted. Then she became weaker and weaker the following evening..." (Mother, Oromia).

Comparison of assessments of illness severity within cases of newborns who died versus cases of newborns who survived showed that, among the former, cases which were deemed to be hopeless were more frequent (4 of 13 cases versus 0 of 16 cases, respectively), cases which were deemed to be initially or ultimately not serious were more frequent (5 of 13 cases versus 2 of 16 cases, respectively), whereas cases which were judged to be serious were less frequent (4 of 13 cases versus 14 of 16 cases, respectively).

Perceived causes

Mothers and witnesses mentioned a number of causes for the observed symptoms. In order of frequency these included fallen uvula – a condition involving a red and swollen uvula and resulting in inability to breastfeed and fever (28%, Amhara only), prolonged labor and common cold (17% each), pregnancy workload and poor hygiene as well as supernatural causes such as God, evil eye or evil spirits (10% each). Causes mentioned in less than 10% of cases included maternal conditions such as bleeding, abdominal cramping, HIV, poor diet or malnutrition, eating bad food, physical sprain and maternal cough, as well as exposure to environmental and metaphysical elements resulting in a local illness known as *mitch* and the use of a scented soap for bathing, evil spirits or pre-term birth resulting in an illness known as *tilla*. Causes also included newborn conditions such as being in a bad position (e.g., breech), being malnourished (e.g., due to twins), being born too soon, having the umbilical cord around the neck as well as improper cord tying. The causes mentioned by mothers and caregivers in 90% of cases might be considered as "physical" or "biological."

Symptoms were sometimes thought to have multiple causes. For example, prolonged labor was associated with maternal twins or a baby that was in a bad position. In turn, prolonged labor was seen by some as a cause for inability to breast feed, continuous crying, difficult breathing or a cold body. A baby born too soon was associated with supernatural forces. Among some Amhara respondents, symptoms such as an inability to breastfeed, vomiting and fever were attributed to a swollen uvula which was, in turn, thought to be a result of natural processes, a heavy workload during pregnancy, bodily sprain or exposure to cold. Among Oromo respondents, these symptoms were thought to be caused by exposure to *mitch*, inadequate diet or poor hygiene. A cough, difficulty breathing and fever were often attributed to a common cold which was, in turn, thought to be a result of exposure to cold weather, a bad smell or lack of hygiene. As one father described,

"I have found out that he had difficulty breathing, fever, coughing and vomiting. I thought the problem was a common cold due to the cold weather and the smell from the cattle we share our house with." (Father, Oromia).

Illness recognition

The MCA bi-plot map (Fig. 2) of the top 11 contributing variable levels for symptoms and causes reported by mothers and witnesses in each case shows that two MCA dimensions explained almost 40% (dimension 1 and 2 explains ~ 24 and 14%) of the variance in the data respectively. The cases are color-coded by two outcome groups: 1 = died within first 28 days, 2 = survived more than 28 days. One can see in the upper left quadrant of the map that symptoms of cough and congestion are correlated with causes common cold and poor hygiene, and that most of these newborns were among those that survived more than 28 days. Similarly, in the lower left quadrant one can see that symptoms of red swollen uvula and fever are associated the condition of fallen uvula, a folk category reported in Amhara only. In the lower right quadrant, symptoms of "weak or no cry," "difficulty breathing," "cold body," and the cause "born too soon" were clustered together, and most of the newborns in this quadrant died within the first 28 days. The cases falling into the two outcome categories (marked by green and brown triangles) appear separated and associated with different kinds of symptoms and causes, and the 95% confidence ellipses drawn around the

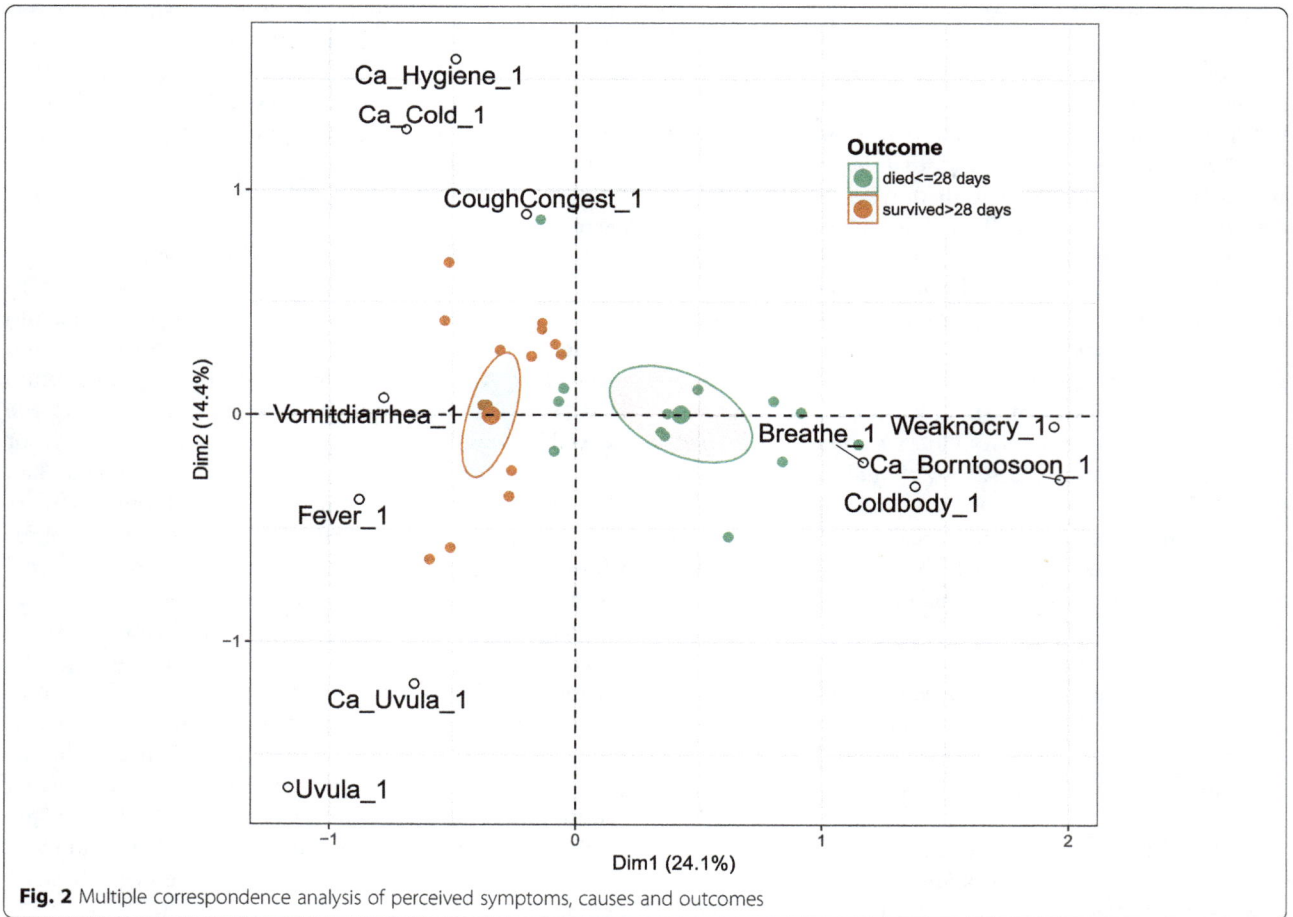

Fig. 2 Multiple correspondence analysis of perceived symptoms, causes and outcomes

mean point of the two groups of individuals do not overlap, indicating that the group means were significantly different. There is heterogeneity in symptoms and causes among the cases in which the newborns survived.

Decision-makers and time to make a decision to seek care

Decision-makers included parents of the newborn as well as other close members of the family such as their parents, a sister, sister-in-law, daughter or neighbor. Although the decision to seek biomedical care was often made in consultation with others, the final decision-makers were often the parents (8 out of 29 cases) or the mother herself (8 cases). Fathers were less often the sole decision maker (4 cases). As one woman commented:

> The baby spent the night crying a lot. It got even worse at night. I then decided that I would take the baby to the health center. Neighbors were complaining that I should not go to the health center before the baby was baptized. They said that an evil spirit would attack me. I ignored them and took the baby to the health center. (Amhara mother).

Of the 16 cases in which biomedical care was pursued, the time from illness recognition to the decision to seek care varied, from less than 12 h (six cases), 12–24 h (five cases), 25–72 h (two cases) to greater than 72 h (three cases, on days 5, 7 and 28).

Delay 2
Care seeking pathways

Mothers and families took different pathways to access care for their newborns. Of the 16 newborns who survived the illness event, twelve families (75%) sought biomedical care (Table 1). Two newborns first received care at a health center. Seven newborns were first treated at home or by a local healer and secondly received care at a hospital, health center, health post or by an HEW who was called-in to the home. One of these newborns was subsequently treated at home and at a health center as third and fourth steps of care. Three newborns received two treatments at home or by a local healer who was called-in before being taken to a health center. One of them was also subsequently treated by a local healer who was called-in as a first step of care. Of the four surviving newborns who did not receive biomedical care (25%), two received treatment at home and two were treated by a local healer who was called-in. One of the former was also subsequently treated by a local healer.

Of the 13 newborns who died, ten families (77%) did not seek biomedical care and were treated or cared for only at home (Table 2). Of the remaining three newborns, two received treatment at a health center and one at a hospital.

For analytical purposes, we chose to define care seeking at a health facility as a first or second step in response to newborn illness symptoms as 'timely

Table 1 Biomedical and non-biomedical care-seeking steps taken by families of 16 surviving newborns

First Step	Second Step	Third Step	Fourth Step
Biomedical care			
Health Center			
($n = 2$)			
Home	Hospital/Health Center/Post	Home	Health Center
($n = 5$)	($n = 5$)	($n = 1$)	($n = 1$)
Home	Home	Health Center	
($n = 1$)	($n = 1$)	($n = 1$)	
Home	Home Call-in	Health Center	Home Call-in
($n = 2$)	($n = 2$)	($n = 1$)	($n = 1$)
Home Call-in	Hospital	Health Center	
($n = 1$)	($n = 1$)	($n = 1$)	
Home Call-in	Home	Health Center	
($n = 1$)	($n = 1$)	($n = 1$)	
Non-Biomedical care			
Home	Home Call-in		
($n = 2$)	($n = 1$)		
Home Call-in			
($n = 2$)			

Table 2 Biomedical and non-biomedicalcare-seeking steps taken by families of 13 newborns who died

First Step	Second Step	Third Step	Fourth Step
Biomedical care			
Health Center			
(n = 2)			
Hospital			
(n = 1)			
Non-Biomedical care			
Home			
(n = 10)			

biomedical care seeking'. According to our definition, 12 of 29 families (41%) sought timely biomedical care in the neonatal period.

Timely biomedical care seeking was more frequent in the case of newborns who survived (8 of 16) compared to newborns who died (4 of 13). It was also associated with some characteristics of families. Timely biomedical care seeking was more frequent among younger mothers aged 19 to 29 years of age versus mothers older than 29 years of age (8 of 17 versus 3 of 10, respectively), mothers who delivered in a health facility as opposed to in a home or on the way to a health facility (10 of 18 versus 2 of 11, repectively), and, to a lesser extent, those who perceived the illness episode to be serious as compared to those who perceived it to be initially or ultimately not serious or hopeless (8 of 12 versus 10 of 17, respectively).

Symptoms and causes that appeared to have triggered biomedical care seeking were coughing, sneezing or stuffy nose associated with the common cold and poor maternal hygiene; and prolonged labor associated with maternal cramping and bleeding. Other symptoms included continuous crying, vomiting, malnutrition and improper cord tying. Symptoms that were as likely to trigger care seeking as not were difficulty breastfeeding and fever, both associated with a number of causes. Finally, symptoms and causes that were not associated with biomedical care seeking included swollen red uvula associated with the folk illness fallen uvula; and difficulty breathing, weak or no crying, and cold body associated with being born too soon or to supernatural causes. Few families relied on local traditional healers and birth attendants as a first or second step of care (6 of 29), in almost all cases for a fallen uvula.

Facilitators, delayers and barriers to care seeking

Respondents reported a number of factors that facilitated, delayed or prevented their use of health facility care. Facilitators included physical and financial accessibility of HEWs or health posts, as well as health education and advice from HEWs, health workers or neighbors. Factors that either delayed or prevented care seeking included postpartum restrictions on women's movement, perceived physical or spiritual vulnerability and weakness of post-natal women and newborns, hopelessness, the hope that the baby will get better, fear of travelling during the day time which may expose one to *mitch*, the evil eye or curious neighbors, or fears of poor treatment at the health facility. Other delaying factors were clinic hours, rain or night time hours, poor communications, distance, lack of transportation and financial constraints, e.g., one family that had to wait several weeks to receive a loan from their funeral association to cover medical costs.

Discussion

Summary of findings

In relation to Delay 1, the study findings suggest that the mothers and witnesses did recognize certain illness symptoms in their newborn. On the one hand, a number of symptoms were reported in clusters and were associated with particular causes such as being born too soon (premature), a common cold or lack of hygiene, or a fallen uvula. On the other hand, frequently mentioned symptoms such as difficulty breastfeeding and fever, important danger signs from a biomedical perspective, were associated with a variety of causes. Although most mothers and witnesses considered the symptoms they observed to be serious, some considered them not serious or only gradually came to believe they were serious, which led to a wait-and-see approach. As mentioned previously, more caretakers who considered their newborns' illnesses symptoms to be hopeless or not serious were among those whose newborns died.

Symptoms or causes perceived as serious, however, did not necessarily lead to care seeking, as evident in the 10 families who did not seek biomedical care or sought late care. It is especially concerning that symptoms such as difficulty breastfeeding, fever, difficulty breathing, weak or no crying, and a cold newborn body did not trigger care seeking in all cases. Although the newborn's parents were the main decision makers, others such as their parents, a sister, sister-in-law, daughter or neighbor were often involved. Their considerations about whether to seek care are consistent with the Delay Model [4] and include cultural norms such as perceived vulnerability and postpartum restrictions on the movement of mothers and newborns, advice from health workers, accessibility of services and perceived quality of care, as well as environmental conditions, economic and logistical issues.

In relation to Delay 2, in spite of the above considerations, 12 of 29 families sought timely bio-medical care, most often after an initial attempt at home-based care. Importantly, 38% of these families made the decision to seek care on the day that they recognized their newborn's illness. And few families relied on local traditional healers and birth attendants as a first or second step of care (10% each), primarily for the traditional illness, fallen uvula. Timely biomedical care seeking was more common among younger mothers, mothers who had delivered in a health facility, babies who survived the neonatal period, and to some extent among families who perceived the illness episode to be serious.

Researchers examining illness recognition and care seeking typically conduct descriptive studies using mixed methods and situated in a variety of settings, often in South Asia and sub-Saharan Africa. Some of these studies found that newborn caretaker recognition of newborn illness symptoms to be poor [9, 10] whereas other studies found that care takers did recognize such symptoms [11, 12]. Findings from our study conform with the latter including symptom clusters associated with the common cold, the folk illness fallen uvula, and preterm babies and those with difficulty breathing, which are associated with different causes and outcomes. Previous studies have shown that perceived causes of newborn illness range from the supernatural to naturalistic which influence whether traditional or modern treatment is utilized [12, 13, 14]. In this study, illness responses exhibited some association with specific types of mostly naturalistic causes. Conceptions and responses related to the fallen uvula illness in Amhara region resemble the local illnesses recognized in other countries which are seen to be best treated with traditional medicine [10, 15]. Illness symptoms that are considered serious have been found to be associated with care seeking in some studies whereas this association was weaker in a study conducted in Ghana and also in our study [10, 16].

Use of biomedical care ranging from 14 to 39% of illness episodes have been reported in various studies as compared to 40% in this study [11, 17, 18]. One of these studies conducted in Nepal reported that half of those who sought medical care did so after the first 48 h from the onset of illness as compared to 38% who sought such care in the first day after symptoms were recognized in our study [14]. The data we have presented on the characteristics of newborn care takers who seek such care are often not available in similar studies and contrast with the findings of one study on characteristics associated with care seeking for children under five [19]. We have also found that newborn survival is associated with facility delivery, the assessment that illness symptoms are serious and with the use of biomedical care.

Previous research has also explicitly identified factors which delay or prevent care seeking for newborn illnesses. Barriers such as aspects of local understanding of illness including symptom recognition, causation and severity, associated use of traditional treatments, wait-and-see attitudes, hopelessnes, negative experiences at health facilities, and lack of physical and financial access have been discussed in various studies [10, 14, 17, 20]. While finding that symptom recognition is not as much of a constraint on care seeking, this study has also identified all these barriers in addition to the role of postpartum restrictions on the movement and perceived vulnerability of women and newborns, reluctance to travel during the day time, limited clinic hours, and environmental factors. Furthermore, enablers such as the physical and financial accessibility of health posts and health counseling and education from health workers and acquaintances have been identified.

Strengths and challenges
The illness narrative method generated data on the actual experience and diverse perspectives of witnesses to the event. The illness event timeline and neutral probes used in the narrative interview stimulate recall and increase validity of the data. The replicability of the narrative interviews is unknown.

Conclusions
The findings of this study show that mothers and other witnesses generally recognize certain newborn illness symptoms and their seriousness. Several of them did initially or ultimately consider symptoms to be not serious or hopeless. Recognition of the seriousness of symptoms does not always lead to timely biomedical care seeking, although in our setting care seeking appears to occur more frequently among younger mothers, as well as those who gave birth in a health facility. The findings thus indicate an urgent need to focus health education and behavior change efforts on the seriousness as well as treatability of illness symptoms and identified local cultural factors that impede care seeking such as traditional postpartum restrictions on women's movement and associated beliefs about the vulnerability of mothers and newborns to harmful metaphysical elements if taken outside of the home, hopelessness and, in the case of Amhara region, the folk illness, fallen uvula. Families must come to understand timely biomedical care will improve the chances of their newborns' survival. Continued efforts to reduce known environmental, logistic and economic barriers to care seeking are also needed.

Abbreviations
FMoH: Federal Ministry of Health; HDA: Health Development Army; HEW: Health Extension Worker; MaNHEP: Maternal and Newborn Health in Ethiopia Partnership; RHB: Regional Health Bureau; URC: University Research Company, LLC; USAID: United States Agency for International Development

Acknowledgements
The authors would like to thank Allisyn Moran, Supria Madhavan, and Neal Brandes of USAID, and Danielle Charlet and Jim Sherry of URC for their vision, technical and financial support to the six country case study teams, including the Ethiopia team. We also thank Abebe Gebremariam Gobezayehu, Solomon Tesfaye, Aynalem H/Michael Frew and Lelisse Tadesse of Emory University Ethiopia and Mulusew Lijalem Belew of the Amhara Regional Health Bureau for their logistic contributions and support in sampling and case identification, as well as Abel Mekonnen, Yeshi Mulatu, Serawit Omer and Getahun Shiferaw of the Consultancy for Social Development for their role in conducting the illness narratives and data coding. Finally, we would like to express our gratitude to the women and families who participated in the illness narratives. While participation sometimes elicited painful memories, the information shared will help to improve our understanding and addressing of factors that facilitate and impede timely biomedical care seeking for others who, in the future, may be faced with complications of pregnancy and childbirth.

Funding
This study was made possible through funding by the United States Agency for International Development Translating Research into Action (TRAction) Project "Systematic Review of Illness Recognition and Appropriate Care Seeking for Maternal and Newborn Complications" through University Research Co., LLC. Both USAID and University Research Company, LLC, contributed to the overall six-country study design and protocol, development and standardization of the illness narrative guide and procedures, and organized data analysis and writing workshops to support six country teams. The views expressed in this manuscript are those of the authors.

Authors' contributions
YA contributed to the development and standardization of the illness narrative guide and procedures, training of interviewers, oversight of data collection and data quality, the analysis, interpretation and write-up of the data. SP contributed to the multiple correspondence analysis, its interpretation and write-up. LS contributed to the overall six-country study design and common protocol, its adaptation to the Ethiopia context, the development and standardization of the illness narrative guide and procedures, the analysis, interpretation and write-up of the data. All authors have read and approve of the final manuscript.

Competing interests
The authors declare that they have no competing interests.

Author details
[1]Consultancy for Social Development, P.O. Box – 70196, Addis Ababa, Ethiopia. [2]Nell Hodgson Woodruff School of Nursing, Emory University, 1520 Clifton Road NE, 30322 Atlanta, Georgia. [3]Nell Hodgson Woodruff School of Nursing and Rollins School of Public Health, Emory University, 1520 Clifton Road NE, 30322 Atlanta, Georgia.

References
1. Central Statistical Agency (CSA) [Ethiopia] and ICF. Ethiopia Demographic and Health Survey 2016. Addis Ababa, Rockville: CSA and ICF; 2016.
2. Department of Evidence, Information and Research (WHO, Geneva) and Maternal Child Epidemiology Estimation (MCEE) 2017. MCEE-WHO methods and data sources for child causes of death 2000-2016. Global Health Estimates Technical Paper WHO/HMM/IER/GHE/2017.1.
3. Sibley LM, Tesfaye S, Desta BF, Frew AH, Kebede A, Mohammed H, Hepburn K, Ethier-Stover K, Dynes M, Barry D, Gobezayehu AG. Improving maternal and newborn health care delivery in rural Amhara and Oromiya regions of Ethiopia through the maternal and newborn health in Ethiopia partnership. J Midwif Womens Health. 2014;59(S1):6–20.
4. Thaddeus S, Maine D. Too far to walk: maternal mortality in context. SocSci Med. 1994;38(8):1091–110.
5. Sibley L, Amare Y. Illness recognition and care seeking for maternal complications of pregnancy and birth in rural Amhara and Oromia regional states of Ethiopia. BMC Pregnancy Childbirth. 2016;17:384.
6. Yount K, Gittelsohn J. Reports of health-seeking behavior from the integrated illness history and a standard child morbidity survey. J Mixed Method Res. 2008;2(1):23–62.
7. Sibley L, Amare Y, Tesfaye S, Belew ML, Shiffra K, Barry D. Appropriateness and timeliness of care-seeking for complications of pregnancy and childbirth in rural Ethiopia: a case study of the maternal and newborn health in Ethiopia partnership. J Health Popul Nutr. 2017;36(Suppl 1):50.
8. The Comprehensive R Archive Network https://cran.r-project.org/. Accessed 2018.
9. Choi Y, El Arifeen S, Mannan I, Rahman SM, Bari S, Darmstadt GL, Black RE, Baqui AH, Projahnmo Study Group. Can mothers recognize neonatal illness correctly? Comparison of maternal report and assessment by community health workers in rural Bangladesh. Tropical Med Int Health. 2010;15(6):743–53.
10. Hill Z, Kendall C, Arthur P, Kirkwood B, Adjei E. Recognizing childhood illnesses and their traditional explanations: Exploring options for care-seeking interventions in the context of the IMCI strategy in rural Ghana. Tropical Med Int Health. 2003;8: 668–76.
11. Awasthi S, Verma T, Agarwal M. Danger signs of neonatal illnesses: perceptions of caregivers and health workers in northern India. Bull World Health Organ. 2006;84:819–26.
12. Engmann C, Adongo P, Akawire Aborigo R, Gupta M, Logonia G, Affah G, Waiswa P, Hodgson A, Moyer CA. Infant illness spanning the antenatal to early neonatal continuum in rural northern Ghana: local perceptions, beliefs and practices. J Perinatol. 2013;33:476–81.
13. Amare Y, Degefie T, Mulligan B. Newborn care seeking practices in central and southern Ethiopia and implications for community-based programming. Ethiop J Health Dev. 2012;27(1):3–7.
14. Mesko N, Osrin D, Tamang S, Shrestha BP, Manandhar DS, Manandhar M, Standing H, Costello AM. Care for perinatal illness in rural Nepal: a descriptive study with cross-sectional and qualitative components. BMC Int Health Hum Rights. 2003;3(1):3.
15. Awasthi S, Srivastava NM, Pant S. Symptom-specific care-seeking behavior for sick neonates among urban poor in Lucknow, northern India. J Perinatol. 2008;28:S69–75.
16. Amarasiri de Silva MW, Wijekoon A, Hornik R, Martines J. Care seeking in Sri Lanka: one possible explanation for low childhood mortality. Soc Sci Med. 2001;53(10):1363–72.
17. Bazzano AN, Kirkwood BR, Tawiah-Agyemang C, Owusu-Agyei S, Adongo PB. Beyond symptom recognition: care-seeking for ill newborns in rural Ghana. Tropical Med Int Health. 2008;13(1):123–8.
18. Chowdhury H, Thompson S, Ali M, Alam N, Yunus M, Streatfield P. Care seeking for fatal illness episodes in neonates: a population-based study in rural Bangladesh. BMC Pediatr. 2011;11:88.
19. Sutrisna B, Kresno S, Utomo B, Sutrisna B, Reingold A, Harrison G. Care-seeking for fatal illnesses in young children in Indramayu, West Java, Indonesia. The Lancet. 1993;342(8874):787–9.
20. Mohan P, Iyengar SD, Agarwal K, Martines JC, Sen K. Care-seeking practices in rural Rajasthan: barriers and facilitating factors. J Perinatol. 2008;28(S2): S31–7.

5

The CANadian Pediatric Weight management Registry (CANPWR): lessons learned from developing and initiating a national, multi-centre study embedded in pediatric clinical practice

Katherine M. Morrison[1,2]*iD, Geoff D. C. Ball[3], Josephine Ho[4], Pam Mackie[2], Annick Buchholz[5], Jean-Pierre Chanoine[6], Jill Hamilton[7], Anne-Marie Laberge[8], Laurent Legault[9], Lehana Thabane[1,2], Mark Tremblay[5] and Ian Zenlea[10]

Abstract

Background: There is increasing recognition of the value of "real-world evidence" in evaluating health care services. Registry-based, observational studies conducted in clinical settings represent a relevant model to achieve this directive. Starting in 2010, we undertook a longitudinal, observational study (the CANadian Pediatric Weight management Registry [CANPWR]), which is embedded in 10 multidisciplinary, pediatric weight management clinics across Canada. The objective of this paper was to share the lessons our team learned from this multi-centre project.

Methods: Data sources included a retrospective review of minutes from 120 teleconferences with research staff and investigators, notes taken during clinical site visits made by project leaders, information from quality control processes to ensure data accuracy and completeness, and a study-specific survey that was sent to all sites to solicit feedback from research team members ($n = 9$). Through an iterative process, the writing group identified key themes that surfaced during review of these information sources and final lessons learned were developed.

Results: Several key lessons emerged from our research, including the (1) value of pilot studies and central research coordination, (2) need for effective and regular communication, (3) importance of consensus on determining outcome measures, (4) challenge of embedding research within clinical practice, and (5) difficulty in recruiting and retaining participants. The sites were, in spite of these challenges, enthusiastic about the benefits of participating in multi-centre collaborative studies.

Conclusion: Despite some challenges, multi-centre observational studies embedded in pediatric weight management clinics are feasible and can contribute important, practical insights into the effectiveness of health services for managing pediatric obesity in real-world settings.

Keywords: Childhood obesity, Treatment, Weight management, Pediatric, Research methodology, Cohort study, Cardiometabolic health outcomes

* Correspondence: kmorrison@mcmaster.ca
[1]Department of Pediatrics, McMaster University, Hamilton, ON, Canada
[2]Population Health Research Institute, McMaster University, Hamilton, ON, Canada
Full list of author information is available at the end of the article

Background

There is evidence to support the effectiveness of family-centred, multi-disciplinary health services for managing pediatric obesity [1, 2]; however, the impact on weight status is modest. Furthermore, there is limited information available on which models of health care delivery are most effective at improving weight and health and for which populations. Given the identified need to improve our evaluation of outcomes in the Canadian pediatric weight management context, our team of clinical researchers developed the CANadian Pediatric Weight management Registry (CANPWR) [3].

CANPWR is a prospective, national, multi-centre, observational cohort study created to evaluate the individual-, family-, and program-level determinants of *(i)* health outcomes (cardiometabolic health and health related quality of life) at baseline, *(ii)* change in health outcomes over a 3-year period, and *(iii)* attrition from multidisciplinary pediatric weight management clinics located across Canada. Results from our pilot study, which included five clinical sites, were reported previously [4]. The main study [3] is ongoing and was designed to enroll 1600 2–17 year-olds with overweight or obesity from 10 clinics over three years. CANPWR includes the systematic collection of a minimal dataset with the intention of documenting the effectiveness of therapies in real-world clinic settings and enhancing our understanding of which children are more likely to benefit from specific interventions [5]. In recent years, similar registries dedicated to the management of pediatric obesity have been undertaken in the US [6], Sweden [7] and Germany [8, 9]. The experience and insights gained in undertaking these projects, including CANPWR, have the potential to strengthen future registry studies as well as inform the structure and delivery of health services for managing pediatric obesity. The purpose of this paper was to document and share the key lessons that we learned from this multi-centre project.

Methods

The history of CANPWR

Our study began as a pilot (2010–2012) that was funded by the Canadian Institutes of Health Research (CIHR) through the Canadian Network and Centre for Trials Internationally program (details available at: www.cannectin.ca). As a pilot, CANPWR included five Canadian tertiary-level, multidisciplinary, pediatric weight management clinics (BC Children's Hospital in Vancouver, BC; Stollery Children's Hospital in Edmonton, AB; Children's Hospital of Eastern Ontario in Ottawa, ON; CHU-Sainte Justine in Montreal, QC; McMaster Children's Hospital in Hamilton, ON). Data collection was supported by a central coordinating site (Population Health Research Institute, McMaster University, Hamilton, ON). Our pilot

study was designed to assess a number of factors that would inform a larger-scale study, including *acceptability* (e.g., Can sites agree on a core set of variables and measurement protocols for data collection? Does data collection for research purposes burden or complement data capture for clinical purposes?) and *feasibility* (e.g., Are sites able to successfully enrol participants into CANPWR from the sample of boys and girls referred to the clinics? Are sites able to retain participants to enable longitudinal research data collection and analysis, regardless of whether individuals discontinue clinical care for weight management?). Data collected during our pilot were compared and contrasted with normative Canadian data, which highlighted the increased health risks present in children referred for weight management [4].

Building on our pilot experience and supported by a CIHR operating grant received in 2012 (Principal Investigator: KMM), CANPWR expanded to eight sites (original five sites, plus The Hospital for Sick Children in Toronto, ON; ICAN clinic in Toronto, ON; Montreal Children's Hospital in Montreal, QC). Two newly established clinics (Alberta Children's Hospital in Calgary, AB; Trillium Health Partners in Mississauga, ON) joined CANPWR in 2016, which brought the total number of sites to 10; subsequently, one site (ICAN clinic) became inactive in 2016 due to changes in the clinical practice.

Monthly teleconferences with research coordinators and investigators were recorded and summarized in minutes. For this manuscript, the research coordinator reviewed these minutes, extracted key themes for each call and summarized the main themes. Based on this, a survey was developed and sent to investigators and research coordinators at each site asking if all key processes and challenges of conducting the study were included (Additional file 1). The final edited survey was circulated electronically to team members at the CANPWR clinics between June and August, 2016. Responses were received from team members at all nine active sites. With these data (see Table 1) and supplemented by information from quality control processes referred to in Lesson 4, our manuscript authorship group summarized the findings as lessons. They used an online communication tool (www.slack.com; SLACK Offices, Vancouver, BC) to facilitate communication and host virtual meetings to author our manuscript. A summary of our results, categorized as lessons learned, is provided below.

Results

Lesson 1: Site-specific regulatory requirements can be managed effectively through the use of a pilot study and central coordinating Centre

The observed challenges of conducting multi-site clinical trials [10] are also relevant to observational studies such as CANPWR. As highlighted, specific requirements and length of time for approval from research ethics boards can

Table 1 Summary of survey responses and corresponding lessons learned from research team members at pilot and main study sites

	Pilot Study (n = 4 sites; % YES)	Main Study (n = 9 sites; % YES)	Comments on lessons learned
Lesson 1: Site-specific regulatory requirements can be managed effectively through the use of a pilot study and central coordinating centre.			
How much time did it take for Research Ethics Board (REB) approval?	Mean number of days: 133	Mean number of days: 38	REB approval was faster in the Main Study. REB approvals from other sites enabled expedited reviews for subsequent sites.
Did your REB require participants to complete a *consent to contact* prior to study recruitment?	0%	33%	The Main Study included a final and refined protocol, so fewer amendments were required over time.
Lesson 2: Effective team communication is essential for study coordination and conduct.			
Did you experience challenges with recruitment?	75%	66%	Pilot Study sites shared recruitment strategies with Main Study sites. Hiring and training new research staff across study sites introduced gaps in recruitment and follow-up.
Lesson 3: Improving clarity and gaining consensus on measures can be time-consuming, but can also enhance study and data quality.			
Were questions of the family difficult for the sites to acquire?	75%	33%	Questionnaires and measures were refined and consensus reached for important data elements, allowing less difficulty with data collection in main study.
Were the questions on family eating patterns challenging for clinical staff or families?	50%	22%	
Lesson 4: Integrating research with clinical practice can create logistical and operational challenges.			
Was the medical history questionnaire difficult to complete?	75%	33%	In the main study, sites were encouraged to integrate research questions and laboratory tests with clinical practice to make it easier to collect data consistently.
Was the physical exam difficult to complete?	25%	22%	When data were not collected during a clinic visit it was difficult to obtain later.
Were labs results difficult to collect?	25%	11%	Incorporating CRF into clinical care helped with data collection.
Were families able to complete all questionnaires at their first visit?	0%	22%	Increased length of CRF to accommodate health outcomes beyond cardiometabolic may have contributed to the observation that there was difficulty in entering data for the Main Study that was not present in the pilot.
Did your first encounter with the family occur at the time of a clinic visit?	100%	77%	
Did you encounter difficulty in entering data?	0%	33%	
Did you experience challenges in collecting clinical data that had been harmonized for the study?	0%	55%	
Were the CANPWR CRF (Case Report Forms) used for clinical purposes, too?	25%	55%	
Most common reasons for study participants choosing to enroll in CANPWR?	-To help others -To improve weight management program		
Clinicians opinions on best reasons to participate in CANPWR?	-Long-term family interactions -Linking weight management programs nationally		
Lesson 5: Study recruitment can be slow; retention is impacted by clinic attrition.			
Did families first learn about CANPWR from clinical team members?	100%	100%	In both the Pilot and Main Studies, clinical staff initially approached families about the study and then connected them with the research coordinators for further details.
Most common reason for families not to agree to recruitment			Lack of time was most commonly noted by the families as a reason not to participate
Did you have difficulty tracking participants over time?	50%	77%	The Main Study extends to three years following the baseline assessment. Sites reported challenges tracking participants (e.g., no longer in clinic; frequent *no-shows* to appointments).

vary site-to-site. As recommended, for our pilot study, we first sought and received research ethics approval at our central coordinating site in Hamilton, ON. The time that each site required to prepare and submit the application to their respective Research Ethics Board (REB) varied considerably (maximum difference of by up to 40 weeks). This delay occurred, in part, due to the requirement of one REB that the documents be translated into both English and French. This step was completed after the wording of the consent form and case report form (CRF) in English had been approved by the other REBs. After approval at the central coordinating site, the time from submission to approval at the other pilot sites varied from 5 to 17 weeks. As we transitioned from the pilot to main study, sites that were part of the original CANPWR pilot study had their REB applications approved in 2 to 10 weeks. The five sites that joined CANPWR for the full study had initial review periods of 1.5 to 12 weeks.

In addition to timelines, REB requirements influenced other study aspects including the type of data that could be collected and transmitted electronically to the central data centre. This was a result of varying definitions of personal identifying information and varying procedures for accessing clinical data for research. REB requirements also influenced study recruitment as three sites required clinicians to serve as intermediaries between families and our research team members, which included clinicians administering a *consent to contact* form with families. In other words, families were required to provide their written consent to be contacted by the research team. Because some site leaders perceived that this step might enhance recruitment, the consent to contact step was added at two additional sites. Other site-specific institutional regulations introduced variability in start-up time, including contract negotiations for accessing clinical data, data ownership, and budget. For instance, CANPWR research funds were received from the CIHR and held at our coordinating site in Hamilton. Individual contracts were then prepared with each site to transfer funds based on site-specific study activities (e.g., recruitment, data collection). At one site, contracts were required with both the academic institution and the regional health authority where the clinic was located, a requirement that delayed study initiation.

Lesson 2: Effective team communication is essential for study coordination and conduct

One of the operational aspects of CANPWR includes monthly teleconference meetings that are led by investigators from our coordinating site in Hamilton. Each month, separate coordinator and investigator teleconferences (duration: 1 h) are held to discuss practical, day-to-day issues as well as broader, academic topics, respectively. This communication has been complemented by an average of one site visit per site so far, made by coordinating site team

members to support individual sites and encourage adherence to study policies and procedures. A second site visit is envisioned. These meetings also provided contextual information, serving to highlight the clinic- and research-related variability between sites. Teleconferences and site visits also enabled data management strategies and kept sites accountable to and engaged with all study team members.

The sites varied in their access to a trained research coordinator, especially at study start-up and staff turnover has been common. Three sites enlisted the help of students as either volunteer helpers or research assistants. This created exceptional learning and teaching opportunities as well as reduced costs. Student activities were always overseen by research staff and the implemented quality control measures ensured high quality data. Some challenges introduced by the use of students included frequent turn-over and less flexible schedules. Thus research staff had to organize recurrent training sessions. Ongoing communication with an available central coordinator through both scheduled and ad hoc communications helped to minimize the impact of staff and student turnover.

Lesson 3: Improving clarity and gaining consensus on outcome measures can be time-consuming, but can also enhance study and data quality

An initial goal of CANPWR was to be the first harmonized, evidence-based registry to identify the key determinants of weight change in pediatric weight management clinics across Canada. The CANPWR investigators designed measures based on the best available evidence at the time. Where strong empirical evidence was lacking, expert, group-level consensus was necessary for measure development. The initial CANPWR measures set was designed along these principles [3]. Through implementation in the pilot sites, we realized that several questions were burdensome and impractical. For example, questions relating to puberty assessment by physician evaluation were discontinued due to challenges in collecting these data. Another example included a narrow focus on cardiometabolic health outcomes in our pilot, so the Main Study included additional data collection on mental health and health-related quality of life. Consensus on unclear definitions of data elements was reached through discussion with research and clinical team members across study sites, facilitated by our monthly teleconferences. A record of all discussions and decisions was maintained by our central research coordinator (PM).

Lesson 4: Integrating research with clinical practice can create logistical and operational challenges

Although integrating research with clinical practice can be beneficial, there are challenges that can arise. For instance, clinicians have busy schedules. Because they are funded to deliver health services, their interest in research can vary. If there is a lack of interest or attention to details, participant data may be missed. In some clinics, having physical space dedicated to research staff can be limited, which can be sub-optimal for participants and families when collecting data. To mitigate these challenges, CANPWR was embedded into clinical practices, which minimized the time needed by clinicians to identify potential participants, enhanced the feasibility of collecting outcome data, and allowed clinicians to focus on caring for their patients while researchers collected the required data [11].

As CANPWR did not require participating sites to modify their clinical practices, variation in the timing and pace of data collection occurred. The 6-month visit was scheduled 6 months after the date the clinical team considered the beginning of the intervention. This may have been beyond 6 months from study recruitment if there were delays in commencing group sessions. To enable flexibility for study participants, the window for conducting the annual study visits was set broadly (6 months on either side of the calculated date).

To ensure the data used to support the research efforts were valid and secure, CANPWR required a robust data management system and related practices. The CANPWR pilot sites learned that integrating the CRF into routine practice improved data collection. Integration of CANPWR data elements into the workflow of clinic visits was accomplished using paper or electronic data collection forms that were shared among sites and modified by each site to meet their local needs. The study sites that integrated the study case report forms into their clinical practice found that, data elements were more consistently collected and available. The requisite data was then extracted from the clinical record and transferred (online) into the electronic case report form. The specific location of the clinical data extracted by each site for each variable on the study CRF was identified at study start-up and reviewed by the central coordinator during the site visit. Sites were expected to use a paper copy to extract the data from the clinical chart as an intermediate step in order that this could be used for verification if the data was questioned through the routine quality control checks either at the time of data entry if outside the variable limits set or in monthly quality control reports.. Using this system, few challenges were identified in entering data into the study web-based data application.

The coordinating centre implemented monthly performance reports to track incomplete data. Reports were used to identify performance gaps, monitor changes over time, and support continuous quality assurance. These reports were valuable to ensure data completeness.

Lesson 5: Study recruitment can be slow; retention is impacted by clinic attrition
The ability of the research team to contact participants is influenced by availability and number of research team members, relationship between researchers and clinic team members, number of other ongoing or competing studies at each clinic, clinic flow, and volume of eligible participants. Researchers commented that recruitment was challenging, in part because potential participants were too tired or overwhelmed to want to hear about the research study or complete the informed consent process after a long clinic assessment. Participants' time pressures and coordination with clinical staff introduced challenges. All sites recruited more slowly than investigators anticipated at study outset. Recruitment was reviewed on monthly teleconference calls to recognize the site personnel for their work, collectively problem-solve challenges, and in some cases, encourage healthy competition (peer pressure) among sites. Additional strategies to improve recruitment included the use of a consent to contact form for all eligible participants, introducing research coordinators at initial clinic orientation sessions, frequent communication with clinicians at clinic meetings to provide study reminders and updates, and having the research coordinator available at clinic times to answer participants' and families' questions.

CANPWR was designed to follow participants for three years, whether or not they were still engaged in clinical care to determine how health outcomes changed once care was completed and to reduce biases introduced by the high attrition rates often seen from weight management clinics [12]. Participants who discontinued attending the clinic, but remained enrolled in CANPWR, were seen at times that accommodated families and the location depended on family preference and space availability (in clinic, in clinic space but out of clinic time or in research space). They were not seen by the clinical team. Continued study participation did not preclude families from re-engaging in clinical care, and our anecdotal experience revealed that for a small number of families, their research engagement facilitated their re-starting clinical care. All laboratory values were shared with the families and their primary care provider. When designing CANPWR, we recognized that including follow-up data collection for three years would be challenging due to high attrition [13] and because follow-up for most childhood obesity treatment studies is ≤24 months [14]. In our communication with families, we were explicit when explaining that their CANPWR participation was separate from their clinical health services; however, at many sites, when families discontinued attending appointments for weight management, it was challenging to engage them in attending CANPWR study visits. When we surveyed our sites, the majority highlighted difficulties in tracking participants longitudinally, noting that increased research personnel time was required as the study progressed to maintain tracking, largely due to attrition from the clinical programs. To mitigate loss to follow-up, the CANPWR investigators gave families unable to attend an in-person visit, the option to complete follow-up study visits by telephone for self-reported measures only (e.g., current health, medication use, health behaviours). While it was intended that this practical option would be effective for collecting data from participants who discontinued clinical care, to date, less than 10% of follow-up visits were carried out that way. Despite having this mode of data collection available for families, attrition remains a substantial issue in our clinics, which highlights the challenges of this issue in successfully managing pediatric obesity [13].

Discussion

In this report, we highlight a number of lessons we learned in developing and implementing the CANPWR study at 10 multidisciplinary, pediatric weight management clinics located across Canada. By surveying our site investigators and research personnel, we learned lessons that we believe may be of interest and relevance to other clinical researchers, both within and beyond our field of study. These lessons highlight the importance of planning, the value of pilot studies, the critical role of rigorous data collection procedures, and an active central coordinating site when conducting "real-world" studies. Finding the balance between rigorous data collection and the flexibility required to accommodate variable inter-clinic procedures is an important challenge that must be addressed prior to study initiation.

The lessons presented in this manuscript are similar to those reported by investigators involved in other registry studies [7, 9, 15–19]. These lessons include the need to train investigators to be able to properly conduct research [17]. Strategies recommended by others, and employed in CANPWR include incorporation of monthly or bi-monthly meetings, development of standard operating procedures, training of team members in data collection and data entry techniques, and variable definition classification to avoid data discrepancies [16, 19]. We, and others, have also identified the need to be creative and adopt alternative strategies to improve study recruitment and retention [15]. While others [18] have suggested flexibility in study design and statistical analyses to mitigate potential bias from missing data, we have utilized standardized approaches but have built in flexibility in timelines to assist sites in collecting as complete a dataset as possible. Further, we have similarly learned that it is important to have regular meetings to discuss the status of the registry and related projects, that meeting minutes be circulated, and that a running list of projects, papers, and abstract deadlines be maintained [19].

In spite of the challenges, investigators and research teams reported that the opportunity to be part of a national network of clinics was the "best thing about CANPWR". Prior to CANPWR, some of the investigators had collaborated on smaller-scale studies related to pediatric obesity in Canada [20]; however, CANPWR represented not only the largest research initiative to date, but the topic and scope of the research had a high degree of clinical relevance to the

day-to-day health services delivery of multidisciplinary care for managing pediatric obesity at clinics across the country. Since most pediatric weight management clinics in Canada were relatively new when CANPWR began [21], there was a high level of interest and collegiality to work collaboratively. Given that few programs at the time were evaluating their clinical services [21], participating in CANPWR provided a built-in procedure to contribute data to examine more general research questions while offering the ability to examine site-specific data, which could be used locally at the hospital or health system level for resource allocation and decision-making. From a practical perspective, there was a general desire to learn with and from one another, which is likely due, at least in part, to the challenges many clinicians face in providing health services to children and youth (and their families) with obesity.

Conclusion

Research studies based in "real-world" settings hold promise to illuminate the efficacy of interventions when implemented in a health care setting. Multiple challenges of conducting such studies have been identified and strategies to address them may improve outcomes. Clinical and research teams highlight the value of participating in such studies to their knowledge and practice.

Abbreviations
CANPWR: CANadian Pediatric Weight management Registry; CIHR: Canadian Institutes of Health Research; CRF: case report form(s); REB: Research Ethics Board

Funding
Funding was received from the Canadian Institutes of Health Research as follows: CANNeCTIN Pilot Project, CIHR #120287, CIHR MOP Grant #FRN 123505.

Authors' contributions
KMM, GDCB, JHO, PM, IZ conceived of this study, developed the questionnaire, interpreted the data, drafted the manuscript, and approved the final manuscript. AB, JPC, MT, JH, AML, LL and LT helped with data collection, provided critical evaluation / edits of the manuscript, and approved the final manuscript.
Written consent was received from the legal guardian of each study participant (all under 18 years of age). In addition, children age 5–17 years provided assent (a common practice with Canadian Children's Hospital Research Ethics Boards).

Competing interests
KM Morrison – No competing financial interests exist.
GDC Ball – No competing financial interests exist.
J Ho – No competing financial interests exist.
P Mackie – No competing financial interests exist.
I Zenlea – No competing financial interests exist.
A Buchholz – No competing financial interests exist.
JP Chanoine – No competing financial interests exist.
M Tremblay – No competing financial interests exist.
J Hamilton – Recipient of unrestricted research funds from the SickKids

University of Toronto Mead Johnson Chair in Child Nutritional Science.
AM Laberge – No competing financial interests exist.
L Legault – No competing financial interests exist.
L Thabane – No competing financial interests exist.

Author details

[1]Department of Pediatrics, McMaster University, Hamilton, ON, Canada. [2]Population Health Research Institute, McMaster University, Hamilton, ON, Canada. [3]Department of Pediatrics, University of Alberta, Edmonton, AB, Canada. [4]Department of Pediatrics, University of Calgary, Calgary, AB, Canada. [5]Children's Hospital of Eastern Ontario, Ottawa, ON, Canada. [6]Department of Pediatrics, University of British Columbia, Vancouver, BC, Canada. [7]The Hospital for Sick Children, Toronto, ON, Canada. [8]Department of Pediatrics, CHU Ste Justine, Montreal, QC, Canada. [9]Department of Pediatrics, McGill University, Montreal, QC, Canada. [10]Credit Valley Hospital, Mississauga, ON, Canada.

References

1. Peirson L, Fitzpatrick-Lewis D, Morrison K, Warren R, Usman Ali M, Raina P. Treatment of overweight and obesity in children and youth: a systematic review and meta-analysis. CMAJ Open. 2015;3:E35–46.
2. Wilfley DE, Staiano AE, Altman M, et al. Improving access and systems of care for evidence-based childhood obesity treatment: conference key findings and next steps. Obesity (Silver Spring). 2017;25:16–29.
3. Morrison KM, Damanhoury S, Buchholz A, et al. The CANadian pediatric weight management registry (CANPWR): study protocol. BMC Pediatr. 2014;14:161.
4. Tremblay MS, Feng M, Garriguet D, et al. Canadian pediatric weight management registry (CANPWR): baseline descriptive statistics and comparison to Canadian norms. BMC Obes. 2015;2:29.
5. Hoque DME, Kumari V, Ruseckaite R, et al. Impact of clinical registries on quality of patient care and health outcomes: protocol for a systematic review. BMJ Open. 2016;6:e010654.
6. Kirk S, Armstrong S, King E, et al. Establishment of the pediatric obesity weight evaluation registry: a National Research Collaborative for identifying the optimal assessment and treatment of pediatric obesity. Child Obes. 2017;13:9–17.
7. Hagman E, Reinehr T, Kowalski J, et al. Impaired fasting glucose prevalence in two nationwide cohorts of obese children and adolescents. Int J Obes. 2014;38:40–5.
8. Flechtner-Mors M, Wiegand S, Gellhaus I, et al. Screening for co-morbidity in 65,397 obese pediatric patients from Germany, Austria and Switzerland: adherence to guidelines improved from the year 2000 to 2010. Obes Facts. 2013;6:360–8.
9. Reinehr T, Wabitsch M, Andler W, et al. Medical care of obese children and adolescents. APV: a standardised multicentre documentation derived to study initial presentation and cardiovascular risk factors in patients transferred to specialised treatment institutions. Eur J Pediatr. 2004;163:308–12.
10. Forjuoh SN, Helduser JW, Bolin JN, et al. Challenges associated with multi-institutional multi-site clinical trial collaborations: lessons from a diabetes self-management interventions study in primary care. J Clin Trials. 2015;5:219.
11. Fiore LD, Lavori PW. Integrating randomized comparative effectiveness research with patient care. N Engl J Med. 2016;374:2152–8.
12. Dumville JC, Torgerson DJ, Hewitt CE. Reporting attrition in randomised controlled trials. BMJ. 2006;332:969–71.
13. Dhaliwal J, Nosworthy NMI, Holt NL, et al. Attrition and the management of pediatric obesity: an integrative review. Child Obes. 2014;10:461–73.
14. Rajjo T, Mohammed K, Alsawas M, et al. Treatment of pediatric obesity: an umbrella systematic review. J Clin Endocrinol Metab. 2017;102(3):763–75.
15. Grape A, Rhee H, Wicks M, et al. Recruitment and retention strategies for an urban adolescent study: lessons learned from a multi-center study of community-based asthma self-management intervention for adolescents. J Adolesc. 2018, Jun;65:123–32.
16. Lavigne J, Sharr C, Ozonoff A, et al. National Down syndrome patient database: insights from the development of a multi-center registry study. Am J Med Genet A. 2015;167A(11):2520–6.
17. Shapiro M, Silva SG, Compton S, et al. The child and adolescent psychiatry trials network (CAPTN): infrastructure development and lessons learned. Child Adolesc Psychiatry Ment Health. 2009;3(1):12.
18. Harambat J, Bonthuis M, Groothoff JW, et al. Lessons learned from the ESPN/ERA-EDTA registry. Pediatr Nephrol. 2016;31(11):2055–64.
19. Siegler JE, Boehme AK, Dorsey AM, et al. A comprehensive stroke center patient registry: advantages, limitations, and lessons learned. Med Student Res J. 2013;2:21–9.
20. Ball GD, Perez GA, Chanoine JP, et al. Should I stay or should I go? Understanding families' decisions regarding initiating, continuing, and terminating health services for managing pediatric obesity: the protocol for a multi-center, qualitative study. BMC Health Serv Res. 2012;12:486.
21. Ball GD, Ambler KA, Chanoine JP. Pediatric weight management programs in Canada: where, what and how? Int J Pediatr Obes. 2011;6:e58–61.

6

Prevalence and determinants of essential newborn care practices in the Lawra District of Ghana

Mahama Saaka*, Fusena Ali and Felicia Vuu

Abstract

Background: There was less than satisfactory progress, especially in sub-Saharan Africa, towards child and maternal mortality targets of Millennium Development Goals (MDGs) 4 and 5. The main aim of this study was to describe the prevalence and determinants of essential new newborn care practices in the Lawra District of Ghana.

Methods: A cross-sectional study was carried out in June 2014 on a sample of 422 lactating mothers and their children aged between 1 and 12 months. A systematic random sampling technique was used to select the study participants who attended post-natal clinic in the Lawra district hospital.

Results: Of the 418 newborns, only 36.8% (154) was judged to have had safe cord care, 34.9% (146) optimal thermal care, and 73.7% (308) were considered to have had adequate neonatal feeding. The overall prevalence of adequate new born care comprising good cord care, optimal thermal care and good neonatal feeding practices was only 15.8%.

Mothers who attained at least Senior High Secondary School were 20.5 times more likely to provide optimal thermal care [AOR 22.54; 95% CI (2.60–162.12)], compared to women had no formal education at all. Women who received adequate ANC services were 4.0 times (AOR = 4.04 [CI: 1.53, 10.66]) and 1.9 times (AOR = 1.90 [CI: 1.01, 3.61]) more likely to provide safe cord care and good neonatal feeding as compared to their counterparts who did not get adequate ANC. However, adequate ANC services was unrelated to optimal thermal care. Compared to women who delivered at home, women who delivered their index baby in a health facility were 5.6 times more likely of having safe cord care for their babies (AOR = 5.60, CI: 1.19–23.30), $p = 0.03$.

Conclusions: The coverage of essential newborn care practices was generally low. Essential newborn care practices were positively associated with high maternal educational attainment, adequate utilization of antenatal care services and high maternal knowledge of newborn danger signs. Therefore, greater improvement in essential newborn care practices could be attained through proven low-cost interventions such as effective ANC services, health and nutrition education that should span from community to health facility levels.

Keywords: Essential newborn care, Newborn danger signs, Neonate feeding, Optimal thermal care, Safe cord care, Lawra District

* Correspondence: mmsaaka@gmail.com
University for Development Studies, School of Allied Health Sciences, P O Box, 1883 Tamale, Ghana

Background

Many countries especially in sub-Saharan Africa were unable to achieve the Millennium Development Goals (MDGs) 4 and 5. In particular, the set target of reducing under-five mortality rates by two-thirds as of 2015 was not met because there was little reduction in neonatal mortality (NMR). Many countries are reported to have made little or no progress towards the child survival target, and that some countries in sub-Saharan Africa had even witnessed a deterioration in child survival rates [1].

Suboptimal newborn care practices still persist and neonatal mortality rates have been resistant to change and now contribute about 40% of all under-five deaths world-wide [2]. In Ghana, neonatal mortality is estimated at 29 /1000 live births and 68% of all deaths among children under age five years take place before a child's first birthday, with 48% occurring during the first month of life [3]. Though there has been a decline of 29% in neonatal mortality since 1993 in Ghana, the decrease was at a slower pace than infant and child mortality. Consequently, the contribution of neonatal deaths to infant deaths had increased from 53% in 1998 to 71% in 2014 [3].

World leaders have launched a renew effort to reduce child mortality under the Sustainable Development Goals (SDGs). One major target of the SDGs is to "end preventable deaths of newborns and children under 5 years of age, with all countries aiming to reduce neonatal mortality to at least 12 per 1,000 live births and under-5 mortality to at least 25 per 1,000 live births by 2030" [4]. To achieve this target, it is important for mothers to adopt essential newborn care practices. To help reduce newborn morbidity, mortality and promote healthy newborn care practices, the World Health Organization (WHO) recommended a package of essential newborn care practices some of which include clean cord care (that is, cutting and tying of the umbilical cord with a sterilized instrument and thread), thermal care (drying and wrapping the newborn immediately after delivery and delaying the newborn's first bath for at least 24 h or several days to reduce hypothermia risk), and initiating breastfeeding within the first hour of birth [5].

It has been estimated globally that over two-thirds of newborns could be saved through existing maternal and child health programmes that relate to cord care to decrease sepsis, temperature control and initiation of early breastfeeding [6–10].

In Ghana, skilled assistance during delivery has increased from 40% in 1988 to 74% in 2014. Facility-based deliveries have increased from 42% in 1993 to 73% in 2014. Despite this modest improvement, more than one-quarter of births occur at home especially in rural areas. In the Upper West Region where this study was conducted, delivery in a health facility was 63% of births [3].

Deliveries at home are usually without the support of skilled birth attendants (SBA). Under such circumstances, babies may not receive the recommended immediate newborn care practices and so become more vulnerable to infection-related risks [11]. There is evidence that suggests that most neonatal deaths in developing countries occur at home, and attended by unskilled health practitioners [2]. However, very little is documented on the traditional newborn care practices in the Lawra District of Ghana where a significant number of deliveries still take place at home. It is in view of this that this study was undertaken. The main aim was to describe the prevalence and determinants of essential newborn care practices.

Methods

Study setting

The study was carried out in the Lawra District hospital. The Lawra District lies in the North-West corner of the upper West Region of Ghana. The total area of the District is 1051.2 km^2. The District has two hospitals located in Lawra and Nandom. They provide clinical and public health services as well as serve as a referral centres for the sub-districts. There are 10 sub-districts which provide primary health care services.

Apart from agriculture, which engages about 80% of the population, there are small scale enterprises such as petty trading, artisanal works, small-scale industry enterprises, hotel/restaurants/chop bar and transport services. There are also those employed as public servants, although wages are low. The dominant economic activity is agriculture which does not yield the required returns necessary for meaningful standards of living. The result is wide spread poverty among the people with severe impact on women and children.

The study design, population, sampling

A cross-sectional study was carried out in June 2014 on a sample of 422 lactating mothers and their children. The primary study population comprised women of reproductive age (15 to 49 years) who have delivered a live baby within the past 12 months prior to the conduct of this study. The 12-month limit was set with the intention of mitigating recall bias by the mother. A systematic random sampling technique was used to select the study participants who attended post-natal clinic in the Lawra District Hospital. The list of mothers contained in the attendance register for mothers who sought post-natal care served as the sampling frame. A sampling interval was calculated by dividing the total number of mothers (800) by the required sample size of 422. A random number between 1 and the sampling interval was selected to be the starting point of the sample extraction. Subsequently, the study participants were selected by adding the sampling interval to the number corresponding to the previous mother chosen on the list. This process was continued until the required number was obtained.

A sample size of 384 was required to ensure that the estimated prevalence of the main outcome variable (coverage of essential new born care practices) was within plus or minus 5% of the true prevalence at 95% confidence level. An additional 10% to adjust for unexpected events (e.g. damaged/incomplete questionnaire) was factored in the sample size determination and so the sample size was 422.

Data collection

A structured questionnaire was administered through face to face interview to obtain information from respondents. The questionnaire comprised different sections including socioeconomic and demographic information, birth preparedness, knowledge of women about newborn danger signs, care during pregnancy and delivery (Additional file 1).

Dependent and independent variables

The women were asked questions on essential newborn care practices including a) type of instrument used to cut the umbilical cord b) whether the newborn was dried and wrapped soon after delivery, c) the number hours or days after birth the newborn was first bathed d) the temperature of the water used in bathing e) whether any pre-lacteal food or drink was given, and f) the number of hours or days after birth breastfeeding was initiated g) whether colostrum was fed to the baby h) whether exclusive breast feeding was practiced.

Three composite indices of essential newborn care practices (safe cord care, optimal thermal care and good neonatal feeding practices) were the main outcome measures used in the study.

Safe cord care was defined as use of a clean cutting instrument to cut the umbilical cord plus clean thread to tie the cord plus no substance applied to the cord. Optimal thermal care was defined as baby wrapped within 10 min of birth plus first bath after 6 or more hours plus using warm water to bath the baby. A child was considered to have received good neonatal feeding, he/she should be breast feeding at the time of the study, initiated breastfeeding within the first 1 hour after birth, not being fed with prelacteals, fed with colostrum and avoidance of bottle-feeding. If one or more of the conditions were not met, then the feeding practice was described as inadequate or bad.

The independent variables included socio-demographic factors, maternal age, educational attainment, ethnicity, religion etc. Socio-economic status (SES) was measured as household wealth index. Principal components analysis (PCA) was used to quantify a proxy measure of SES based on ownership of specified durable goods (television, radio,

car, mobile telephone, etc.) and housing characteristics (access to electricity, source of drinking water, type of toilet facilities, type of flooring material and type of cooking fuel) [12]. Utilization of antenatal care services and maternal knowledge on newborn danger signs were also assessed as explanatory variables.

Data analysis

Descriptive and inferential statistics were done using the predictive analytic software (PASW) for Windows version 18.0 and statistical significance was taken when $p < 0.05$. Chi-square statistics were performed to compare the levels of each of the dependent variables with the explanatory variables. A multiple logistic regression was used to identify socio-demographic, mothers' knowledge of specific newborn danger signs, attendance at delivery by skilled birth attendant, antenatal and delivery care factors that were associated with the three newborn care practices (that is, safe cord care, optimal thermal care and good neonatal breastfeeding). Explanatory variables which were significant at bivariate analysis at a p-value of 0.05 or less were fed into the regression model after confirming the absence of multi-collinearity between these independent variables.

Ethical considerations

The study protocol was approved by the Scientific Review and Ethics Committee of the School of Allied Health Sciences, University for Development Studies, Ghana.

Informed consent was also obtained after needed information and explanation. In situations, where the respondent could not write or read, verbal informed consent was sought from all the study participants before the commencement of any interview. Data were analyzed and presented anonymously.

Results

In all 422 women were recruited for the study, but due to incomplete responses to questionnaires, the valid responses obtained from respondents was 418, giving a response rate of 99.1%.

Socio-demographic characteristics of study sample

The 418 respondents were mothers who were residents in rural settings. The mean age was 28.5 (SD 5.6) years with a range of 16–49 years. The details of the sample characteristics including maternal educational level, marital status, religion of mothers, occupation of mothers, and maternal age distribution are shown in Table 1. About 29 (6.9%) of the mothers had no formal education and 75 (17.9%) attained tertiary level of education. The majority of the mothers 333 (79.7%) were married. Most of the mothers 239 (57.2%) were Christians.

Table 1 Socio-demographic and reproductive characteristics of respondents (N = 418)

Age category	Frequency n (%)
Under 20 years	14 (3.3)
20–34 years	349 (83.5)
At least 35 years	55 (13.2)
Religion	
Christianity	239 (57.2)
Islam	179 (42.8)
Marital Status	
Married	333 (79.7)
Single	81 (19.4)
Divorced	1 (0.2)
Widowed	3 (0.7)
Educational Level	
None	29 (6.9)
Primary	54 (12.9)
JHS	113 (27.0)
SHS/Vocational/Technical	147 (35.2)
Tertiary	75 (17.90
Occupational Level	
Unemployed	69 (16.5)
Petty trader	182 (43.5)
Farmer	18 (4.3)
Civil / Public Servant	50 (12.0)
Others	99 (23.7)
Maternal Knowledge of dangers of newborn care signs	
1–3	229 (54.8)
At least 4	189 (45.2)
Total	418 (100.0)
Gravidity	
Primigravidae	166 (39.7)
Secundigravidae	132 (31.6)
Multigravidae	120 (28.7)
Parity	
Primiparous	211 (50.5)
Secundiparous	111 (26.6)
Multiparous	96 (23.0)
Timing of first ANC visit	
First trimester	372 (89.0)
Second trimester	41 (9.8)
Third trimester	5 (1.2)

Most 182 (43.5%) of the mothers were petty traders and only 18 (4.3%) mothers were farmers. More than half 263 (62.9%) of the infants were females.

Coverage of essential newborn care practices
Of the 418 respondents, 215 (51.4%) reported their babies were wrapped 5 min after delivery and 12(2.9%) were wrapped between 30 and 60 min after birth. In 85.4% of the deliveries, scissors were used to cut the cord and 39.7% (166) of the babies were bathed within 1–6 h of delivery. Shea- butter was commonly applied to the umbilical stump in 60.3% (252) of the babies and 51.4% were wrapped immediately after delivery. The main reasons given by mothers for applying substances to the cord stump were to prevent infection and aid healing (Table 2).

Three composite indices of essential newborn care practices (safe cord care, optimal thermal care and good neonatal feeding practices) were created. The coverage of these composite newborn care measures was generally low. Of the 418 newborns, only 36.8% (154) were judged to have had safe cord care, 34.9% (146) optimal thermal care, and 73.7% (308) were considered to have had adequate neonatal feeding. The overall prevalence of adequate newborn care comprising good cord care, optimal thermal care and good neonatal feeding practices was only 15.8% (Table 3).

Women who were classified as high ANC content had a significantly higher prevalence of good infant feeding compared to women who received low ANC content (75.5% versus 58.7%) (Chi-squared = 6.0, $p = 0.014$). Similarly, women whose ANC attendance was adequate were more likely to provide optimal thermal care (37.9% versus 10.9%) (Chi-squared = 13.2, $p < 0.001$). Adequate ANC attendance was also associated with safe cord care ($\chi2 = 15.0$, $p < 0.001$).

Determinants of essential newborn care practices
We tested whether the composite newborn care practices (safe cord care, optimal thermal care and good neonatal feeding) were related to socio-demographic factors, socio-economic status, and adequacy of antenatal services and mothers' knowledge of specific newborn danger signs.. The predictors were common for the newborn care practices. Overall, the findings show that good neonatal feeding practices, optimal thermal care and good cord care were commonly adopted among women aged 25–34 years, women who had adequate ANC attendance (that is, ANC early initiated in first trimester and at least 4 ANC visits), and those who could mention at least 4 danger signs of the newborn (Tables 4, 5, 6).

In logistic regression analysis, the main predictors of essential new born care practices were maternal educational attainment, maternal age, and adequacy of antenatal care (ANC) attendance and maternal knowledge of newborn danger signs.

Maternal age at interview showed an independent association with essential newborn care practices. Compared to women aged at least 35 years, women under 20 years

Table 2 Newborn Care Practices (N = 418)

New born care practice	Frequency n (%)
Instrument used to cut the umbilical cord	
New blade	48 (11.5)
Any available blade	5 (1.2)
Scissors	357 (85.4)
Others	8 (1.9)
Total	418 (100)
Material used to clamp tie cord	
Thread	18 (4.3)
Cord tie	14 (3.3)
Cord clamp	385 (92.1)
Others	1 (0.2)
Total	418 (100.0)
What was applied to cord	
Nothing	12 (2.9)
Shea butter	252 (60.3)
Spirit	147 (35.2)
Shea butter with powder	3 (0.7)
String	1 (0.2)
Others	3 (0.7)
Total	418 (100.0)
Time baby was wrapped	
Immediately (< 5 min)	215 (51.4)
5–10 min	155 (37.1)
30–60 min	12 (2.9)
Unknown	36 (8.6)
Total	418 (100.0)
Timing of newborn's first bath	
Soon after birth	29 (6.9)
1–6 h	166 (39.7)
More than 6 h but less than 24 h	148 (35.4)
More than 24 h	4 (1.0)
Can't tell	71 (17.0)
Total	418 (100.0)
Reasons for applying substances to the cord stump	
Prevent infection	109 (26.1)
To aid healing	281 (67.2)
Keep it dry	4 (1.0)
Prevent water from entering the stomach	8 (1.9)
Midwifes advised me to used	8 (1.9)
Not Applicable	8 (1.9)
Total	418 (100.0)

Table 3 Composite measures of newborn care practices

New born care practice	Frequency n (%)
Safe cord care	
No	264 (63.2)
Yes	154 (36.8)
Total	418 (100.0)
Optimal thermal care	
No	272 (65.1)
Yes	146 (34.9)
Total	418 (100.0)
Good neonatal feeding	
No	110 (26.3)
Yes	308 (73.7)
Total	418 (100.0)
Adequate total neonatal care	
No	352 (84.2)
Yes	66 (15.8)
Total	418 (100.0)

were 6.6 times more likely to provide safe cord care to their babies (AOR = 6.57, CI: 1.71–25.31), $p = 0.006$. Compared to women aged at least 35 years, their counterparts aged 20–34 years were 3.3 times (AOR = 3. 28 [CI: 1.34, 8.04]), 2.0 times (AOR = 2.02 [CI: 1.11, 3.70]) and 7.3 times (AOR = 7.31 [CI: 1.65, 32.44]) more likely to provide optimal thermal care, good neonatal feeding and overall adequate new born care practices respectively (Table 7). Compared to women who delivered at home, women who delivered their index baby in a health facility were 5.6 times more likely to have safe cord care for their babies (AOR = 5.60, CI: 1.19–23.30).

Women who received adequate ANC services were 4.0 times (AOR = 4.04 [CI: 1.53, 10.66]) and 1.9 times (AOR = 1.90 [CI: 1.01, 3.61]) more likely to provide safe cord care and good neonatal feeding as compared to their counterparts who did not get adequate ANC. However, adequate ANC services was unrelated to optimal thermal care.

Compared to primiparous women, multiparous women were 2.7 times (AOR = 2.67 [CI: 1.41, 5.05]) more likely to provide optimal thermal care whilst secondi-parous were 2 times (AOR = 2.05 [CI: 1.08, 3.89]) more likely to provide overall adequate new born care.

Mothers who attained at least Senior High Secondary School were 20.5 times more likely to provide optimal thermal care [AOR 22.54; 95% CI (2.60–162.12)], compared to women had no formal education at all.

Maternal knowledge of at least four key newborn danger signs was significantly associated with increased probability of providing good neonatal feeding to babies (AOR = 2.0, 95% CI: 1.26–3.17). Furthermore, mothers who could recall at least 4 new born danger signs were at least 2 times more likely to provide overall adequate

Table 4 Predictors of good cord care (Bivariate analysis)

Variable	N	Good cord care?		Test statistic
		No n (%)	Yes n (%)	
Age (years)				
Under 20 years	14	5 (35.7)	9 (64.3)	Chi-square (χ^2) = 11.6, p = 0.003
20–34 years	349	215 (61.6)	134 (38.4)	
At least 35 years	55	44 (80.0)	11 (20.0)	
Adequacy of ANC attendance				
No	46	41 (89.1)	5 (10.9)	Chi-square (χ^2) = 15.0, p < 0.001
Yes	372	223 (59.9)	149 (40.1)	
Knowledge of dangers of newborn care signs				
1–3	229	156 (68.1)	73 (31.9)	Chi-square (χ^2) = 5.4, p = 0.02
At least 4	189	108 (57.1)	81 (42.9)	
Mothers' education				
None	29	25 (86.2)	4 (13.8)	Chi-square (χ^2) = 14.0, p = 0.001
Low	167	115 (68.9)	52 (31.1)	
High	222	124 (55.9)	98 (44.1)	

new born care practices than their counterparts who knew less than 4 new born danger signs.

Discussion

This study is the first that has assessed the prevalence and determinants of newborn care practices in the Lawra District of Ghana. Though some studies conducted in Ghana have highlighted on optimal thermal care and clean delivery practices for newborns [13–15], issues regarding neonatal feeding practices have received less attention. Furthermore, this present study has used composite indices which give a better reflection of safe

Table 5 Relationship between optimal thermal care and socio-demographic/antenatal care factors (N = 418)

Variable	N	Optimal thermal care?		Test statistic
		No n (%)	Yes n (%)	
Age (years)				
Under 20 years	14	10 (64.3	5 (35.7)	Chi-square (χ^2) = 10.1, p = 0.006
20–34 years	349	216 (61.9)	133 (38.1)	
At least 35 years	55	46 (83.6)	9 (16.4)	
Total				
Mothers education				
None	29	24 (82.8)	5 (17.2)	Chi-square (χ^2) = 45.4, p < 0.001
Low	167	131 (78.4)	36 (21.6)	
High	222	113 (50.9)	109 (49.1)	
Religion of mother				
Christianity	239	167 (69.9)	72 (30.1)	χ^2 = 5.7, p = 0.02
Islam	179	105 (58.7)	74 (41.3)	
Knowledge of newborn danger signs				
1–3	229	165 (72.1)	64 (27.9)	χ^2 = 10.9 p = 0.001
At least 4	189	107 (56.6)	82 (43.4)	
Adequacy of ANC attendance				
No	46	41 (89.1)	5 (10.9)	Chi-square (χ^2) = 13.2, p < 0.001
Yes	372	231 (62.1)	141 (37.9)	

Table 6 Relationship between good neonatal feeding and socio-demographic/antenatal care factors ($N = 418$)

Variable	N	Good neonatal feeding?		Test statistic
		No n (%)	Yes n (%)	
Age (years)				
Under 20 years	14	5 (35.7)	9 (64.3)	Chi-square (χ^2) = 6.2, $p = 0.05$
20–34 years	349	85 (24.4)	264 (75.6)	
At least 35 years	55	22 (40.0)	33 (60.0)	
Adequacy of ANC attendance				
No	46	19 (41.3)	27 (58.7)	Chi-square (χ^2) = 5.9, $p = 0.014$
Yes	376	91 (24.5)	281 (75.5)	
Mothers' education				
None	29	10 (34.5)	19 (65.5)	$\chi^2 = 5.5$, $p = 0.06$
Low	167	52 (31.1)	115 (68.9)	
High	222	48 (21.6)	174 (78.4)	
Knowledge of newborn danger signs				
1–3	229	74 (32.3)	155 (67.7)	$\chi^2 = 9.4$ $p = 0.002$
At least 4	189	36 (19.0)	153 (81.0)	

cord, optimal thermal care and neonatal feeding. The findings of our study remain relevant because they confirm that of earlier studies and also fill a knowledge gap by showing that using single practice indicators could be less informative in the magnitude of essential newborn practices. For example, optimal thermal care as assessed in the present study included summing up scores for wrapping the baby within 10 min of birth, delaying for at least 6 h and using warm water. A study that uses only one of these indicators will present a different situation from one that uses a combination of these variables.

Prevalence of essential newborn care practices
Three composite newborn care practices (safe cord care, optimal thermal care, and good neonatal breastfeeding) were investigated and the coverage of these was found to be generally low. These composite variables give a better reflection of safe cord, optimal thermal care and neonatal feeding. The three newborn care practices were associated with socio-demographic, antenatal and delivery care factors.

As in other studies, safe cord care was defined as use of a clean cutting instrument to cut the umbilical cord plus clean thread to tie the cord plus no substance applied to the cord [16–18]. Cord cutting with safe instruments such as new razor blades and scissors was commonly practiced (96.9%) but then when one takes a closer and more holistic approach to safe cord care (that is using composite indicators), only 36.8% actually received that. This means assessing the situation using single practice indicators could be misleading. Poor cord

care was driven mainly by putting substances on the cord.

Most mothers applied various things like shea-butter, methylated spirit, shea-butter mixed with powder to the cord stump. The reasons given for applying substances to the cord stump include hastening the healing process, prevent cord stump from smelling and infections and also to prevent water from entering into newborn's stomach. Since these substances are coming from unsterile sources the likelihood of contamination is high and may thus be harmful to newborns. Similar findings have been reported in the Asante Akim North District in Southern Ghana [19] and in Bangladesh where unhygienic cord care practices were prevalent [20].

Optimal thermal care (defined as baby wrapped within 10 min of birth plus first bath after six or more hours plus using warm water to bath the baby) is an essential intervention for the survival of the newborn especially during the first 24 h of birth. Though most babies were wrapped soon after delivery and were also bathed with hot water, poor thermal care was caused mainly by early bathing. In this study, 46.7% of the newborns were given a bath in less than 6 hours of delivery. Apart from exposing newborns to hypothermia, early bathing removes maternal bacteria and the vernix caseosa (a potent inhibitor of *Escherichia coli*) [21], and eliminates the crawling reflex [22]. Aside its role as a protective barrier from liquids while in the uterus, vernix serves as an antioxidant, skin cleanser, moisturizer, temperature regulator, and a natural, safe antimicrobial for the new baby post-delivery [5, 23]. These are some of the reasons why WHO recommended delay bathing up to at least 24 h.

Table 7 Determinants of safe cord care, optimal thermal care and good neonatal feeding

Variable	AOR (95% CI) safe cord care	AOR (95% CI) optimal thermal care	AOR (95% CI) good neonatal feeding	AOR (95% CI) [a]Overall adequacy of new born care practices
Maternal Age (years)				
≥ 35	Reference	Reference	Reference	Reference
Under 20 years	6.57 (1.71, 25.31)**	3.65 (0.79, 16.86)	2.22 (0.55, 9.0)	7.41 (0.85, 64.91)
20–34 years	2.01 (0.98, 4.12)	3.28 (1.34, 8.04)**	2.02 (1.11, 3.70)*	7.31 (1.65, 32.44)**
Adequacy of ANC attendance				
No	Reference	Reference	Reference	Reference
Yes	4.04 (1.53, 10.66)**	2.74 (1.01, 7.55)	1.90 (1.01, 3.61)*	Not significant
Place of delivery				
Home	Reference	Reference	Reference	Reference
Health facility	5.60 (1.19, 26.30)**	Not significant	Not significant in final model	Not significant in final model
Mother could recall at least 4 new born danger signs?				
1–3	Reference	Reference	Reference	Reference
At least 4	Not significant in final model	Not significant	2.00 (1.26, 3.17)**	2.51 (1.41, 4.47)**
Maternal Educational level				
No education	Reference	Reference	Reference	Reference
Low (Primary to JHS)	Not significant in final model	6.76 (0.85, 53.89)	Not significant in final model	Not significant in final model
High (At least SHS)	Not significant in final model	20.54 (2.60, 162.12)**	Not significant in final model	Not significant in final model
Type of religion				
Christianity	Reference	Reference	Reference	Reference
Islam	Not significant in final model	1.72 (1.09, 2.72)*	Not significant in final model	Not significant
Parity				
Primiparous	Reference	Reference	Reference	Reference
Secundiparous	Not significant	1.19 (0.70, 2.02)	Not significant	2.05 (1.08, 3.89)*
Multiparous	Not significant	2.67 (1.41, 5.05)**	Not significant	2.04 (0.97, 4.30)

AOR (95% CI): Adjusted odds ratio at 95% confidence level
*significant at $p < 0.05$; **significant at $p < 0.01$; ***significant at $p < 0.001$
[a]Overall adequacy of new born care practices was defined to comprise safe cord care, optimal thermal care and good neonatal feeding

This notwithstanding, many societies have some reasons why babies are bathed early after delivery.

For a normal uncomplicated vaginal birth in a health facility, it is recommended that healthy mothers and newborns should receive care in the facility for at least 24 h after birth [5]. In Ghana, women who deliver in health facilities are detained for a minimum of 6 h and not 24 h. Women who for some reasons deliver at home do not even wait for the 6 h before bathing the newborn. This is why in our study, we limited waiting period to at least 6 h. Early bathing of the baby is a cultural practice and so asking for a waiting time of 24 h appears to be something that is impossible at least for now. Our data showed that only 4 (1%) of the newborns in our sample will have received optimal thermal care if the 24-h cutoff was used instead of 6 h.

In an intervention trial in Ghana that used home visits to promote positive behavior change regarding thermal care, only 41% of mothers delayed bathing for more than 6 h in the intervention areas compared to 29% in the comparison areas [24].

The timing of bathing the newborn appears inconsistent as reported in some earlier studies conducted in Ghana [13, 15]. Whereas some mothers reported bathing their newborns shortly after delivery, others mentioned waiting until later in the day but the exact waiting period has not been more than a few hours after delivery. As reported in one of these studies, early bathing was commonly practiced in Ghana as a measure to reduce body odour in later life, shaping the baby's head, and to make the baby sleep and feel clean [15].

Some studies conducted on thermal practices in many countries including Ghana, Tanzania, Uganda and India have reported strong cultural beliefs in the benefits of early bathing [15, 25–30], which largely promotes the practice. The practice of early bathing is rooted in the firm belief that the birth process is dirty and that the baby is dirty after birth. This is particularly the case if there is an obvious sign of vernix which is regarded as dirty.

The problem of early bathing of the newborn appears to be widespread across the world. A study in Nepal reported that newborn babies are considered dirty since they came out of their mother's womb, so almost all newborn babies are bathed within the first hour of birth [31]. Another study conducted in low socioeconomic settlements of Karachi, Pakistan, revealed that newborns were bathed immediately after delivery as the vernix was considered "dirty looking" and it was felt it should be removed [32].

A composite index comprising good neonatal feeding showed that more than 70% of respondents practiced adequate feeding behaviours. For example, timely initiation of breastfeeding (TIBF) rate was 97%.

There are a number of benefits associated with early initiation of breastfeeding including stimulation of breast milk production and the release of oxytocin, which helps the contraction of the uterus and reduces post-partum blood loss [33].

The analysis from this study showed that the expected essential newborn care practices are not available to a greater proportion of the newborns. Poor newborn care practices together with poor maternal care and staff shortages in rural health facilities are major contributing factors of newborn mortality in developing countries [34]. The fact that a greater number of newborns are not getting adequate care suggests the need to extend these essential newborn care practices to the rural areas through rigorous training of community health workers in newborn care practices and sustained educational campaigns by the Ghana Health Service and other health related non-governmental agencies.

It is important to note that about 50% of newborn deaths occur within 24 h of birth [2].

Furthermore, though hypothermia contributes to neonatal morbidity and mortality in low-income countries [35, 36], yet the Ghana National Newborn Strategy and Action Plan (2014–2018) is silent on the specifics on the WHO recommendation on delay bathing of the newborn. The preventive basic essential newborn care specified in the action plan document mentioned drying and provision of warmth through skin to skin contact with the mother. The intervention package for the newborn in this strategy and action plan appears to focus on complication of prematurity and low birth weight, adverse intrapartum events including birth asphyxia and infection.

Predictors of essential newborn care practices

In logistic regression analysis, the main predictors of essential new born care practices were maternal educational attainment, maternal age, and adequacy of antenatal care (ANC) attendance and maternal knowledge of newborn danger signs. Adequacy of antenatal care in particular was a consistent determinant of safe cord care, optimal thermal care and good neonatal feeding.

Maternal education of secondary school level or higher was one of the strongest socio-demographic factors that determined safe cord care, optimal thermal care practice and good neonatal feeding. This association has been reported from several countries including India and Nepal [37, 38].

The educational attainment of the mother was positively associated with the adequacy level of ANC attendance ($\chi 2 = 59.1$, $p < 0.001$) and maternal knowledge of newborn danger signs ($\chi 2 = 16.7$, p < 0.001). The effect of maternal education on essential newborn care practices was therefore mediated through ANC attendance and knowledge of newborn dangers.

We observed very strong association between use of antenatal and delivery care and the newborn care practices. This may be explained by the fact that when pregnant women make contact with health workers during ANC, they are provided with health information and made aware of proper newborn care practices. Clean cord care practice and thermal care have found to be positively associated with receiving antenatal care [37].

Mothers' knowledge of newborn care danger signs

Poor knowledge of newborn danger signs delays care seeking and ultimately greater risk of death and so early detection of neonatal danger signs is an important step towards improving newborn survival [39, 40]. Overall, the mothers' knowledge of newborn care issues was not satisfactory in the sample population. In our study sample, only 45.2% of the mothers knew at least four newborn danger signs out of the seven. Knowledge on critical newborn danger signs other than high body temperature, diarrhoea, excessive crying was inadequate and similar findings have earlier been reported in the Asante Akim North District Ghana [19].

The low mothers' knowledge of newborn care practices reported in the present study confirmed what has been reported in some other developing countries including Sri Lanka, Kenya, Uganda and Nepal had unsatisfactory level of knowledge in the recognition of newborn danger signs [34, 41–44]. Available evidence from the literature shows that the maternal knowledge is an important intermediate factor that may lead to good practices and child survival outcomes child survival outcomes [34, 41].

Though maternal knowledge of newborn danger signs was positively associated with the odds of optimal thermal care, only a small proportion of mothers were knowledgeable in newborn danger signs. This means the majority of the women lacked adequate knowledge of good newborn care practices, so their newborn practices were likely to be adversely affected. The low knowledge levels of mothers may be due to inadequate messages received on newborn care practices at the ANC. This calls for strengthening of focused health education on newborn care practices especially during prenatal care to mitigate these problems. By integrating health education on newborn care practices into routine antenatal care services, it may increase a woman's knowledge and the ability to practice safe newborn care behaviours.

Conclusions

The analysis from this study showed that the expected essential newborn care practices are not getting to a greater proportion of the newborns. Early bathing, non-immediate drying and application of substances to cord stump were commonly practiced. This may be depriving newborns of basic protections against infection and death.

Overall, the findings show that good neonatal feeding practices, optimal thermal care and overall adequate newborn care practices were commonly adopted by women aged 20–34 years. The results also showed that essential newborn care practices are positively associated with high maternal educational attainment, adequate utilization of antenatal care services and high maternal knowledge of newborn danger signs.

Policy implications and recommendations

Greater improvement in essential newborn care practices could be attained through modifiable proven low-cost interventions such as effective ANC services, health and nutrition education that should span from community to health facility levels.

Of the three-composite essential newborn services indicators, optimal thermal care was the least provided to babies. Unfortunately, uptake of adequate ANC services in this study population was unrelated to optimal thermal care. This finding has important implications for the implementation of focused ANC to improve essential newborn care practices, especially that of thermal care. Therefore, ANC interventions should lay emphasis on the promotion and provision of thermal care for all newborns to prevent hypothermia (that is, immediate drying, warming, skin to skin, delayed bathing).

Limitations of the study

There are some limitations of the findings of this study. The recall period was limited to the past 1 year in order to avoid recall bias over a longer period of time. This notwithstanding, some amount of recall bias cannot be completely ruled out. During the interviews, the women had to recall a number of events including antenatal care visits and neonatal practices. So, recall bias and misclassification might happen. In order to reduce misclassification errors, the women were required to present their antenatal records booklet for confirmation of verbal information provided.

Our design was a cross sectional study and as with all such studies, the strength of causality is weak. The cross-sectional nature of the data limits our ability to draw any causal conclusions on the relationships found in the current study. Despite these limitations, our results have shed more light on critical areas of newborn care practices that need urgent pragmatic intervention.

Abbreviations
ANC: Antenatal care; AOR: Adjusted odds ratio; MDGs: Millennium Development Goals; NMR: Neonatal mortality; PASW: Predictive analytic software; SBA: Skilled birth attendants; SDGs: Sustainable Development Goals; SES: Socio-economic status; TIBF: Timely initiation of breastfeeding

Acknowledgements
The authors would like to gratefully acknowledge with gratitude the effort of the data collection teams, without their participation, the quality of the data presented in this report would not have been possible. Their commitment to improving maternal and newborn health is commendable.
We very much appreciate the input and support received from the Lawra District Health Management team (DHMT) that granted the research team audience. We also fully appreciate the involvement of all the women and community leaders whose co-operation led to a successful data collection experience.

Authors' contribution
MS conceived the idea and designed the study, coordinated data collection, performed analysis, interpretation of data and drafted the manuscript. FV coordinated the collection of data from the field, designed the study, interpreted data analysis and critical review and obtained funding. FA helped in the data collection, instrument development, assisted in data collection and manuscript writing, and critically commented on the draft manuscript. All authors gave final approval of the version to be published.

Competing interest
The authors declare that they have no competing interests.

References
1. Countdown Coverage Writing Group, Countdown to 2015 Core Group, Bryce J, Daelmans B, Dwivedi A, Fauveau V, Lawn JE, Mason E, Newby H, Shankar A, et al. Countdown to 2015 for maternal, newborn, and child survival: the 2008 report on tracking coverage of interventions. Lancet. 2008;371:1247–58.
2. Lawn JE, Cousens S, Zupan J. 4 million neonatal deaths: when? Where?Why? Lancet. 2005;365(9462):891–900.
3. Ghana Statistical Service (GSS), Ghana Health Service (GHS), ICF International: 2015. Ghana demographic and health survey 2014. Rockville: GSS, GHS, and ICF International; 2015.
4. United Nations: Sustainable Development Goals (SDGs). United Nations sustainable development summit 2015, vol. 2015. New York: United Nations.
5. WHO. WHO recommendations on postnatal care of the mother and newborn. Geneva: World Health Organization; 2013.
6. Gary LD, Bhutta ZA, Cousens S, Taghreed A, Walker N, de Bernis L. Team ftLNSS: evidence-based, cost-effective interventions: how many newborn babies can we save? Lancet. 2005;365:977–88.
7. Lawn J, Kerber K. Opportunities for Africa's newborns: practical data, policy and programmatic support for newborn care in Africa. PMNCH: Cape Town, South Africa; 2006.
8. The Partnership for Maternal NaCH. A global review of the key interventions related to reproductive, maternal, newborn and child health. Geneva: The Partnership for Maternal, Newborn and Child Health; 2011.
9. WHO. Neonatal & Perinatal Mortality; country, regional and global estimate. Geneva: World Health Organization; 2006.
10. McCall EM, Alderdice F, Halliday HL, Jenkins JG, Vohra S. Interventions to prevent hypothermia at birth in preterm and/or low birthweight infants. Cochrane Database Syst Rev. 2010;3(3).
11. WHO. Protecting, promoting and supporting breast-feeding: the special role of maternity services, a joint WHO/UNICEF statement. Geneva: World Health Organization/UNICEF; 2002.
12. Vyas S, Kumaranayake L. Constructing socio-economic status indices: how to use principal components analysis. Health Policy Plan. 2006;21:459–68.
13. Moyer CA, Aborigo RA, Logonia G, Affah G, Rominski S, Adongo PB, Williams J, Hodgson A, Engmann C. Clean delivery practices in rural northern Ghana: a qualitative study of community and provider knowledge, attitudes, and beliefs. BMC Pregnancy and Childbirth. 2012;12:50.
14. Hill Z, Tawiah-Agyemang C, Okeyere E, Manu A, Fenty J, Kirkwood B. Improving hygiene in home deliveries in rural Ghana: how to build on current attitudes and practices. Pediatr Infect Dis J. 2010;29(11):1004–8.
15. Hill Z, Tawiah-Agyemang C, Manu A, Okeyere E, Kirkwood B. Keeping newborns warm: beliefs, practices and potential for behaviour change in rural Ghana. TMIH. 2010;15(10):1118–24.
16. Osuchukwu EC, Ezeruigbo CSF, Eko JE. Knowledge of standard umbilical cord management among mothers in Calabar south local government area, cross river state Nigeria. Int J Nurs Sci. 2017;7(3):57–62.
17. Saaka M, Aryee P, Kuganab-lem R, Ali M, Masahudu AR. The effect of social behaviour change communication package on maternal knowledge on obstetric danger signs among mothers in east Mamprusi District of Ghana. Glob Health. 2017;13(19)
18. Afolaranmi TO, Hassan ZI, Akinyemi OO, Sule SS, Malete MU, Choji CP, Bello DA. Cord care practices: a perspective of contemporary African setting. Front Public Health. 2018;6(10) https://doi.org/10.3389/fpubh.2018.00010.
19. Marah A. Assessing household practices that influence neonatal survival in the Asante-Akim North District of Ashanti region - Ghana. Kumasi, Ghana: Kwame Nkrumah University Science and Technology; 2011.
20. Awasthi S, Verma T, Agarwal M: Danger signs of neonatal illnesses: perceptions of caregivers and health workers in northern India 2006. Available at: http://www.who.int/entity/bulletin/volumes/84/10/05-029207.pdf. Accessed on 20th Dec 2013.
21. Tollin M, Bergsson G, Kai-Larsen Y, Lengqvist J, Sjövall J, Griffiths W, et al. Vernix caseosa as a multicomponent defense system based on polypeptides, lipids and their interactions. Cell Mol Life Sci. 2005;62:2390–9.
22. Righard L, Alade M. Effect of delivery room routines on success of first breastfeed. Lancet. 1990;336:1105–7.
23. World Health Organization. Essential newborn care: a report of a technical working group. Geneva: WHO; 1996.
24. Kirkwood BR, Manu A, ten Asbroek AH, Soremekun S, Weobong B, Gyan T, Danso S, Amenga-Etego S, Tawiah-Agyemang C, Owusu-Agyei S, et al. Effect of the Newhints home-visits intervention on neonatal mortality rate and care practices in Ghana: a cluster randomised controlled trial. Lancet. 2013;381(9884):2184–92.
25. Waiswa P, Kemigisa M, Kiguli J, Naikoba S, Pariyo GW, Peterson S. Acceptability of evidence-based neonatal care practices in rural Uganda – implications for programming. BMC Pregnancy Childbirth. 2008;8:21.
26. Iyengar SD, Iyengar K, Martines JC, Dashora K, Deora KK. Childbirth practices in rural Rajasthan, India: implications for neonatal health and survival. J Perinatol. 2008;28:S23–30.
27. Kesterton AJ, Cleland J. Neonatal care in rural Karnataka: healthy and harmful practices, the potential for change. BMC Pregnancy Childbirth. 2009;9:20.
28. Shamba D, Schellenberg J, Penfold S, Mashasi I, Mrisho M, Manzi F, Marchant T, Tanner M, Mshinda H, Schellenberg D, et al. Clean home delivery in rural southern Tanzania: barriers, influencers and facilitators. J Health Popul Nutr. 2013;1:1107–870.
29. Baqui AH, Williams EK, Darmstadt GL, Kiran TU, Panwar D, Sharma RK, Ahmed S, Sreevasta V, Ahuja R, Santosham M, et al. Newborn care in rural Uttar Pradesh. Indian J Pediatics. 2007;74:241–7.
30. Shamba D, Schellenberg J, Hildon ZJL, Mashasi I, Penfold S, Tanner M, Marchant T, Hill Z. Thermal care for newborn babies in rural southern Tanzania: a mixed-method study of barriers, facilitators and potential for behaviour change. BMC Pregnancy and Childbirth. 2014;14:267.
31. Yadav S. Newborn care: traditional practices in Nepal. Student BMJ. 2007;15: 293–336.
32. Fikree FF, Tazeen SA, Jill MD, Rahbar MH. Newborn care practices in low socioeconomic settlements of Karachi, Pakistan. Social Science Direct and Medicine. 2005;60:911–21.
33. Gartner LM, Morton J, Lawrence RA, Naylor AJ, O'Hare D, Schanler RJ, Eidelman AI. Breastfeeding and the use of human milk. Pediatrics. 2005; 115(2):496–506.
34. Sharan M. Determinants of safe motherhood and newborn care behaviors in rural India. Johns Hopkins University. 2004;
35. Darmstadt GL, Bhutta ZA, Cousens S, Adam T, Walker N, Bernis L. Evidence based, cost-effective interventions: how many newborn babies can we save? Lancet. 2005;365:977–88.
36. Kumar V, Shearer JC, Kumar A, Darmstadt GL. Neonatal hypothermia in low resource settings: a review. J Perinatol. 2009;29:401–12.
37. Baqui AH, Williams EK, Dramstadt GL, Kumar V, Kiran TU, Panwar D, et al. Newborn care in rural Uttar Pradesh. Indian J Pediatr. 2006;74(3):241–7.

38. Ministry of Health and Population (MoHP), New ERA, Macro International Inc. Nepal demographic and health survey 2006. Kathmandu, Nepal: Ministry of Health and Population, New ERA, Macro International Inc; 2007.

39. Choi Y, El Arifeen S, Mannan I, Rahman SM, Bari S, et al. Can mothers recognize neonatal illness correctly? Comparison of maternal report and assessment by community health workers in rural Bangladesh. Tropical Med Int Health. 2010;15(6):743–53.

40. Hill Z, Kendall C, Arthur P, Kirkwood B, Adjei E. Recognizing childhood illnesses and their traditional explanations: exploring options for care-seeking interventions in the context of the IMCI strategy in rural Ghana. Tropical Med Int Health. 2003;8(7):668–76.

41. Senarath U, Fernando D, Vimpani G, Rodrigo I. Factors associated with maternal knowledge of newborn care among hospital-delivered mothers in Sri Lanka. Trans R Soc Trop Med Hyg. 2007;101(8):823–30.

42. Obimbo E, Musoke RN, Were F. Knowledge, attitudes and practices of mothers and knowledge of health workers regarding care of the newborn umbilical cord. East Afr Med J. 1999;76(8):425–9.

43. Tuladhar S. The determinants of good newborn care practices in the rural areas of Nepal. Australia: University of Canterbury; 2010.

44. Sandberg J, Odberg Pettersson K, Asp G, Kabakyenga J, Agardh A. Inadequate knowledge of neonatal danger signs among recently delivered women in southwestern rural Uganda: a community survey. PLoS One. 2014;9(5):e97253.

7

Incidence of obesity and its predictors in children and adolescents in 10 years of follow up

Maryam Barzin[1], Shayan Aryannezhad[1], Sara Serahati[1], Akram Beikyazdi[1], Fereidoun Azizi[2], Majid Valizadeh[1], Maryam Ziadlou[1] and Farhad Hosseinpanah[1*]

Abstract

Background: Childhood obesity is one of the most challenging public health issues of twenty-first century. While we know that there is an increase in prevalence of childhood and adolescence obesity, incidence studies must be carried out. The main objective of this study was to determine childhood obesity incidence and its potential predictors in Tehranian urban population.

Methods: This study was conducted within the framework of the Tehran Lipid and Glucose Study (TLGS), addressing incidence and risk factors of obesity throughout several phases from 1999–2001 to 2009–2011 among Tehranian urban population. Total study subjects were 1033 non-obese children, aged between 7 to 11 years, with a median 8.7 years of follow-up. Body mass Index (BMI) was used to define obesity and overweight based on World Health Organization (WHO) criteria, and definition of metabolic syndrome (MetS) for children was based on the Cook survey. Cumulative incidence of obesity and obesity incidence rates were calculated for each gender. Cox proportional hazard models was used to estimate potential risk factors of obesity.

Results: Our Participants had a mean age of 9.2 ± 1.4 years, mean BMI of 16.1 ± 2.2 kg/m^2 and mean waist circumference (WC) of 57.2 ± 6.7 at baseline. Total cumulative incidence of obesity was calculated to be 17%, CI =14.1–20.4 for whole population (19.6%, CI =15.4–24.8 for boys and 14.5%,CI = 10.9–19.1 for girls). Participants which were in the age group of 7–9 years at baseline experienced higher rate of cumulative obesity incidence compared to those who were in the age group of 10–11 years at baseline (22% vs 10.8%).

In addressing risk factors, 5 parameters were significantly associated with obesity incidence: being overweight at baseline (HR = 14.93 95%CI: 9.82–22.70), having higher WC (HR = 5.05 95%CI: 3.01–8.48), suffering from childhood MetS (HR: 2.77 95%CI: 1.57–4.89) and having a obese father (HR: 2.69 95%CI: 1.61–4.50) or mother (HR: 3.04 95%CI: 1.96–4.72).

Conclusion: Incidence of obesity is significantly high in Tehranian children, especially the age group 7–9 years. Best predictors of childhood obesity incidence are childhood overweight, WC above 90th percentile, childhood MetS and parental obesity.

Keywords: Obesity, Childhood, Adolescents, Incidence, Predictors

* Correspondence: fhospanah@endocrine.ac.ir
[1]Obesity Research Center, Research Institute for Endocrine Sciences, Shahid Beheshti University of Medical Sciences, Tehran, Iran
Full list of author information is available at the end of the article

Background

Based on World Health Organization (WHO) reports, childhood obesity is one of the most serious global health challenges of the twenty-first century which is steadily affecting many low- and middle-income countries [1]. It has also been stated that overweight or obese children are more likely to remain overweight or obese in adulthood [2]. This persistency of obesity into the adulthood is associated with increased morbidity risk in later life, leading to development of adult diabetes, coronary heart disease and a range of cancers [3].

Increase in the prevalence of overweight and obesity has been detected among children and adolescents worldwide, making obesity one of the most common chronic disorders in this age group [4]. In a 2017 systematic review; global and regional prevalence of obesity among 5–19 years old children and adolescents was published. The study showed an increasing trend of obesity worldwide; prevalence of obesity in 1975 was 0.7% in girls and 0.9% in boys, rising to 5.6% in girls and 7.8% in boys in 2016. The Middle East and north Africa (MENA) region was among the regions with the largest absolute increase in the number of children and adolescents with obesity globally (around or above 20%, in some countries). These findings highlight the growing concern of the rising prevalence of childhood overweight and obesity in this region [5].

A national based study in Iran, a developing country in Middle East region, showed prevalence of overweight and obesity among children and adolescents to be high, 14.5 and 6% respectively [6]. Estimations of childhood and adolescence obesity prevalence reported by Tehran Lipid and Glucose Study (TLGS) are comparable with this previously published national based study: prevalence of overweight and obesity, were demonstrated be 13.3 and 4.3% respectivly (for 3–19 years old) in TLGS population at phase I of study (1999–2001) [7].

Findings of a recent systematic review and meta-analysis study of Iranian children and adolescents revealed an alarming increase in the trend of excess weight in children aged below 11 years compared with older children. [8]. Although prevalence of childhood obesity has been reported in many studies, incidence studies are needed to determine potential risk factors for developing obesity. Despite its importance, there is limited knowledge regarding childhood obesity incidence. Studies carried out based on nationally representative data in the U.S and England, investigated different childhood ages to ascertain as the most probable for incidence of obesity and the results are rather conflicting [9, 10], with the effects of different risk factors on the age of obesity incidence still being under question.

This longitudinal population based cohort study aimed to determine childhood obesity incidence in a Tehranian urban population, and to evaluate the potential predictors of obesity incidence in this sample.

Methods

Study setting and participants

This prospective study was conducted within the framework of the Tehran Lipid and Glucose Study (TLGS), a population based cohort study aimed at determining the risk factors of non-communicable diseases among Tehranian population. Details of this study protocol are available elsewhere [11]. Tehran, the capital of the Islamic Republic of Iran, is a metropolitan city composed of 22 urban districts, which make up a population of more than 8.6 million people (based on Iran National Census 2016). All participants were chosen from the urban District 13 of Tehran via multistage cluster random sampling method and were given a written invitation form. Rational for choosing district 13 as a representative of the overall population of Tehran is its high stability of the residing population and its age distribution which is similar to whole Tehran. Based on the written data, every family was contacted, invited, and then recruited to participate in the study and was referd to one of the three chosen medical health centers in district 13 for the measurements and next follow-ups. TLGS consists of several phases, phase I (1999–2001), a cross-sectional prevalence study of cardiovascular risk factors, in which, 15,005 people, aged ≥3 years were selected; then a prospective follow up study was conducted with phases II (2002–2005), III (2006–2008) and IV (2009–2011) by means of approximately 3 years intervals between assessments. Moreover, during phase II, 3500 new participants were recruited.

This study has been approved by the National Research Council of the Islamic Republic of Iran (No. 121) and has been performed with the approval of the Human Research Review Committee of the Endocrine Research Center, Shahid Beheshti University (M. C.).

In the current study, participants aged between 7 to 11 years entered study at first 2 phases, total 1507 participants from phase I ($N = 1257$) and II ($N = 250$) were selected. After exclusion of those who were obese at baseline and those with consumption of glucocorticoids or other hormonal drugs (total number of exclusions $N = 106$); 1401 participants remained. Of these participants, 368 had no further follow-up. Final analysis were performed on 1033 participants for a median of 8.7 years [dropout rate about 26.3% (368 of 1401)] (Fig. 1).

Measurements and definitions

Trained interviewers collected information regarding demographics, education, medical and drug history. All measurements were taken by trained technicians in order to reduce subjective errors.

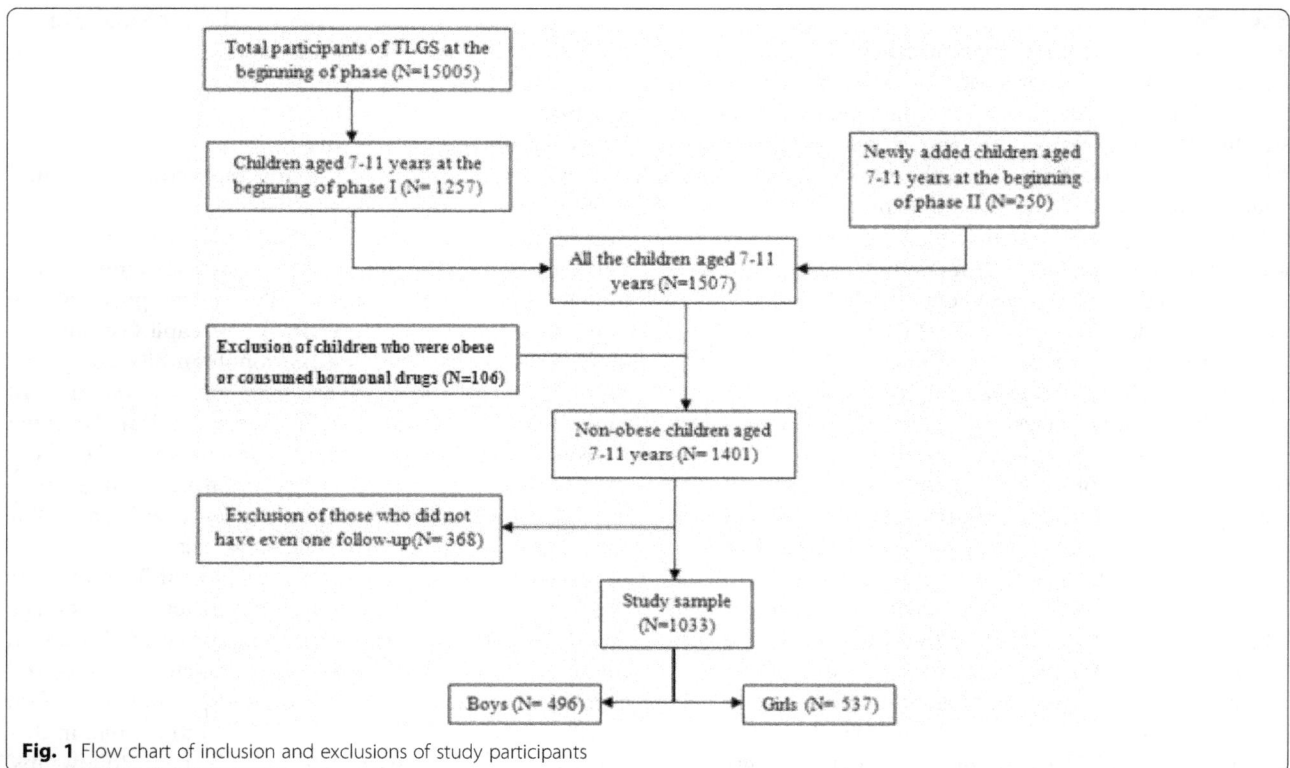

Fig. 1 Flow chart of inclusion and exclusions of study participants

Anthropometric parameters: Weight was measured according to standard protocols with an accuracy of up to 100 g, with subjects minimally clothed without shoes using digital scales. Height was measured in a standing position, without shoes, using a tape measure while the shoulders were in a normal position. BMI was calculated as weight in kilograms divided by the height in squared meters (kg/m^2). Waist circumference (WC) was measured at the narrowest level over light clothing, using an un-stretched tape meter, without any pressure to body surface, and measurements were recorded to the nearest 0.1 cm. Based on BMI-for-age standards of WHO, obesity for children was defined as BMI-for-age > 2SD and overweight was defined as 1SD < BMI-for-age ≤ 2SD in each gender [12]; parental obesity was defined as BMI ≥30.

Blood pressure and metabolic parameters: A qualified physician, using a standard mercury sphygmomanometer, measured systolic and diastolic blood pressure two times on the right arm, with the subject in a seated position, asked to rest for 15 min period between measurements. The mean of two measurements was considered to be the participant's blood pressure. Blood samples were drawn from all the study participants after an overnight fasting of 12–14 h. All blood analyses were performed at the TLGS research laboratory on the day of blood collection. Fasting plasma glucose (FPG) was measured by the enzymatic colorimetric method using glucose oxidase. Plasma total cholesterol (TC) and triglyceride (TG) levels were measured by enzymatic colorimetric kits using cholesterol esterase/cholesterol oxidase and glycerol phosphate oxidase respectively. High-density lipoprotein cholesterol (HDL-C) was measured after precipitation of the apolipoprotein B–containing lipoproteins with phosphotungstic acid. Definition of metabolic syndrome (MetS) for children was based on the Cook et al. survey [13]. This definition is based on criteria analogous to that of the National Cholesterol Education Program Expert Panel on Detection, Evaluation and Treatment of High Blood Cholesterol in Adult Treatment Panel III [14] and it defines MetS as three or more of the following: Fasting TG ≥ 110 mg/dl; HDL cholesterol < 40 mg/dl; WC ≥ 90th percentile for age and gender, according to national reference curves [15]; systolic blood pressure (SBP) and/or diastolic blood pressure (DBP) ≥90th percentile for gender, age and height according to Heart, Lung, and Blood Institute standards and FPG ≥ 100 mg/dl [16].

Education: Parental educational levels were assessed using a questionnaire and were categorized into two groups, >high school diploma and ≤ high school diploma. In Iran, it took 12 years of education to receive a high school diploma.

Statistical analysis

Normality of distributions was checked using the Kolmogorov-Smirnov test for all continuous variables. Normally distributed and skewed continuous variables are illustrated as mean ± SD and median (IQ 25–75), respectively. Categorical variables are reported as frequency (percentages). To assess the significance of differences for categorical and continuous variables in the baseline characteristics of all participants at follow-up, Pearson chi square test, t-test and Mann-Whitney test were used, when appropriate.

In this study, as the exact time of obesity incidence was not known, it was considered as interval-censored data. Considering alternate interval censoring approaches, results were investigated using mid-point censoring, which converts interval-censored data to the right-censored data problems. Mid-point censoring was set to the mid-point between the last negative and the most recent positive event time minus the first positive observation for the incidence of obesity and to the time span between the first and the last observation for censored subjects. End points were considered as the time of incidence of obesity and censoring was defined as lost to follow up or end of the follow up.

Cumulative incidence of obesity with 95% (CI) was calculated for each gender as the number of new cases of obesity over the total number of subjects in that group minus half of the censored population. The person-year method was used to obtain obesity incidence rates (IRs); IR is reported as number of cases per 1000 person years. Cox proportional hazard modeling was used to estimate unadjusted and age adjusted hazard ratios (HRs) along with 95% (CI) for baseline components of MetS, parental obesity and educational level. The proportionality assumption was verified by assessing the correlation between the Schoenfield residuals and person-days along with observing log minus log plots (considering different groups as strata variables). All proportionality assumptions were generally appropriate. All analyses were performed using IBM SPSS for Windows version 20 and STATA version 12 SE (STATA Inc., TX, USA), with a two-tailed P-value, 0.05 being considered significant.

Results

Total of 1033 non-obese participants (496 males, 537 females) with a mean age of 9.2 ± 1.4 years, mean BMI 16.1 ± 2.2 kg/m^2 and mean WC 57.2 ± 6.7 cm at baseline were followed up for a median of 8.7 (IQ = 5.5–10.4) years. Prevalence of overweight was 14.9% ($n = 154$) at baseline, 16.3% ($n = 81$) in boys and 13.6% ($n = 73$) in girls. Baseline characteristics of the study participants separated by gender are shown in Table 1 indicating a non-significant difference between different genders in their demographic and biochemical characteristics except for WC, mother's BMI, FPG, TG and SBP.

At the end of follow up, 4.0% ($n = 35$) of the normal weight subjects and 39.6% ($n = 61$) of overweight subjects at baseline, became obese contributing to a cumulative incidence of 17.0% (CI 14.1–20.4%). Gender striated cumulative incidence was 19.6% (CI 15.4–24.8%) and 14.5% (CI 10.9–19.1%) for boys and girls, respectively. For the whole

population, incidence density rate was 11.8 (9.7–14.4) per 1000 person year, and corresponding incidence density rates among boys and girls were 14.3 (10.9–18.7) and 9.7 (7.2–13.1) per 1000 person year, respectively. Kaplan-Meier curve (Fig. 2a) shows that boys are at increased risk of obesity, compared to girls, also it is not statistically significant. (Log-rank test: 3.05 $P = 0.081$). As shown in Table 2, contributions of different candidate predictor of incidence of obesity were analyzed and corresponding HRs were calculated for the whole population. Once the adjustments for baseline age were performed, Being overweight and having WC of ≥90th percentile at baseline had significant association with incidence of obesity; (HR = 14.93 95%CI:9.82–22.70) and HR = 5.05 95%CI: 3.01–8.48) respectively. Childhood MetS (HR: 2.77 95% CI: 1.57–4.89) and parental obesity (HR: 2. 69 95% CI: 1.61–4.50 and HR: 3.04 95% CI: 1.96–4.72 for paternal and maternal obesity, respectively), also had a significant association with incidence of obesity. However, other parameters including HDL cholesterol, hypertension, fasting blood sugar and parental educational levels showed no significant association with developing obesity in the whole population. After separating data by gender (Tables 3 and 4) the same pattern was observed for all the covariates except for paternal obesity in girls which had a non-significant association with obesity incidence.

Table 5 presents the cumulative incidence and incidence density rate over the whole population, stratified by different age groups i.e. 7–9 ($N = 559$) and 10–11 ($N = 474$) years old; cumulative incidence was 22 and 10.8% in these age subgroups, respectively. Kaplan-Meier curve (Fig. 2b) also shows that children in the 7–9 year old group compared to their counterparts in 10–11 year old group are at increased risk of obesity (Log-rank test: 12.6, $P < 0.001$). Table 5 and Kaplan-Meier curves (Figs. 2c and d) are further stratified by gender and different age groups (7–9 and 10–11 years old) indicating that both boys and girls in 7–9 year age group are at greater risk of incidence of obesity in comparison to their 10–11 year old counterparts (Log-rank test: 10.91, P < 0.001 and Log-rank test: 2.65, $P = 0.103$, respectively). In cox regression models after adjustment for relevant confounders, age group 7–9 years had higher risk for development of obesity compared to age group 10–11 years. Corresponding adjusted HRs for whole population, boys and girls were 7.40 (CI 95%, 4.32–12.56), 11.76 (CI 95% 5.35–26.31) and 6.06 (CI 95% 2.69–13.69), respectively (reference category, age group 10–11 years).

Discussion

This longitudinal cohort study shows a relatively high incidence of childhood obesity (17%) after over 10 years of follow-up in an urban population of the Tehranian children, which was higher in boys than in girls. Younger non-obese children (7–9 years old) are at greater risk of

Table 1 Baseline characteristics of study participants

Characteristic	Boys (N = 496)	Girls (N = 537)	Total (N = 1033)	P-value[b]
Age (years)	9.1 ± 1.5	9.2 ± 1.4	9.2 ± 1.4	NS
BMI (kg/m²)	16.1 ± 2.0	16.0 ± 2.3	16.1 ± 2.2	NS
Overweight n(%)	81 (16.3)	73 (13.6)	154 (14.9)	< 0.05
WC (cm)	56.4 ± 6.0	57.9 ± 7.1	57.2 ± 6.7	< 0.05
WC ≥90th (cm) n(%)	32 (6.5)	32 (6.0)	64 (6.2)	NS
FPG (mg/dl)	88.2 ± 8.8	86.4 ± 7.7	87.3 ± 8.3	< 0.05
FPG ≥ 100 (mg/dl) n(%)	44 (9.3)	24 (4.6)	69 (6.9)	< 0.05
HDL-C (mg/dl)	47.6 ± 11.4	46.3 ± 11.2	46.9 ± 11.3	NS
HDL-C < 40 (mg/dl) n(%)	126 (27.0)	161 (31.1)	287 (29.2)	NS
TG[a] (mg/dl)	80.0 (61.0–103.0)	88.0 (70.0–118.0)	84.0 (64.0–111.2)	< 0.05
TG ≥ 110 (mg/dl) n(%)	101 (21.5)	160 (30.7)	261 (26.4)	< 0.05
Paternal BMI (kg/m²)	26.4 ± 3.6	25.7 ± 3.7	26.0 ± 3.8	NS
Paternal obesity n(%)	51 (14.5)	52 (13.6)	103 (14.0)	NS
Maternal BMI (kg/m²)	27.7 ± 4.8	27.6 ± 3.0	27.5 ± 4.6	< 0.05
Maternal obesity n(%)	120 (28.2)	113 (24.1)	233 (26.1)	NS
Paternal educational level				
Higher than diploma n(%)	71 (18.0)	67 (16.1)	138 (17.5)	NS
Maternal educational level				
Higher than diploma n(%)	55 (11.7)	48 (9.5)	103 (10.5)	NS
MetS n(%)	26 (5.5)	40 (7.7)	66 (6.7)	NS
SBP (mmHg)	102.7 ± 11.6	100.2 ± 12.1	101.3 ± 11.9	< 0.05
DBP(mmHg)	70.2 ± 10.2	69.3 ± 10.2	69.8 ± 10.2	NS
Hypertension n(%)	163 (33.6)	180 (33.8)	343 (33.7)	NS

BMI body mass index, Overweight, 1SD < BMI-for-age ≤ 2SD based on WHO criteria; WC waist circumference, FPG fasting plasma glucose, HDL-C high-density lipoprotein cholesterol, TG triglycerides, Father's obesity, Father's BMI ≥ 30 kg/m²; Mother's obesity, Mother's BMI ≥ 30 kg/m²; SBP systolic blood pressure, DBP diastolic blood pressure, Hypertension, SBP and/or DBP ≥90th percentile for gender and age
[a]median IQ 25–75
[b]between genders differences

obesity, compared to older non-obese children (10–11 years old), supported by a cumulative incidence of obesity equal to 22.0% vs 10.8% respectivley. Moreover, four parameters are associated with obesity incidence, including being overweight, having higher WC, childhood MetS and parental obesity.

Although many studies have reported the prevalence of childhood obesity before, there is paucity of data regarding incidence of obesity in childhood. Few studies have investigated this subject in developed countries. Cunningham et al. [10] reported a cumulative obesity incidence of 11.9% in the U.S children (aged 5–14) which was significantly lower than what we roported, they also showed the incidence of obesity is more likely to occur at a younger age, particulary among overweight 5-year-old children. Moreover, a study from United Kingdom (UK) carried out in a large contemporary cohort of English children, compared childhood obesity incidence in a subsample of children and reported the incidence of obesity to be 5.1, 6.7, 1.6% in early-childhood (3–7 years), mid-childhood (7–11 years)

and late-childhood (11–15 years), respectively; with the highest peak in the mid-childhood age group [9]. Compared to results of these two studies we demonstrated higher incidence of childhood obesity (17%), which can be explained by differences in inclusion and exclusion criteria, study sample size, geographical location and population characteristics of the study samples. For example, exclusion of overweight children at the baseline in a cohort of English children might be a reason of this lower incidence reported for childhood obesity, whereas we only excluded obese children at baseline. Morover, both the above mentioned studies [9, 10] had larger sample sizes than this study (US: 7738 and UK: 4283 subjects vs. this study: 1033). Another reason for discrepancies between this study results and these two previously mentioned studies is employing different definition of childhood obesity; while we applied the definition of WHO, Cunningham et al. used Centers for Disease Control and Prevention (CDC) definitions and the UK's study used The International Obesity Task Force(IOTF) definitions. As noted by Kelishadi et al., the

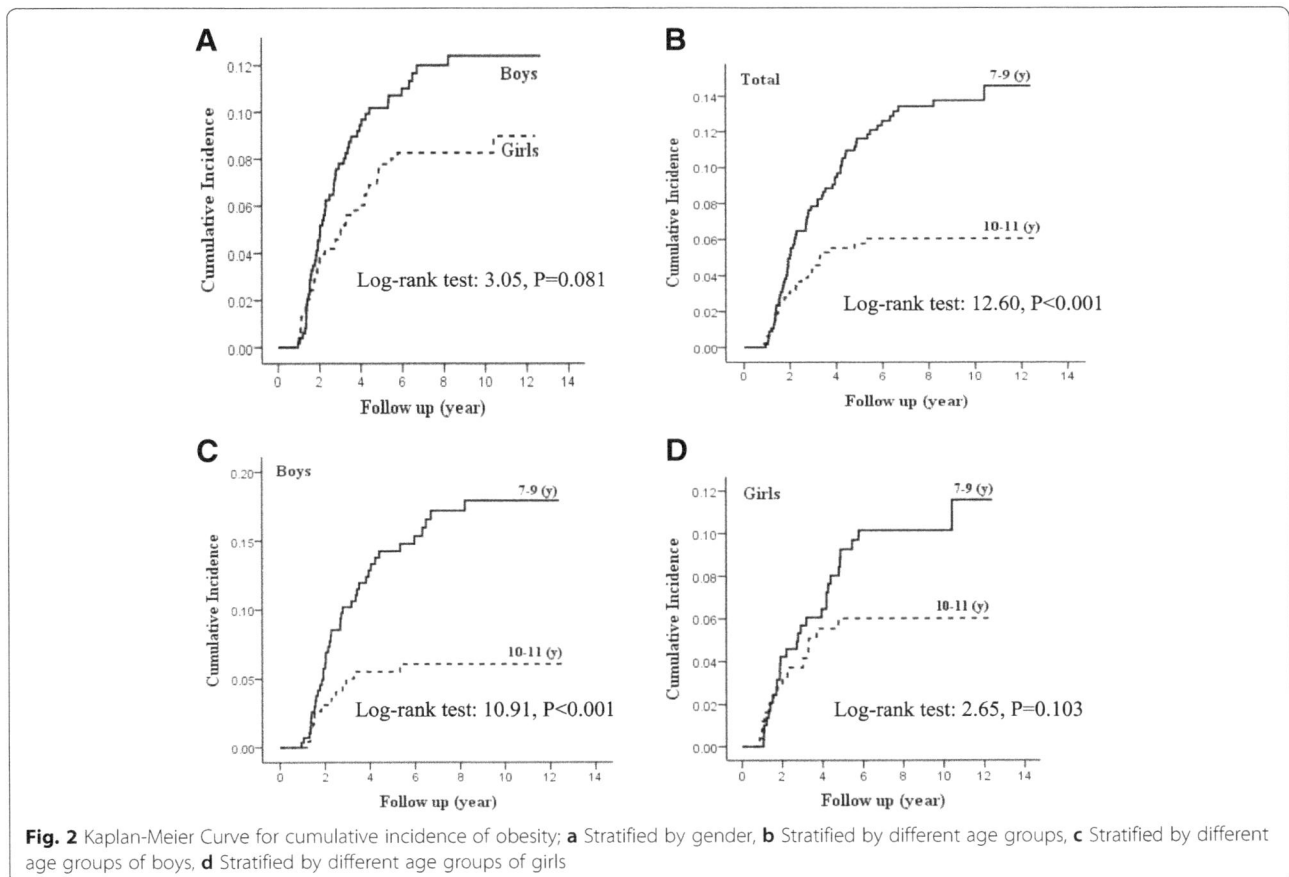

Fig. 2 Kaplan-Meier Curve for cumulative incidence of obesity; **a** Stratified by gender, **b** Stratified by different age groups, **c** Stratified by different age groups of boys, **d** Stratified by different age groups of girls

definition of obesity (e.g., WHO, CDC, IOTF) may contribute to an over or under-estimation of obesity and make comparisons across studies difficult [8]. Other important factors are globalization and epidemiologic transition, currently occurring in Iran - a developing country. The key aspect of this epidemiologic transition is an increase in the incidence and prevalence of chronic non-communicable diseases (obesity, diabetes, hypertension and cardiovascular disease) [17]. This change is the consequent of the "nutritional transition"; which is occurring rapidly in Iran. This phenomenon is the result of overconsumption of simple sugars, saturated oil and processed food [18].

Findings of incidence studies can help health policy makers to focus implementation of preventative strategies on high risk subgroups. For reducing the burden of childhood obesity, results of current study could guide national program implementers to find best targets for anti-obesity interventions. Based on this study's analysis [and in line with previously mentioned findings [9, 10]]; younger non-obese children (7–9 years old) have the highest risk for obesity development. The higher incidence of obesity at younger ages emphasizes the importance of prevention of obesity in the earlier years of childhood, a critical time to promote healthier eating behavior and life style that would prevent obesity [19] .

In agreement with Cunningham et al.'s findings, current study also demonstrated that boys had a relatively higher incidence of obesity than girls [10]. However, in our study while boys showed higher level of cumulative incidence in the 7–9 year age group, compared with girls, both genders had similar incidence for obesity in the 10–11 year old group. Moreover, in line with our results, a meta-analysis study reported higher trend in prevalence of obesity in boys than girls in Iran [8]. There are several possible explanations for this higher incidence of obesity in boys; it might be a reflection of changing body composition that occurs during puberty and is earlier and more continuous in girls, as well as some behavioral differences in the two genders [20, 21].

Regarding the prevalence and incidence of childhood obesity in TLGS population, recently, a study was carried out by Mottaghi et al., children aged 3–7 yr. at baseline were followed up for 10 years [22]. Using CDC's definition of obesity, Mottaghi et al. reported a 18.8% cumulative incidence of obesity for normal weight children over 10 years of follow-up, which was much greater than what we observed for this group of children with same time of follow-up (7.7%). This discrepancy is probably because of age difference of study populations, while mean age of

Table 2 Hazard ratios and 95% confidence intervals of potential risk factors in whole population

Variables	Cumulative Incidence of Obesity (95% CI)	Incidence rate (in 1000 person year)	Un-adjusted HR (95% CI)	Adjusted HR[a] (95% CI)
Total	17.0 (14.1–20.4)	11.8 (9.7–14.4)	–	
Gender				
Boys	19.6 (15.4–24.8)	14.3 (10.9–18.7)	1	1
Girls	14.5 (10.9–19.1)	9.7 (7.2–13.1)	0.70 (0.47–1.05)	0.72 (0.48–1.07)
Weight groups				
Normal weight	7.7 (5.6–10.5)	4.8 (3.5–6.7)	1	1
Overweight	56.7 (47.6–66.2)	68.8 (53.5–88.4)	13.48 (8.88–20.46)	14.93 (9.82–22.70)
WC ≥ 90th				
No	14.9 (12.1–18.3)	10.1 (8.1–12.6)	1	1
Yes	43.9 (30.4–60.3)	50.3 (32.7–79.8)	4.49 (2.68–7.50)	5.05 (3.01–8.48)
FPG ≥ 100 (mg/dl)				
No	16.8 (13.8–20.4)	11.7 (9.5–14.5)	1	1
Yes	18.7 (9.4–35.2)	14.7 (6.5–28.8)	1.13 (0.52–2.44)	1.25 (0.57–2.69)
TG ≥ 110 (mg/dl)				
No	16.6 (13.3–20.6)	11.6 (9.1–14.7)	1	1
Yes	17.5 (12.2–24.8)	12.1 (8.2–17.9)	1.07 (0.68–1.70)	1.17 (0.74–1.86)
HDL-C < 40 (mg/dl)				
No	16.1 (12.8–20.2)	11.2 (8.7–14.4)	1	1
Yes	18.9 (13.6–25.9)	13.3 (9.3–19.1)	1.21 (0.78–1.87)	1.20 (0.77–1.86)
Hypertension				
No	14.8 (11.6–18.9)	10.4 (7.9–13.5)	1	1
Yes	21.8 (16.6–28.3)	15.2 (11.2–20.6)	1.53 (1.02–2.29)	1.35 (0.90–2.03)
MetS				
No	15.5 (12.6–19.0)	10.6 (8.5–13.3)	1	1
Yes	35.0 (22.4–51.8)	31.28 (18.0–52.8)	2.84 (1.61–5.02)	2.77 (1.57–4.89)
Paternal obesity				
Non-obese	14.1 (10.8–18.3)	9.1 (6.9–12.1)	1	1
Obese	33.9 (23.6–47.1)	26.8 (17.5–41.1)	2.83 (1.70–4.72)	2.69 (1.61–4.50)
Maternal obesity				
Non-obese	12.2 (9.2–16.1)	7.7 (5.7–10.4)	1	1
Obese	28.0 (21.3–36.4)	21.6 (15.7–29.7)	2.69 (1.74–4.16)	3.04 (1.96–4.72)
Paternal educational level				
Diploma or lower than diploma	17.1 (13.6–21.4)	11.9 (9.3–15.3)	1	1
Higher than diploma	18.4 (11.3–29.1)	12.7 (7.5–21.5)	1.07 (0.60–1.90)	1.11 (0.62–1.99)
Maternal educational level				
Diploma or lower than diploma	17.1 (14.0–20.8)	11.7 (9.4–14.5)	1	1
Higher than diploma	19.3 (11.2–32.1)	16.3 (9.1–29.5)	1.25 (0.67–2.35)	1.20 (0.64–2.26)

Overweight, 1SD < BMI-for-age ≤ 2SD based on WHO criteria; *WC* waist circumference; *FPG* fasting plasma glucose; HDL-C, high-density lipoprotein cholesterol; *TG* triglycerides; Paternal obesity, Father's BMI ≥ 30 kg/m^2; Maternal obesity, Mother's BMI ≥ 30 kg/m^2; Hypertension, SBP and/or DBP ≥90th percentile for gender and age; MetS, Metabolic syndrome for children based on the definition of Cook et al. work
[a] Adjusted for age at baseline

Table 3 Hazard ratios and 95% confidence intervals of potential risk factors in boys

Variables	Cumulative Incidence of Obesity (95% CI)	Incidence rate (in 1000 person year)	Un-adjusted HR (95% CI)	Adjusted HR[a] (95% CI)
Weight groups				
Normal weight	10.5 (7.1–15.3)	6.9 (4.6–10.4)	1	1
Overweight	55.4 (43–68.6)	66.8 (47–94.9)	9.16 (5.33–15.47)	10.42 (6.04–17.97)
WC ≥ 90th				
No	16.6 (12.6–21.8)	11.6 (8.5–15.6)	1	1
Yes	54.6 (35.7–75.6)	82.3 (46.8–145.0)	5.93 (3.11–11.32)	9.31 (4.62–18.73)
FPG ≥ 100 (mg/dl)				
No	19.0 (14.6–24.7)	13.8 (10.3–18.4)	1	1
Yes	20.4 (9.0–42.2)	16.0 (6.7–38.5)	1.10 (0.44–2.77)	1.32 (0.45–2.85)
TG ≥ 110 (mg/dl)				
No	20.0 (15.1–26.2)	14.8 (10.9–20.2)	1	1
Yes	14.7 (7.6–27.2)	9.9 (5.0–19.8)	0.70 (0.32–1.48)	0.72 (0.34–1.54)
HDL-C < 40 (mg/dl)				
No	17.7 (12.9–24.0)	12.8 (9.0–18.0)	1	1
Yes	22.5 (14.5–34.1)	16.7 (10.2–27.3)	1.32 (0.73–2.40)	1.18 (0.65–2.15)
Hypertension				
No	18.0 (13.1–24.6)	13.2 (9.3–18.7)	1	1
Yes	23.8 (16.3–33.8)	17.4 (11.5–26.5)	1.37 (0.80–2.36)	1.24 (0.72–2.14)
MetS				
No	18.0 (13.7–23.4)	12.9 (9.6–17.4)	1	1
Yes	37.5 (18.9–65.1)	32.5 (15.8–87.4)	2.58 (1.10–6.06)	2.33 (1.00–5.48)
Paternal obesity				
Non-obese	14.8 (10.1–21.3)	9.8 (6.5–14.6)	1	1
Obese	47.8 (32.6–65.7)	46.5 (28.5–76.0)	4.41 (2.34–8.30)	3.93 (2.08–7.42)
Maternal obesity				
Non-obese	15.1 (10.5–21.5)	10.0 (6.7–14.8)	1	1
Obese	26.0 (17.3–38.1)	19.8 (12.5–31.5)	1.92 (1.05–3.52)	2.14 (1.66–3.94)
Paternal educational level				
Diploma or lower than diploma	19.6 (14.4–26.1)	14.2 (10.2–19.8)	1	1
Higher than diploma	22.5 (12.4–38.8)	17.0 (8.8–32.6)	1.16 (0.56–2.41)	1.15 (0.55–2.34)
Maternal educational level				
Diploma or lower than diploma	20.2 (15.6–26.0)	14.4 (10.9–19.2)	1	1
Higher than diploma	16.7 (7.3–35.5)	14.3 (6.0–34.4)	0.87 (0.35–2.19)	0.68 (0.55–0.83)

Overweight, 1SD < BMI-for-age ≤ 2SD based on WHO criteria; *WC* waist circumference, *FPG* fasting plasma glucose, *HDL-C* high-density lipoprotein cholesterol, *TG* triglycerides, Paternal obesity, Father's BMI ≥ 30 kg/m^2; Maternal obesity, Mother's BMI ≥ 30 kg/m^2; Hypertension, SBP and/or DBP ≥90th percentile for gender and age; MetS, Metabolic syndrome for children based on the definition of Cook et al. work
[a]Adjusted for age at baseline

children entering their study was 5.3 years, in this study it was 9.2 years. In addition to Mottaghi et al's results regarding incidence of obesity, we provided age subgroup analysis of obesity incidence allowing us to claim that age group itself is an important risk factor for obesity incidence, independent of any other variable including time.

Prevalence-based cross-sectional data in developing countries have addressed unhealthy nutrition, physical inactivity, socioeconomic status, area of residence, socio-cultural factors and genetic as risk factors associated with childhood obesity [23]. Other than age group and gender discussed earlier, this study reports childhood overweight, having higher WC, MetS and parental obesity as the best predictors of obesity incidence. It is already well known that childhood overweight increases the probability of incidence of obesity [24]; consistent to

Table 4 Hazard ratios and 95% confidence intervals of potential risk factors in girls

Variables	Cumulative Incidence of Obesity (95% CI)	Incidence rate (in 1000 person year)	Un-adjusted HR (95% CI)	Adjusted HR[a] (95% CI)
Weight groups				
Normal weight	5.0 (2.9–8.7)	3.0 (1.7–5.4)	1	1
Overweight	58.2 (45.3–71.7)	71.0 (49.7–101.5)	21.8 (11.14–42.67)	23.42 (11.93–45.96)
WC ≥ 90th				
No	13.3 (9.8–18.0)	8.7 (6.3–12.1)	1	1
Yes	31.6 (15.6–57.2)	28.3 (12.7–62.9)	3.09 (1.30–7.33)	3.12 (1.31–7.41)
FPG ≥ 100 (mg/dl)				
No	14.9 (11.2–19.8)	10.0 (7.3–13.6)	1	1
Yes	10.0 (4.1–48.8)	10.1 (2.5–40.4)	1.01 (0.21–4.19)	1.23 (0.29–5.14)
TG ≥ 110 (mg/dl)				
No	13.0 (9.0–18.6)	8.5 (5.8–12.6)	1	1
Yes	19.2 (12.4–29.1)	13.5 (8.4–21.7)	1.60 (0.86–2.96)	1.77 (0.95–3.29)
HDL-C < 40 (mg/dl)				
No	14.5 (10.3–20.4)	9.7 (6.7–14.1)	1	1
Yes	16.0 (9.8–25.5)	10.8 (6.4–18.3)	1.12 (0.59–2.13)	1.87 (0.62–2.26)
Hypertension				
No	11.8 (7.9–17.3)	7.9 (5.2–12.0)	1	1
Yes	20.0 (13.4–29.2)	13.3 (8.6–20.7)	1.77 (0.96–3.24)	1.60 (0.86–2.96)
Mets				
No	13.2 (9.6–18.0)	8.7 (6.2–12.1)	1	1
Yes	33.3 (18.2–55.7)	28.8 (14.4–57.7)	3.22 (1.49–6.96)	3.55 (1.51–7.03)
Paternal obesity				
Non-obese	13.5 (9.3–19.5)	8.6 (5.8–12.8)	1	1
Obese	17.5 (7.7–37.0)	11.4 (4.7–27.4)	1.32 (0.50–3.47)	1.33 (0.51–3.49)
Maternal obesity				
Non-obese	9.7 (6.2–14.9)	5.9 (3.7–9.4)	1	1
Obese	30.0 (20.6–42.6)	23.6 (15.2–36.5)	3.85 (2.04–7.29)	4.43 (2.33–8.45)
Paternal educational level				
Diploma or lower than diploma	14.8 (10.5–20.7)	10.0 (6.9–14.4)	1	1
Higher than diploma	13.9 (6.0–20.2)	8.8 (3.6–21.0)	0.91 (0.35–2.35)	0.96 (0.37–2.51)
Maternal educational level				
Diploma or lower than diploma	14.2 (10.4–19.2)	9.3 (6.7–12.9)	1	1
Higher than diploma	22.2 (10.7–42.9)	18.6 (8.3–41.3)	1.81 (0.76–4.30)	1.82 (0.77–4.34)

Overweight, 1SD < BMI-for-age ≤ 2SD based on WHO criteria; *WC* waist circumference; *FPG* fasting plasma glucose, *HDL-C* high-density lipoprotein cholesterol, *TG* triglycerides; Paternal obesity, Father's BMI ≥ 30 kg/m^2; Maternal obesity, Mother's BMI ≥ 30 kg/m^2; Hypertension, SBP and/or DBP ≥90th percentile for gender and age; Mets, Metabolic syndrome for children based on the definition of Cook et al. work
[a]Adjusted for age at baseline

Table 5 Cumulative incidence and incidence rate (in 1000 person year) stratified by gender and age groups

Age Group	7–9 years old (N = 559)			10–11 years old (N = 474)		
	Boys	Girls	Total	Boys	Girls	Total
Cumulative incidence	26.4 (20.2–34.1)	17.6 (12.5–24.5)	22.0 (17.8–27)	10.8 (6.4–17.9)	10.7 (6.5–17.4)	10.8 (7.5–15.3)
Incidence rate (in 1000 person year)	20.4 (15.0–27.7)	12,0 (8.2–17.3)	15.9 (12.5–20.1)	7.3 (4.2–12.6)	7.0 (4.1–11.8)	7.1 (4.9–10.4)

this, in current study a positive correlation of high childhood BMI and WC with obesity incidence was detected. As demonstrated earlier, there is a risk of an increased adverse cardiovascular outcomes and obesity in children with MetS [25], an association supported by this study's findings, suggesting a 2.77 HR for obesity incidence in children with MetS.

There are numbers of strengths in this study. To the best of our knowledge, this study is the first population-based representative cohort which reports childhood obesity incidence and its associated demographic, anthropometric, metabolic, and socioeconomic risk factors in Iran and the middle east and north africa (MENA) region. The longitudinal design and having a relatively long follow-up period allowed us to assess the gender stratified incidence of obesity and its risk factors. Last but not least, is the use of direct measurements, instead of self-reported data for both children and parents.

We are also aware that our study has several limitations; first, our subjects were selected from TLGS, an urban-based population cohort in district 13 area of Tehran, with limited potential of generalization to the whole population of Iran, especially in rural areas. Second, taking account some variables and cofounders like dietary habits, socioeconomic status, physical activity, maternal smoking status during pregnancy, and psychological factors was beyond the scope of this study, even though they also could play a role in obesity incidence. Third, the drop out rate of 26.3%; importantly, our loss to follow-up participants had statistically significant higher baseline BMI and WC, suggesting that our results might even underestimate rates of obesity incidence in Tehranian children and adolescents.

Conclusion

This study shows a significantly high childhood obesity incidence in Tehran, capital city of a developing country. To prevent incidence of obesity, we suggest earlier weight control plans in childhood, particularly before the age of 7. Moreover young children who suffer from overweight, WC above 90th percentile, MetS and parental obesity are the best targets for intervention against childhood obesity. However, further cohort studies with larger sample sizes and wider age group coverages are needed for better identification of high risk groups by exploring more risk factors involved in the development of obesity in children.

Abbreviations
BMI: Body mass Index; FPG: Fasting plasma glucose; HDL-C: High -density lipoprotein cholesterol; HRs: Hazard ratios; MetS: Metabolic syndrome; TC: Total cholesterol; TG: Triglyceride; TLGS: Tehran Lipid and glucose Study; WC: Waist circumference

Acknowledgments
We would like to acknowledge Ms. Niloofar Shiva for critical editing of English grammar and syntax of the manuscript, and also the staff and participants in the TLGS Study for their important contribution.

Authors' contributions
FH study design. MB and SA, AB, literature review, data analysis, interpretation and manuscript preparation. SS and MZ data collection and analysis. MV, FA and FH manuscript review, critical appraisal and specialist advice. All authors read and approved the manuscript.

Competing interests
The authors declare that they have no competing interest.

Author details
[1]Obesity Research Center, Research Institute for Endocrine Sciences, Shahid Beheshti University of Medical Sciences, Tehran, Iran. [2]Endocrine Research Center, Research Institute for Endocrine Sciences, Shahid Beheshti University of Medical Sciences, Tehran, Iran.

References
1. Childhood overweight and obesity. World Health Organization. (WHO Media centre URL: http://www.who.int/mediacentre/factsheets/fs311/en/ [accessed 2015-12-24]).
2. Simmonds M, Burch J, Llewellyn A, Griffiths C, Yang H, Owen C, et al. The use of measures of obesity in childhood for predicting obesity and the development of obesity-related diseases in adulthood: a systematic review and meta-analysis. Health technology assessment (Winchester, England). 2015;19(43):1–336.
3. Llewellyn A, Simmonds M, Owen CG, Woolacott N. Childhood obesity as a predictor of morbidity in adulthood: a systematic review and meta-analysis. Obesity Reviews. 2015; n/a-n/a
4. de Onis M, Blossner M, Borghi E. Global prevalence and trends of overweight and obesity among preschool children. Am J Clin Nutr. 2010; 92(5):1257–64.
5. Trends in adult body-mass index in 200 countries from 1975 to 2014: a pooled analysis of 1698 population-based measurement studies with 19.2 million participants. Lancet (London, England). 2016;387(10026):1377–96.
6. Mansourian M, Marateb HR, Kelishadi R, Motlagh ME, Aminaee T, Taslimi M, et al. First growth curves based on the World Health Organization reference in a nationally-representative sample of pediatric population in the Middle East and North Africa (MENA): the CASPIAN-III study. BMC Pediatr. 2012;12:149.
7. Azizi F, Rahmani M, Emami H, Mirmiran P, Hajipour R, Madjid M, et al. Cardiovascular risk factors in an Iranian urban population: Tehran lipid and glucose study (phase 1). Sozial- und Praventivmedizin. 2002;47(6):408–26.
8. Kelishadi R, Haghdoost AA, Sadeghirad B, Khajehkazemi R. Trend in the prevalence of obesity and overweight among Iranian children and adolescents: a systematic review and meta-analysis. Nutrition (Burbank, Los Angeles County, Calif). 2014;30(4):393–400.
9. Hughes AR, Sherriff A, Lawlor DA, Ness AR, Reilly JJ. Incidence of obesity during childhood and adolescence in a large contemporary cohort. Prev Med. 2011;52(5):300–4.
10. Cunningham SA, Kramer MR, Venkat NK. Incidence of childhood obesity in the United States. N Engl J Med. 2014;370(5):403–11.
11. Azizi F, Ghanbarian A, Momenan AA, Hadaegh F, Mirmiran P, Hedayati M, et al. Prevention of non-communicable disease in a population in nutrition transition: Tehran lipid and glucose study phase II. Trials. 2009;10:5.
12. BMI-for-age (5–19 years). World Health Organization. 2006.
13. Cook S, Weitzman M, Auinger P, Nguyen M, Dietz WH. Prevalence of a metabolic syndrome phenotype in adolescents: findings from the third National Health and nutrition examination survey, 1988-1994. Archives of pediatrics & adolescent medicine. 2003;157(8):821–7.
14. Executive Summary of The Third Report of The National Cholesterol Education Program (NCEP) Expert Panel on Detection, Evaluation, And Treatment of High Blood Cholesterol In Adults (Adult Treatment Panel III). Jama. 2001;285(19):2486–97.
15. Kelishadi R, Gouya MM, Ardalan G, Hosseini M, Motaghian M, Delavari A, et al. First reference curves of waist and hip circumferences in an Asian population of youths: CASPIAN study. J Trop Pediatr. 2007;53(3):158–64.

16. The fourth report on the diagnosis, evaluation, and treatment of high blood pressure in children and adolescents. Pediatrics. 2004;114(2 Suppl 4th Report):555–76.

17. Reddy KS, Yusuf S. Emerging epidemic of cardiovascular disease in developing countries. Circulation. 1998;97(6):596–601.

18. Ghassemi H, Harrison G, Mohammad K. An accelerated nutrition transition in Iran. Public Health Nutr. 2006;5(1a):149–55.

19. Karnik S, Kanekar A. Childhood obesity: a global public health crisis. Int J Prev Med. 2012;3(1):1–7.

20. Lobstein T, Baur L, Uauy R. Obesity in children and young people: a crisis in public health. Obesity reviews : an official journal of the International Association for the Study of Obesity. 2004;5(Suppl 1):4–104.

21. Govindan M, Gurm R, Mohan S, Kline-Rogers E, Corriveau N, Goldberg C, et al. Gender differences in physiologic markers and health behaviors associated with childhood obesity. Pediatrics. 2013;132(3):468–74.

22. Mottaghi A, Mirmiran P, Pourvali K, Tahmasbpour Z, Azizi F. Incidence and prevalence of childhood obesity in Tehran, Iran in 2011. Iranian Journal of Public Health. 2017;46(10):1395–403.

23. Gupta N, Goel K, Shah P, Misra A. Childhood obesity in developing countries: epidemiology, determinants, and prevention. Endocr Rev. 2012;33(1):48–70.

24. Wright CM, Parker L, Lamont D, Craft AW. Implications of childhood obesity for adult health: findings from thousand families cohort study. BMJ (Clinical research ed). 2001;323(7324):1280–4.

25. Weiss R, Dziura J, Burgert TS, Tamborlane WV, Taksali SE, Yeckel CW, et al. Obesity and the metabolic syndrome in children and adolescents. N Engl J Med. 2004;350(23):2362–74.

8

Epidemiology and clinical characteristics of acute respiratory tract infections among hospitalized infants and young children in Chengdu, West China, 2009–2014

Jiayi Chen[1,2], Pengwei Hu[1,3], Tao Zhou[1], Tianli Zheng[1], Lingxu Zhou[1,4], Chunping Jiang[1] and Xiaofang Pei[1*]

Abstract

Background: Acute respiratory infection (ARI) is the leading cause of morbidity and mortality in pediatric patients worldwide and imposes an intense pressure on health care facilities. Data on the epidemiology profiles of ARIs are scarce in the western and rural areas of China. The purpose of the current study is to provide data on the presence of potential pathogens of ARIs in hospitalized children in Chengdu, west China.

Methods: Respiratory specimens were obtained from hospitalized patients (under 6 years old) with ARIs in a local hospital in Chengdu. Eight respiratory viruses were identified by PCR and 6 respiratory bacteria by biochemical reactions and Analytical Profile Index (API). Pathogens profiles, clinical characteristics and seasonality were analyzed.

Results: Fifty-one percent of patients were identified with at least one respiratory pathogen. Human rhinovirus (HRV) (23%), Respiratory syncytial virus (RSV) (22.7%) was the most commonly identified viruses, with *Klebsiella pneumoniae* (11.5%) the most commonly identified bacterium in the study. The presences of more than one pathogen were found, and multiple viral, bacterial, viral/bacterial combinations were identified in 14.9, 3.3 and 13.9% of patients respectively. Respiratory viruses were identified throughout the year with a seasonal peak in December–February. Pathogens profiles and clinical associations were different between infants (< 1 year of age) and older children (> 1 year of age). Infants with ARIs were more likely to have one or more viruses than older children. Infants identified with multiple pathogens had significantly higher proportions of tachypnea than infants that were not.

Conclusions: This study demonstrated that viral agents were frequently found in hospitalized children with ARI in Chengdu during the study period. This study gives us better information on the pathogen profiles, clinical associations, co-infection combinations and seasonal features of ARIs in hospitalized children, which is important for diagnoses and treatment of ARIs, as well as implementation of vaccines in this area. Moreover, future efforts in reducing the impact of ARIs will depend on programs in which available vaccines, especially vaccines on RSV, HRV and *S. pneumoniae* could be employed in this region and new vaccines could be developed against common pathogens.

Keywords: Acute respiratory infections, Epidemiology, Clinical characteristics, Pediatrics, West China

* Correspondence: xxpeiscu@163.com
[1]Department of Public Health Laboratory Sciences, West China School of Public Health (No.4 West China Teaching Hospital), Sichuan University, 16#, Section 3, Renmin Road South, Chengdu 610041, Sichuan, People's Republic of China
Full list of author information is available at the end of the article

Background

Acute respiratory infections (ARIs) remain one of the most common major public health threats [1]. There were approximate 11.9 million episodes of severe acute lower respiratory infections (ALRI) resulted in hospital admissions in young children worldwide [2], and ARIs-related pneumonia was one of the leading cause of death that due to infectious disease in China (> 30,000 deaths annually) as well as globally (935,000 in 2013) [3, 4]. There were, as have been suggested, associations of several viral agents with ARIs, such as: respiratory syncytial virus (RSV), human rhinovirus (HRV), human metapneumovirus (HMPV), influenza virus (IFV), parainfluenza virus (PIV), adenovirus (ADV) and human bocavirus (BoV), accounting for about 35–87% of children with ARI [5]. Viral co-infections occurred in 4–33% of children hospitalized with ARIs, and may indicate an increasing risk for clinical outcome [6, 7]. Further, bacterial infections such as: *Streptococcus pneumoniae*, *Haemophilus influenzae*, *Staphylococcus aureus*, *Pseudomonas aeruginosa* and *Klebsiella pneumoniae*, et al., were commonly observed in the later stage of diseases due to immune-compromised viral infections [8].

Similarities among ARI symptoms hampers the diagnostic and therapeutic efficacy among infected children, and inappropriate medication options may lead to the potential of viral escape mutants or bacterial resistance [8]. The composition of ARIs is geographically diverse and is largely associated with the epidemic status of each ARIs and climate conditions [9, 10]. The prevalence of ARIs varies from 14.6 to 94.3% among hospitalized children with respiratory infections in some metropolitan cities such as Beijing, Shanghai and Shenzhen in China [11–14]. However, in the underdeveloped interior areas of China, epidemiology profiles of ARIs are seldom reported. Chengdu is a mega-city in the southwest of China and has a population of more than 15 million people. Flu vaccination rates were pretty low in this area, which were 2.18, 1.69, 1.82 and 1.63% respectively from 2010 to 2013 [15]. The purpose of the current study is to investigate the profiles of respiratory pathogens and epidemiology characteristics of ARIs in hospitalized children in Chengdu. The results were expected to help improve diagnosis and optimization of therapeutic regimens of ARIs in this area.

Methods

Study design and patient population

The cross-sectional study was conducted monthly at a sentinel tertiary women's and children's hospitals in Chengdu, West China, from September 2009 to February 2014. A total of 1992 hospitalized children younger than 6 years old that presented symptoms of ARIs were recruited. Inclusion criteria for cases were (i) acute infection, for example fever, WBC anomaly, shivering; (ii) respiratory

symptoms such as cough, rhinorrhea, pharyngalgia, expectoration, nose/throat congestion, shortness of breath, abnormal breathing sounds or dyspnea. The study protocol was approved by the Medical Ethics Committee of Sichuan University and written informed consents were obtained from the parents or the caregiver before collecting samples.

Samples including nasopharyngeal aspirates, sputum, throat swabs, blood and bronchoalevlar lavage fluid were collected by qualified medical personnel. The demographic information and medical records of the participated patients were also collected. All samples were delivered to the Microbiology Laboratory of Department of Public Health Laboratory Sciences, Sichuan University immediately after collection samples via cold chain transportation and stored at − 80 °C.

Pathogen analysis

Nasopharyngeal aspirates, sputum, throat swabs and bronchoalevlar lavage fluid were used for respiratory virus analyses. Viral RNA and DNA were extracted by Viral Nucleic Acid Extraction Kit (Geneaid, Taiwan District) according to the manufacturer's instructions. cDNA were synthesized with reverse transcription kit (BIO-RAD, California, US). Primers and multiplex PCR conditions for IFV [16], RSV [16], PIV [17], ADV [18], HMPV [13], human coronavirus (HCoV) [19], HBoV [20] and HRV [17] have been described previously. Primers were synthesized by Life Technology Corp. (Shanghai, China) and PCRs were performed using PCR Mastermix (Tiangen Company, China) and the S1000™ Thermal Cycler (BIO-RAD, California, US). Respiratory viruses were initially identified by the size of PCR products following agarose gel electrophoresis, with confirmation by DNA sequencing (Life Technology Corp., Shanghai, China).

Nasopharyngeal aspirates, sputum, blood and bronchoalevlar lavage fluid were used for bacterial analyses. For isolation of bacteria, specimens were cultured on sheep blood agar, chocolate agar and MacConkey's agar plates. Isolated bacteria were primarily evaluated by colonial morphology, Gram staining, and were finally identified by biochemical reactions and API system. *S. pneumoniae* were differentiated by Optochin sensitivity and *Group A streptococcus* were identified by bacitracin sensitivity. *P. aeruginosa* and *K. pneumoniae* were identified by API 20E. *H. influenzae*, *S. aureus* were differentiated by API HN, API Staph respectively.

Statistical analysis

The collected data were analyzed through SPSS version 19.0. Descriptive statistics were done in the form of means, frequencies and ranges of the variables. Continuous variables were expressed as means with their standard deviations. Categorical variables such as age groups and their associations with proportions of certain pathogens were analyzed using the chi-square test or the Fisher's exact test. Significant differences, associations and interrelationships of the variables were assessed at a level of $P < 0.05$.

Results

Profile of enrolled patients

The median age of the patients was 9 months (ranged from 1 days to 6 years old), with 54% of patients under 1 year of age. Of 1992 enrolled children, 1185 were boys and 807 were girls (gender ratio of 1.47: 1). Cough was found in 1354 (68.0%) of the children, followed by fever (51.9%, 1033) and expectoration (29.0%, 578). The median number of days between symptom onset and hospitalization was 10 days. 52.5% (1045/1992) of the patients were diagnosed with pneumonia by chest X-ray. Among all the cases, 9 children died during the study period, including 8 boys and 1 girl.

Results of pathogen analysis

Respiratory viruses were analyzed in 1764 samples. HRV testing was added in 2012 and HRV was analyzed in 795 samples. One or more respiratory viruses were identified in 51.0% of the patients (Table 1). HRV (23.0%, 183/795) and RSV (22.7%, 401/1764) were the most commonly identified viruses in hospitalized children, followed by PIV (13.4%, 236/1764), HBoV (8.4%, 149/1764) and ADV (6.2%, 110/1764). Other viruses such as IFV (4.4%), HMPV (2.2%) and HCoV (0.6%) were identified in small proportions. Multiple viral combinations in samples were found, including 223 dual, 37 triple and 3 quadruple combinations. Common combinations are listed in Table 2.

Six respiratory bacteria were analyzed among 1816 samples. One or more respiratory bacteria were identified in 26.2% (475/1816) of the patients. The most commonly detected bacteria were *K. pneumoniae* (11.5%, 209/1816), *S. pneumoniae* (9.5%, 173/1816) and *S. aureus* (4.0%, 73/1816), followed by *H. influenzae* (2.5%), *P. aeruginosa* (1.9%), and *Group A streptococcus* (0.4%). Multiple bacterial combinations in samples were found, including 52 dual and 8 triple bacterial combinations. *K. pneumoniae/S. pneumoniae* co-infection was the most frequent combination. Eight viruses and 6 bacteria were tested in 1728 samples, among which 883 (51.1%) were identified with at least one respiratory pathogen. 240 (27.2%, 240/883) were viral/bacterial combination among positive cases.

Among 9 death cases, 6 patients were identified with at least 1 respiratory pathogen, including 2 boys with single virus (IFV, HRV respectively), 2 boys with dual virus (PIV/HRV, PIV/HBoV respectively), 1 boy with triple virus (RSV/PIV/HRV) and 1 girl with both virus and bacteria (PIV/*S.pneumoniae*). None of the pathogens was identified in the rest of 3 boys.

Respiratory pathogens and clinical characteristics

A univariate analysis was conducted to find associations between demographic and clinical characteristics with infection (Table 3). Infants tended to have a higher proportion of virus infection than older children ($P < 0.001$), with those from 6 to 12 months of age having the highest proportion (67.4%) ($P < 0.001$). Infants identified with viruses had higher proportion of fever ($P < 0.001$), cough ($P < 0.001$), runny nose ($P = 0.007$), expectoration ($P < 0.001$) and diarrhea ($P = 0.031$) than infants that were not. Older children with viral infections had a higher proportion of tachypnea

Table 1 Pathogen profiles and distributions of viral agents among age groups

	< 6 months, n = 799		6 months-1 year, n = 193		1-3 years, n = 351		> 3 years, n = 421		All ages, n = 1764	
	No.%	Mixed	No.%	Mixed	No.%	Mixed	No.%	Mixed	No.%	Mixed
Positive	414 (51.8)[a]		130 (67.4)		194 (55.3)		162 (38.5)		900 (51.0)[a]	
Single	297 (33.0)[b]		92 (10.2)		127 (14.1)		121 (13.4)		637 (70.8)[b]	
Mixed	117 (13.0)[c]		38 (4.2)		68 (7.6)		40 (4.4)		263 (29.2)[b]	
IFV	29 (3.2)[b]	21 (72.4)[c]	11 (1.2)	8 (72.7)	18 (23.1)	15 (83.3)	20 (25.6)	8 (40.0)	78 (4.4)[a]	52 (66.7)
RSV	212 (23.6)	69 (32.5)	61 (6.8)	27 (44.3)	82 (9.1)	29 (35.4)	46 (5.1)	24 (52.2)	401 (22.7)	149 (37.2)
PIV	91 (10.1)	47 (51.6)	42 (4.7)	23 (48.9)	61 (6.8)	30 (49.2)	42 (4.4)	16 (38.1)	236 (13.4)	116 (49.2)
ADV	29 (3.2)	22 (75.9)	25 (2.8)	10 (40.0)	33 (3.7)	20 (60.6)	23 (2.6)	9 (39.1)	110 (6.2)	61 (55.5)
HPMV	20 (2.2)	10 (50.0)	4 (0.4)	3 (75.0)	8 (0.9)	7 (87.5)	6 (0.7)	1 (16.7)	38 (2.2)	21 (55.3)
CoV	7 (0.8)	6 (85.7)	1 (0.1)	0 (0.0)	1 (0.1)	1 (100.0)	2 (0.2)	1 (50.0)	11 (0.6)	8 (72.7)
HBoV	62 (6.9)	26 (41.9)	19 (2.1)	10 (52.6)	44 (4.9)	23 (52.3)	24 (2.7)	13 (54.2)	149 (8.4)	72 (48.3)
HRV	95 (20.4)[d]	47 (49.4)	17 (3.7)	7 (41.2)	27 (5.8)	22 (81.5)	44 (9.5)	14 (31.8)	183 (23.0)[e]	90 (49.2)

[a]Case number and percentage by age group
[b]Case number and percentage among all positive cases
[c]Co-infection cases of each virus detected and percentages of number of positive cases
[d]Positive cases in the group that were analyzed for HRV was 465
[e]HRV was analyzed in 795 samples (HRV testing was added in 2012)

Table 2 Common combinations of analyzed pathogens

	No.
Virus Combinations	
RSV + PIV	40
RSV + ADV	25
RSV + HRV	23
PIV + HBoV	18
HBoV+HRV	14
RSV + PIV + HRV	9
Virus/Bacteria Combinations	
RSV + S. pneumoniae	22
RSV + K. pneumoniae	16
IFV + S. pneumoniae	12
HRV+ S. pneumoniae	11
HRV+ K. pneumoniae	10

($P = 0.007$) than younger children (less than 1 year of age). In the virus-positive group, infants with viral co-infections had a significantly higher proportion of tachypnea ($P = 0.033$) than that with single viral infections.

Demographic and clinical features for each analyzed respiratory virus were also examined. PIV and ADV were usually recognized in children aged from 6 to 12 months, whereas HBoV was mostly found in 1 to 3 years group, while HRV was found in all age groups (Table 1). PIV was associated with fever, cough and expectoration while HRV with cough, expectoration and diarrhea (Data not shown).

Among children tested for respiratory bacteria, older children had higher proportion of bacterial infections than infants ($P = 0.010$). K. pneumoniae was usually detected in infants and S. pneumoniae, H. influenzae were more common in older children. Infants with bacterial infections had higher proportion of cough ($P < 0.001$) and expectoration ($P = 0.048$).

Among 1728 children (with complete viral and bacterial workups), infants identified with any pathogen (Table 4) had higher proportions of fever ($P < 0.001$),

cough ($P < 0.001$), runny nose ($P = 0.011$), expectoration ($P < 0.001$) and diarrhea ($P = 0.009$) than infants that were not. Pathogen-positive older children had a higher proportion of chest pain ($P = 0.037$). In the pathogen positive group, infants with viral/bacterial co-infection had significantly higher proportions of cough ($P = 0.007$) and tachypnea ($P = 0.025$).

Considering diagnoses and etiology, pneumonia was taken into consideration. Older children had significantly higher proportion of pneumonia ($P < 0.001$) than infants, with the highest rate observed in children 1 to 3 years of age. Infants identified with bacterial had a higher proportion of pneumonia than older children, and S. aureus ($P = 0.004$) and S. pneumonia ($P = 0.009$) were associated with pneumonia.

Seasonal distributions

Seasonal distributions of respiratory pathogens were estimated by admission dates for the included children. The seasonal detection rates ranged from 7.4 to 79.7% with a mean rate of 49.5%. Overall, viral infections were more likely to occur in winter months (December to February) with a decline in summer months (June to August) (Fig. 1). The same distribution was observed for ADV (Fig. 2). PIV and HRV were detected all year, with their detection peaks often in autumn. HBoV infections showed a peak in the summer season of 2010 and 2012. No regular seasonal variations with IFV and HPMV were observed during the study period.

Discussion

To the best of our knowledge, this study is the first study to investigate the role of 8 respiratory viruses and 6 respiratory bacteria in ARIs among hospitalized children in Chengdu district, west China over a 5-year period. Therefore, these findings may be useful nationally and internationally equally.

The results confirmed a frequent viral etiology among 51% of children aged < 6 years presenting ARIs. A review of studies on positive proportions of respiratory viruses among

Table 3 Clinical characteristics in infants with viral or bacterial workups

Clinical characteristics	Any Virus n = 544	No Virus n = 448	P Value	Any Bacteria n = 241	No Bacteria n = 773	P Value
Fever (> 37.5 °C)	208 (38.2)	108 (24.1)	0.000**	85 (35.3)	239 (30.9)	0.235
Cough	366 (67.3)	177 (39.5)	0.000**	171 (71.0)	379 (49.0)	0.000**
Runny nose	71 (13.1)	34 (7.6)	0.007**	28 (11.6)	76 (9.8)	0.465
Expectoration	146 (26.8)	66 (14.7)	0.000**	63 (26.1)	154 (19.9)	0.048*
Tachypnea	95 (17.5)	66 (14.7)	0.261	35 (14.5)	126 (16.3)	0.546
Dyspnea	93 (17.1)	94 (21.0)	0.122	47 (19.5)	145 (18.8)	0.851
Diarrhea	70 (12.9)	38 (8.5)	0.031*	27 (11.2)	85 (11.0)	1.000
Pneumonia	279 (51.3)	211 (47.1)	0.189	143 (59.3)	361 (46.7)	0.001**

* $P < 0.05$, ** $P < 0.01$

Table 4 Clinical characteristics in infants with complete viral and bacterial workups

Clinical characteristics	Any Pathogen n = 332	No Pathogen n = 653	P Value	Virus Alone n = 412	Bacteria Alone n = 113	Virus/Baccteria Co-infection n = 128	P Value
Fever (> 37.5 °C)	69 (20.8)	243 (37.2)	0.000**	158 (38.3)	37 (32.7)	48 (37.5)	0.559
Cough	105 (31.6)	433 (66.3)	0.000**	262 (63.6)	71 (62.8)	100 (78.1)	0.007**
Runny nose	23 (6.9)	80 (12.3)	0.011*	52 (12.6)	10 (8.8)	18 (14.1)	0.455
Expectoration	44 (13.3)	166 (25.4)	0.000**	103 (25.0)	22 (19.5)	41 (32.0)	0.077
Tachypnea	57 (17.2)	104 (15.9)	0.649	69 (16.7)	9 (8.0)	26 (20.3)	0.025*
Dyspnea	69 (20.8)	117 (17.9)	0.301	70 (17.0)	25 (22.1)	22 (17.2)	0.445
Diarrhea	24 (7.2)	83 (12.7)	0.009**	56 (13.6)	13 (11.5)	14 (10.9)	0.680
Pneumonia	341 (52.2)	146 (44.0)	0.014*	198 (48.1)	64 (56.6)	79 (61.7)	0.002**

* $P < 0.05$, ** $P < 0.01$

patients with ARIs in different parts of China, such as Beijing [14] Shanghai [11], Shenzhen [12], Wuhan [21], Lanzhou [22], indicated high variability. Different incidences may be attributed to different age groups, samples collected, inclusion criteria, diagnostic methods, target pathogens and seasonality.

IFV, RSV, HPMV and HRV were the most commonly detected viruses in most regions. HRV and RSV were equally predominant in our study period. RSV is a major respiratory virus that causes respiratory illness including bronchiolitis, pneumonia, and wheezing [23]. RSV may bring about annual epidemics worldwide because of virus variability [24]. It is reported that RSV epidemic was associated with the alternate circulation of multiple genotypes and with the change of G protein [25]. HRV are usually associated with upper respiratory tract infections and are responsible for one half of all "common colds" [26]. The implementation of molecular methods has revealed HRV

as an etiologic agent in lower respiratory tract infections (LRTI), associated with recurrent wheezing and asthma in infancy [26, 27].

Clinical presentations of respiratory infections may be overlapping and could not discriminate between respiratory viruses. However, infants identified with respiratory virus tended to have more severe symptoms, particularly those in the 7–12 months of age group. Age and exposure were two crucial factors for infection [8]. Immune status of infants is different from adults, and the amount of maternal antibodies attenuate distinctly, which would make infants susceptible to respiratory viral infections. The onset of disease is an interplay of immune pathology and viral pathology and prevention measures need to be taken into account [28].

It has been suggested that multiplex PCR techniques demonstrate a high detection rate of viral co-infections [29]. In this target population, mixed respiratory virus had

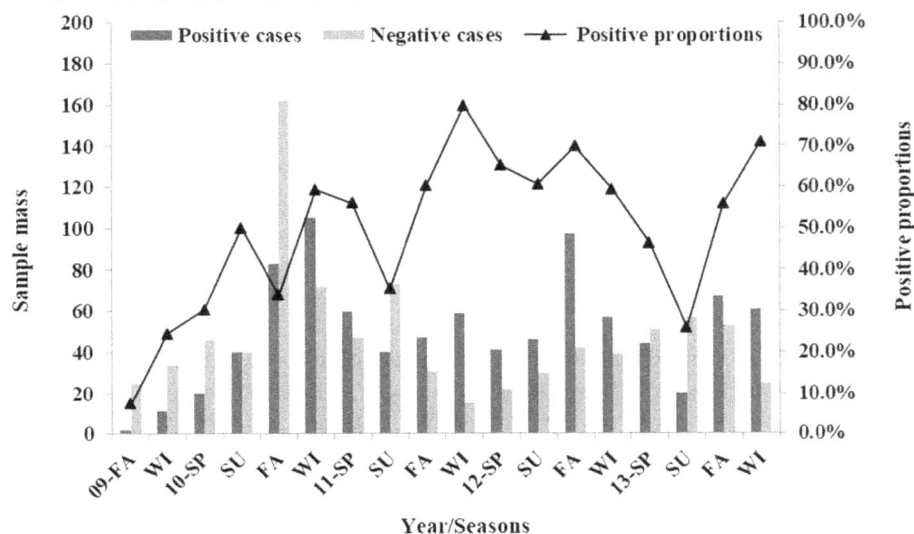

Fig. 1 Seasonal distribution of ARIs in hospitalized children, Nov 2009 - Feb 2014. Spring (SP); Summer (SU); Fall (FA); Winter (WI)

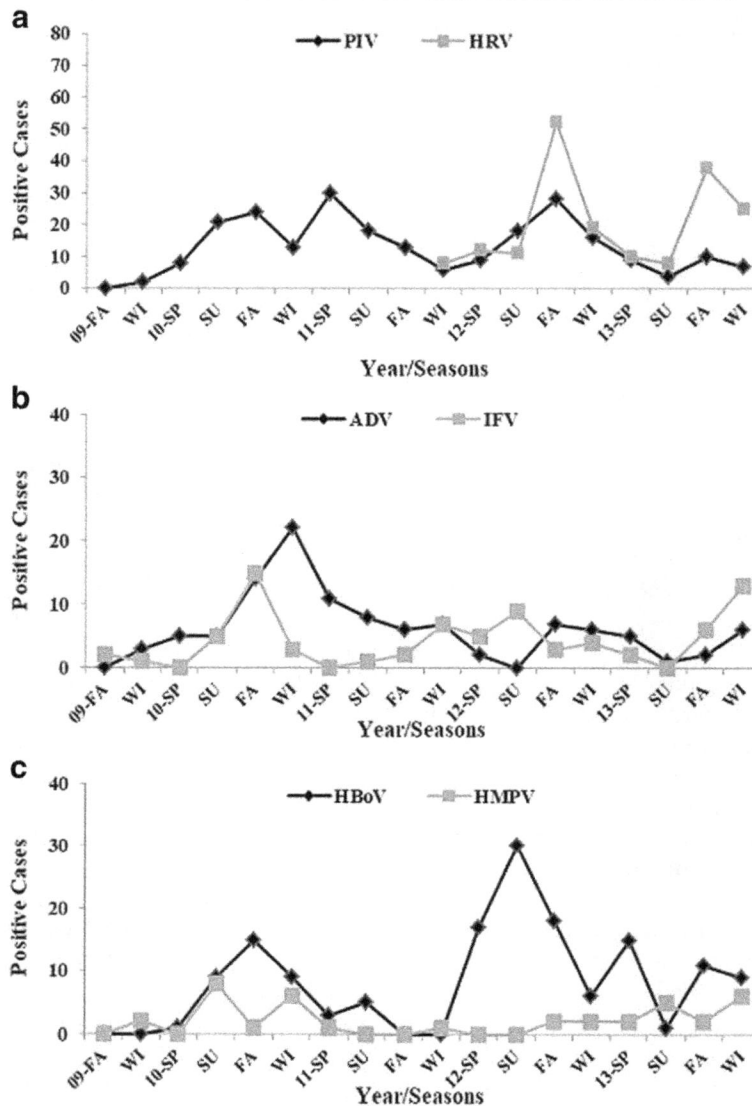

Fig. 2 Seasonal distributions of respiratory viruses in hospitalized children, Nov 2009- Feb 2014. Spring (SP); Summer (SU); Fall (FA); Winter (WI)

a proportion of 14.9%, with RSV/PIV the most frequent combination. Previous research showed proportions of viral co-infection ranged from 4.0 to 24.7%, with RSV, IFV, HPMV the common viruses present in co-infections. Different incidence of co-infection may be due to high single infection rates of certain viruses, overlapping epidemic seasons, target pathogens as well as methodology. Evidence for increased clinical severity of viral single infections versus co-infections is controversial [30–33]. The impact of co-infection on clinical presentations may rely on the specific agent involved, as well as viral load [32, 33]. Experimental studies of simultaneous respiratory infections are scarce. However, one study showed by mathematical modeling, found that one virus can block replication of another due to competition for resources, which may

have implications for the treatment regimens of simultaneous viral infections [34].

Despite vaccination, pneumonia still remains a serious public health issue in the world [35]. In this study, children > 1 year seemed to suffer more from bacterial infections than younger children. The WHO reports that pneumonia is the forgotten killer of children and one of the main disease burdens worldwide [36]. Pneumonia is the most serious result of ARIs and is often due to bacterial infection [37]. *S. pneumoniae, H. influenzae type b* are the leading causes of bacterial pneumonia in children worldwide [38, 39]. Under-nutrition, lack of breast-feeding, crowding, exposure to indoor air pollution, low birth weight and diarrhea have been identified as risk factors for pneumonia [40, 41]. Etiologic studies could provide information on the prevalence of bacterial infections, which may help achieve a reduction in child mortality.

The incidence of respiratory viral/bacterial co-infection in young children ranged from 1 to 44% [42]. In the current study, we observed a respiratory viral/bacterial co-infection proportion of 13.9% (240/1728). *S.pneumoniae*, *S. aureus*, *H. influenzae* and *Pseudomonas* species were common bacterial co-pathogens. Influenza pandemics over the last 100 years have strengthened the association of bacterial super-infection and influenza infection [42, 43]. There are mounting data indicating that virus infection can predispose to bacterial colonization and overgrowth, which adversely affect the pathogenesis of respiratory infections [44, 45]. Disruption of the epithelial barrier, up regulation of adhesion proteins, production of viral factors and alterations in immune responses are several known mechanisms [44, 45]. Increased morbidity with bacterial co-infections was found in children, leading to increased duration of mechanical ventilation, longer hospital stays and admission to pediatric intensive care units [42, 46]. However, the statistical association was weak and sporadic in some studies, and additional longitudinal cohort studies may be needed to reveal the contribution of bacterial to viral ARIs.

There was a paucity of study that was conducted for etiologies of ARIs among hospitalized children in this area. Including 14 different respiratory pathogens (both viruses and bacteria), recruiting almost 2000 hospitalized children, over 5-year period, this current study revealed pathogens profiles, co-infection pattern, clinical features, and seasonality among hospitalized children with ARIs in Chengdu, west China. There are however some limitations in this study. Outpatients were not recruited and the study lacked an asymptomatic control group. Positive rates may be somewhat lower as other potential viral pathogens were not included (e.g. enteroviruses, HCoV NL63 and HKU1). In addition, virus genotyping and strain identification (such as HRV A/B/C) would be helpful for understanding viral epidemics and associated disease severity.

Conclusions

In conclusion, this 5-year consecutive surveillance research confirmed that respiratory viruses, especially RSV and HRV, were the leading potential cause of ARIs in hospitalized children in Chengdu, west China. Co-infections were associated with severity of illness in infants, who tended to have increased risks of ARIs. This study gives us better information on the pathogen profiles, clinical association, co-infection combinations, and seasonal features of ARIs in hospitalized children in this area. Moreover, future efforts in reducing the impact of ARIs will depend on a commitment to fund and implement programs to utilize available vaccines, especially vaccines on RSV, HRV and *S. pneumoniae* in in this region, and to develop new vaccines against common pathogens.

Abbreviations
ADV: Human adenovirus; ARI: Acute respiratory infection; HBoV: Human bocavirus; HCoV: Human coronavirus; HMPV: Human metapneumovirus; HRV: Human rhinovirus; IFV: Influenza virus; LRTI: Lower respiratory tract infection; PCR: Polymerase chain reaction; PIV: Parainfluenza virus; RSV: Respiratory syncytial virus

Acknowledgements
We gratefully thank to all patients who participated in this study, and to Research Center for Public Health and Preventive Medicine, West China School of Public Health, Sichuan University for providing experimental resources.

Funding
This study was supported by National Mega Projects of Science and Technology in 13th Five-Year Plan of China: Technical Platform for Communicable Disease Surveillance Project (2017ZX10103010–002).

Authors' contributions
PXF and CJY designed the research; CJY, HPW, ZT, ZTL, ZLX, JCP performed the research and acquired data; CJY, HPW, ZT, ZTL analyzed the data; CJY, HPW, ZT, ZTL, JCP and PXF wrote the paper; JCP and PXF revised the manuscript; PXF approved the final version to be published. All authors read and approved the final manuscript.

Competing interests
The authors declare that they have no competing interests.

Author details
[1]Department of Public Health Laboratory Sciences, West China School of Public Health (No.4 West China Teaching Hospital), Sichuan University, 16#, Section 3, Renmin Road South, Chengdu 610041, Sichuan, People's Republic of China. [2]Research Center for Occupational Respiratory Diseases, West China School of Public Health (No.4 West China Teaching Hospital), Sichuan University, 16#, Section 3, Renmin Road South, Chengdu 610041, Sichuan, China. [3]Shenzhen Nanshan Center for Disease Control and Prevention, 95#, Nanshang Road, Shenzhen 518054, Guangdong, China. [4]Chongqing Yuzhong District Center for Disease Control and Prevention, 254#, Heping Road, Yuzhong District, Chongqing 400010, China.

References
1. Shi T, McLean K, Campbell H, Nair H. Aetiological role of common respiratory viruses in acute lower respiratory infections in children under five years: A systematic review and meta-analysis. J Glob Health. 2015;5:010408.
2. Nair H, Simões EAF, Rudan I, Gessner BD, Azziz-Baumgartner E, et al. Global and regional burden of hospital admissions for severe acute lower respiratory infections in young children in 2010: a systematic analysis. Lancet. 2013;381:1380–90.
3. Rudan I, Chan KY, Zhang JSF, Theodoratou E, Feng XL, et al. Causes of death in children younger than 5 years in China in 2008. Lancet. 2010;375:1083–9.
4. Liu L, Oza S, Hogan D, Perin J, Rudan I, et al. Global, regional, and national causes of child mortality in 2000–13, with projections to inform post-2015 priorities: an updated systematic analysis. Lancet. 2015;385:430–40.
5. Doan Q, Enarson P, Kissoon N, Klassen TP, Johnson DW. Rapid viral diagnosis for acute febrile respiratory illness in children in the Emergency Department. Cochrane Database Syst Rev. 2014;15(9):CD006452.
6. Sung RY, Chan PK, Tsen T, Li AM, Lam WY, et al. Identification of viral and atypical bacterial pathogens in children hospitalized with acute respiratory infections in Hong Kong by multiplex PCR assays. J Med Virol. 2009;81:153–9.
7. Ruuskanen O, Lahti E, Jennings LC, Murdoch DR. Viral pneumonia. Lancet. 2011;377:1264–75.
8. Tregoning JS, Schwarze J. Respiratory viral infections in infants: causes, clinical symptoms, virology, and immunology. Clin Microbiol Rev. 2010;23: 74–98.
9. Zhang Y, Yuan L, Zhang Y, Zhang X, Zheng M, et al. Burden of respiratory syncytial virus infections in China: Systematic review and meta-analysis. J Glob Health. 2015;5:020417.

10. Nair H, Brooks WA, Katz M, Roca A, Berkley JA, et al. Global burden of respiratory infections due to seasonal influenza in young children: a systematic review and meta-analysis. Lancet. 2011;378:1917–30.

11. Dong W, Chen Q, Hu Y, He D, Liu J, et al. Epidemiological and clinical characteristics of respiratory viral infections in children in Shanghai. China Arch Virol. 2016;161:1907–13.

12. Wang H, Zheng Y, Deng J, Wang W, Liu P, et al. Prevalence of respiratory viruses among children hospitalized from respiratory infections in Shenzhen. China Virol J. 2016;13:39.

13. Cai X, Wang Q, Lin G, Cai Z, Lin C-X, et al. Respiratory Virus Infections Among Children in South China. J Med Virol. 2014;86:1249–55.

14. Zhang C, Zhu N, Xie Z, Lu R, He B, et al. Viral etiology and clinical profiles of children with severe acute respiratory infections in China. PLoS One. 2013;8: e72606.

15. Jiao W. Analysis on Influenza Vaccination Status in Chengdu, 2010–2013. J Prev Med Inf. 2015;31:688–90.

16. Coiras M, Pérez-Breña P, García M, Casas I. Simultaneous detection of influenza A, B, and C viruses, respiratory syncytial virus, and adenoviruses in clinical samples by multiplex reverse transcription nested-PCR assay. J Med Virol. 2003;69:132–44.

17. Coiras MT, Aguilar JC, García ML, Casas I, Pérez-Breña P. Simultaneous detection of fourteen respiratory viruses in clinical specimens by two multiplex reverse transcription nested-PCR assays. J Med Virol. 2004;72:484–95.

18. Allard A, Girones R, Juto P, Wadell G. Polymerase chain reaction for detection of adenoviruses in stools samples. J Clin Microbiol. 1991;29:2683.

19. Woo PCY, Lau SKP, Chu C-M, Chan K-H, Tsoi H-W, et al. Characterization and complete genome sequence of a novel coronavirus, coronavirus HKU1, from patients with pneumonia. J Virol. 2005;79:884–95.

20. Kapoor A, Simmonds P, Slikas E, Li L, Bodhidatta L, et al. Human Bocaviruses Are Highly Diverse, Dispersed Recombination Prone, and Prevalent in Enteric Infections. J Infect Dis. 2010;201:1633–43.

21. Liu J, Ai H, Xiong Y, Li F, Wen Z, et al. Prevalence and correlation of infectious agents in hospitalized children with acute respiratory tract infections in Central China. PLoS One. 2015;10:e0119170.

22. Jin Y, Zhang RF, Xie ZP, Yan KL, Gao HC, et al. Newly identified respiratory viruses associated with acute lower respiratory tract infections in children in Lanzou, China, from 2006 to 2009. Clin Microbiol Infect. 2012;18:74–80.

23. Nair H, Nokes DJ, Gessner BD, Dherani M, Madhi SA, et al. Global burden of acute lower respiratory infections due to respiratory syncytial virus in young children: a systematic review and meta-analysis. Lancet. 2010;375:1545–55.

24. Agoti CN, Mwihuri AG, Sande CJ, Onyango CO, Medley GF, et al. Genetic relatedness of infecting and reinfecting respiratory syncytial virus strains identified in a birth cohort from rural Kenya. J Infect Dis. 2012;206:1532–41.

25. Hu P, Zheng T, Chen J, Zhou T, Chen Y, et al. Alternate circulation and genetic variation of human respiratory syncytial virus genotypes in Chengdu, West China, 2009–2014. J Med Virol. 2017;89:32–40.

26. Jacobs SE, Lamson DM, St George K, Walsh TJ. Human rhinoviruses. Clin Microbiol Rev. 2013;26:135–62.

27. Message SD, Laza-Stanca V, Mallia P, Parker HL, Zhu J, et al. Rhinovirus-induced lower respiratory illness is increased in asthma and related to virus load and Th1/2 cytokine and IL-10 production. Proc Natl Acad Sci U S A. 2008;105:13562–7.

28. Gern JE, Brooks GD, Meyer P, Chang A, Shen K, et al. Bidirectional interactions between viral respiratory illnesses and cytokine responses in the first year of life. J Allergy Clin Immunol. 2006;117:72–8.

29. Cilla G, Onate E, Perez-Yarza EG, Montes M, Vicente D, et al. Viruses in community-acquired pneumonia in children aged less than 3 years old: High rate of viral coinfection. J Med Virol. 2008;80:1843–9.

30. Asner SA, Science ME, Tran D, Smieja M, Merglen A, et al. Clinical disease severity of respiratory viral co-infection versus single viral infection: a systematic review and meta-analysis. PLoS One. 2014;9:e99392.

31. Franz A, Adams O, Willems R, Bonzel L, Neuhausen N, et al. Correlation of viral load of respiratory pathogens and co-infections with disease severity in children hospitalized for lower respiratory tract infection. J Clin Virol. 2010; 48:239–45.

32. Martin ET, Kuypers J, Wald A, Englund JA. Multiple versus single virus respiratory infections: viral load and clinical disease severity in hospitalized children. Influenza Other Respir Viruses. 2012;6:71–7.

33. Goka EA, Vallely PJ, Mutton KJ, Klapper PE. Single, dual and multiple respiratory virus infections and risk of hospitalization and mortality. Epidemiol Infect. 2015;143:37–47.

34. Pinky L, Dobrovolny HM. Coinfections of the Respiratory Tract: Viral Competition for Resources. PLoS One. 2016;11:e0155589.

35. Nohynek H, Madhi S, Grijalva CG. Childhood bacterial respiratory diseases: past, present, and future. Pediatr Infect Dis J. 2009;28:S127–32.

36. UNICEF. Pneumonia The Forgotten Killer of Children. New York and Geneva: UNICEF/WHO; 2006.

37. Ma HM, Lee KP, Woo J. Predictors of viral pneumonia: The need for viral testing in all patients hospitalized for nursing home-acquired pneumonia. Geriatr Gerontol Int. 2013;13:949–57.

38. Watt JP, Wolfson LJ, o'Brien KL, Henkle E. knoll MD, et al. Burden of disease caused by Haemophilus influenzae type b in children younger than 5 years: global estimates. Lancet. 2009;374:903–11.

39. O'Brien KL, Wolfson LJ, Watt JP, Henkle E, Deloria-Knoll M, et al. Burden of disease caused by Streptococcus pneumoniae in children younger than 5 years: global estimates. Lancet. 2009;374:893–902.

40. Walker CLF, Rudan I, Liu L, Nair H, Theodoratou E, et al. Global burden of childhood pneumonia and diarrhoea. Lancet. 2013;381:1405–16.

41. Poll Tvd OSM. Pathogenesis, treatment, and prevention of pneumococcal pneumonia. Lancet. 2009;374:1543–56.

42. Thorburn K, Riordan A. Pulmonary bacterial coinfection in infants and children with viral respiratory infection. Expert Rev Anti-Infect Ther. 2012;10:909–16.

43. McCullers JA. The co-pathogenesis of influenza viruses with bacteria in the lung. Nat Rev Microbiol. 2014;12:252–62.

44. Bosch AA, Biesbroek G, Trzcinski K, Sanders EA, Bogaert D. Viral and bacterial interactions in the upper respiratory tract. PLoS Pathog. 2013;9:e1003057.

45. Hendaus MA, Jomha FA, Alhammadi AH. Virus-induced secondary bacterial infection: a concise review. Ther Clin Risk Manag. 2015;11:1265–71.

46. Nguyen T, Kyle UG, Jaimon N, Tcharmtchi MH, Coss-Bu JA, et al. Coinfection with Staphylococcus aureus increases risk of severe coagulopathy in critically ill children with influenza A (H1N1) virus infection. Crit Care Med. 2012;40: 3246–50.

9

Prevalence and predictors of metabolically healthy obesity in adolescents

Lara Nasreddine[1†], Hani Tamim[2†], Aurelie Mailhac[2] and Fadia S. AlBuhairan[3,4*]

Abstract

Background: Obese children and adolescents may vary with respect to their health profile, an observation that has been highlighted by the characterization of metabolically healthy obesity (MHO). The objectives of this study were to examine the prevalence of MHO amongst obese adolescents in Saudi-Arabia, and investigate the anthropometric, socio-demographic, and lifestyle predictors of MHO in this age group.

Methods: A national cross-sectional school-based survey (*Jeeluna*) was conducted in Saudi-Arabia in 2011–2012 ($n = 1047$ obese adolescents). Anthropometric, blood pressure and biochemical measurements were obtained. A multicomponent questionnaire covering socio-demographic, lifestyle, dietary, psychosocial and physical activity characteristics was administered. Classification of MHO was based on two different definitions. According to the first definition, subjects were categorized as MHO based on the absence of the following traditional cardiometabolic risk (CR) factors: systolic blood pressure (SBP) or diastolic blood pressure (DBP) >90th percentile for age, sex, and height; triglycerides (TG) > 1.25 mmol/L; high density lipoprotein-cholesterol (HDL-C) ≤1.02 mmol/L; glucose ≥5.6 mmol/L. The second definition of MHO was based on absence of any cardiometabolic risk factor, according to the International Diabetes Federation (IDF) criteria.

Results: The prevalence of MHO ranged between 20.9% (IDF) and 23.8% (CR). Subjects with MHO were younger, less obese, had smaller waist circumference (WC) and were more likely to be females. Based on stepwise logistic regression analyses, and according to the IDF definition, body mass index (BMI) (OR = 0.89, 95% CI: 0.84–0.93) and WC (OR = 0.97, 95% CI: 0.96–0.98) were the only significant independent predictors of MHO. Based on the CR definition, the independent predictors of MHO included female gender (OR = 1.76, 95% CI: 1.29–2.41), BMI (OR = 0.97, 95% CI: 0.94–1.00), and weekly frequency of day napping (OR = 1.06, 95% CI: 1.00–1.12). Analysis by gender showed that vegetables' intake and sleep indicators were associated with MHO in boys but not in girls.

Conclusion: The study showed that one out of five obese adolescents is metabolically healthy. It also identified anthropometric factors as predictors of MHO and suggested gender-based differences in the association between diet, sleep and MHO in adolescents. Findings may be used in the development of intervention strategies aimed at improving metabolic heath in obese adolescents.

Keywords: Obesity, Adolescents, Metabolically healthy obesity, Prevalence, Predictors, Saudi Arabia, Middle-East

* Correspondence: falbuhairan@aldaramed.com
†Lara Nasreddine and Hani Tamim contributed equally to this work.
3Department of Pediatrics and Adolescent Medicine, AlDara Hospital and Medical Center, P.O. Box 1105, Riyadh 11431, Saudi Arabia
4Department of Population, Family, and Reproductive Health, Bloomberg School of Public Health, Johns Hopkins University, Baltimore, MD, USA
Full list of author information is available at the end of the article

Background

Pediatric obesity has become a global challenge in health care, plaguing both high and low-income nations and jeopardizing their ability to cope with the increasing cost of obesity management and treatment [1]. The Eastern Mediterranean Region (EMR), and particularly countries of the Gulf Cooperation Council (GCC), harbor one of the highest burdens of childhood obesity worldwide, with reported estimates exceeding 25% in some countries [2–4]. Childhood obesity is associated with numerous adverse health consequences, with both immediate and longer-term complications [5]. Among the immediate health risks are cardiometabolic abnormalities including insulin resistance, dyslipidemia, increased glucose levels, metabolic syndrome, and hypertension [5–7]. On the long term, childhood obesity tends to track into the adult years, increasing the risk for non-communicable diseases (NCDs), such as type 2 diabetes, cardiovascular diseases (CVDs), and certain types of cancer, while also being associated with mental health problems, such as low self-esteem and depression [8, 9].

Obesity is however being increasingly recognized as a "heterogeneous condition", a fact that has been emphasized by the identification and characterization of metabolically healthy obesity (MHO) amongst adults [10–12]. Despite being obese, these individuals do not present any of the traditional cardiometabolic risk factors that are usually associated with obesity [10, 11]. It has been argued that this subgroup of obese subjects may have a lower mortality risk and a healthier medical prognosis, compared to their non-metabolically healthy obese counterparts [13–17]. Available studies have indicated that, amongst obese adults, the prevalence of MHO may range between 6 and 40% [10, 11, 18, 19]. Similarly, it has been suggested that obese children may also vary in terms of their health profile [12, 20–22], but MHO in the pediatric population has not been well-characterized [12]. The investigation of MHO amongst children is important for several reasons. First, given the increasing need for weight management care, it may be necessary to prioritize specialized service delivery for those individuals with the greatest cardiometabolic risk [12]. By characterizing obese individuals according to their relative health risks, those at lower cardiometabolic risk may be directed towards less intensive management services (e.g. outpatient dietitian counseling, behavioral modification etc.), while their peers at higher risk may require more intensive health services (e.g., multidisciplinary obesity treatment or drug-based management) [12]. The recognition of childhood obesity as a heterogeneous condition implies that "a menu of therapeutic options" for children (and their caregivers) would be available to address their individual health needs, an approach that is in harmony with treating obesity as a chronic disease [12, 23]. Second, given the possible protective effects of MHO on disease risk, when compared to metabolically unhealthy obese (MUO), it would be crucial to investigate and identify the characteristics that are associated with the MHO status in youth and to foster our understanding of the factors that could prevent obese subjects from developing metabolic abnormalities [24–26].

In the Kingdom of Saudi-Arabia (KSA), like in several other countries of the EMR, the rate of obesity amongst children and adolescents is following an escalating secular trend [27]. A recent national study (*Jeeluna*) conducted in KSA showed that 15.9% of adolescents were obese [28], a proportion that is considerably higher than what was reported in the early 1990s, where the prevalence of obesity was estimated at 6% in boys and 6.7% in girls aged 1–18 years [29]. This alarming trend coupled with the probable protective effect of MHO on morbidity, highlights the need to investigate and better characterize MHO in the pediatric years. This study builds on the "Jeeluna" national study to examine the proportions of obese adolescents who are metabolically healthy in KSA and to investigate socio-demographic, anthropometric, and lifestyle predictors of MHO in this age group. Due to the lack of a universal definition for MHO, two commonly used definitions will be adopted in this study to assess the prevalence and factors associated with MHO in this population [12, 30]. The selected definitions are based on traditional cardiometabolic risk factors that are easily measured and are routinely obtained in clinical practice.

Methods

Study design

This study is based on the national cross-sectional school-based survey (*Jeeluna*) that was conducted in KSA in 2011–2012 [28]. Details on the design, sampling protocol and data collection are published elsewhere [28]. In brief, a nationally representative sample ($n = 12{,}575$) of students attending intermediate/secondary schools in KSA participated in the "*Jeeluna*" study [28]. A stratified, cluster random sampling procedure was adopted with sampling occurring in all of the 13 administrative regions in the country. Within each region, several school districts exist, with a total of 42 districts in the country. Sampling occurred at the district level, ensuring that both rural, as well as urban/suburban areas were covered. Based on the student population per region, district, gender, and school level (intermediate vs. secondary), proportionate sampling was performed. For the selection of the schools, any male/female, intermediate/secondary, public/private school in a city/town in the KSA that operates during the day was eligible. Evening schools and schools that only cater for students with special needs were excluded from this study. Using a computer-based randomized sampling, schools were drawn from the list of intermediate and secondary schools enlisted with the Ministry of Education. Within the selected schools, classes were randomly chosen. Sampling was clustered whereby all students within a selected class were invited to participate in the study. An information letter describing the study objectives and protocol was sent to students and their parents.

The study protocol was approved by the institutional review board (IRB) and ethics committee at King Abdullah International Medical Research Center (KAIMRC) and the Ministry of Education (MOE). Prior to accessing the selected schools, permission was obtained from the schools' principals. Written parental consent and student assent were obtained prior to subjects' enrollment in the study [28]. Students were given the choice of opting out of blood sampling. Students were assured that all the responses that they provided on the questionnaire would remain anonymous and confidential.

Study participants

For the present study, the selection of subjects from the original survey participants ($n = 12,575$) was undertaken according to the following criteria: 1) having provided blood samples; 2) not exceeding 19 years of age; and 3) being obese.

Of the total sample of 12,575 subjects, 7329 had consented to blood withdrawal and provided blood samples (response rate: 58.3%). Of those, 51 were above 19 years old and were thus excluded, yielding a sample of 7278 subjects. According to the World Health Organization (WHO) new growth standards [31], obesity was defined based on sex and age, as + 2 body mass index (BMI) z-scores [31]; the WHO AnthroPlus software (WHO, Geneva, Switzerland) was utilized to calculate BMI z-scores. To allow for comparisons with previous studies conducted in KSA, prevalence rates of obesity were also determined using the Centers for Disease Control and Prevention (CDC) 2000 criteria [32]. Accordingly, of the 7278 subjects who have provided blood samples and who were aged less than 19 years, 1179 (16.20%) were obese based on the WHO criteria and 1176 (16.16%) were obese based on the CDC criteria. For the remaining analyses, the WHO criteria were retained. In addition, subjects with missing information on blood pressure measurements, waist circumference or biochemical assessment (lipid profile; fasting glucose), were excluded ($n = 132$). Consequently, the final sample for this study included 1047 subjects.

Data collection

Data collection included: (1) completion of self-administered multi-component questionnaire; (2) anthropometric and blood pressure measurements; and (3) blood sampling and biochemical assessment. Data collection was conducted by trained personnel who received standardized and structured training prior to the initiation of the study. Other quality control measures were implemented, including the pre-testing of the questionnaire, equipment, and data collection protocols as well as the field monitoring of data collection.

Completion of the multi-component questionnaire

The study questionnaire was developed based on the Youth Risk Behavior Survey [33] and the Global School-based Student Health Survey [28, 34]. Since Arabic is the native language in KSA, the Arabic version of the GSHS questionnaire was used [35]. In addition, questions adopted from the YRBS were translated to Arabic and reviewed for translational appropriateness. Cultural adaptation was introduced to the questionnaire. For instance, questions that were considered culturally inappropriate such as sexual behaviors and sexually transmitted diseases, were not included. In addition, questions related to the subject's family, lifestyle, sleep, and health status were added. The questionnaire was reviewed for content validity by an expert panel, which included an adolescent medicine physician, a pediatrician, an epidemiologist, a public health professional, and a school health professional [36]. It is worth noting that previous investigations that were based on the same tools (Arabic version of GSHS and Arabic translation of YRBS) have reported a high internal consistency, with a Cronbach Alpha of 0.84 [37].

The questionnaire was pilot-tested on a sample of adolescents and questions or statements that were found difficult, unclear, or ambiguous to the participating adolescents were further refined or modified [36]. For instance, examples were added to clarify some questions, such as examples of main meals, snacks, vegetables, or energy drinks. In addition, the option to choose more than one response if needed was added to some questions. None of the items included in the questionnaire were found to be inappropriate or distressing to the pilot sample of adolescents and thus, none of the questions were completely eliminated [36]. The final amended version of the questionnaire was adopted for data collection (http://kaimrc.med.sa/?page_id=5036).

As such, the final version of the questionnaire covered several domains, including socio-demographic, dietary practices, sleep habits, sedentary, physical activity, behaviors that contribute to unintentional injuries and violence, tobacco use, alcohol and substance use, history of bullying, mood, health status, and access to health services. The questionnaire was self-administered.

Anthropometric measurements

Anthropometric measurements were taken using standardized protocols [38] and calibrated equipment. Height was measured to the nearest 0.5 cm (cm) and body weight to the nearest 0.1 kg (kg) using an electronic scale (Omron SC100 digital scale; Omron Healthcare, Inc., Lake Forest, IL), in light indoor clothing and with bare feet or stockings [28]. BMI was calculated as the ratio of weight (kilograms) to the square of height (meters). Waist circumference was measured at the midpoint between the costal margin and iliac crest at the end of expiration using a non-elastic flexible tape measure and was recorded to the nearest millimeter (mm) [39]. Measurements were taken twice and the average was adopted.

Blood pressure measurements

Blood pressure (BP) was measured in the supine position by a digital BP monitor (Omron M2, Netherlands) on the right arm. After a period of rest, measurements were taken twice a few minutes apart and recorded as an average using appropriate cuff size.

Biochemical assessment

Licensed phlebotomists/nurses collected blood samples from the students who consented to blood withdrawal, after an 8- h fast. Blood samples were collected in serum separator tubes (BD, USA), labeled, transported at cool temperature to the hospital lab upon collection, allowed to clot for more than 15 min and then centrifuged for 10 min at 3000 rpm using a Multifuge 35R centrifuge at room temperature. The serum samples were either immediately assayed by an Architect 8000c clinical chemistry analyzer (Abbott, USA) or stored in the freezer at − 70 °C for further testing. The specimens were not stored for longer than three months due to the instability of lipids in vitro. Lipid tests were performed. In addition, glucose level was also measured on the same analyzer using the hexokinase method. Three levels of quality control were performed for each assay (Bio-Rad, USA). The patient results were stored in the Laboratory Information System (LIS) (Cerner, USA), which was interfaced with the Architect 8000c clinical chemistry analyzer. The data were then retrieved from the LIS and integrated within the *Jeeluna* database.

Definition of metabolically healthy obesity (MHO)

We applied two different definitions to examine the prevalence and factors associated with MHO. The first definition was the one proposed by Prince et al. [12], according to which subjects were categorized as MUO or MHO, based on the presence or absence of the following four traditional cardiometabolic risk (CR) factors (MHO: 0 risk factor; MUO: >1 risk factors): systolic blood pressure (SBP) or diastolic blood pressure (DBP) >90th percentile

for age, sex, and height [40]; triglycerides (TG) > 1.25 mmol/L [41, 42]; high density lipoprotein-cholesterol (HDL-C) ≤ 1.02 mmol/L; and glucose ≥5.6 mmol/L [12].

The second definition of MHO was based on the International Diabetes Federation (IDF) criteria. Accordingly, participants were dichotomized as MHO or MUO based on the presence or absence of the following risk factors: amongst those aged between 10 and 16 years old: SBP ≥130 or DBP ≥85 mmHg; TG ≥1.7 mmol/L; HDL-C < 1.03 mmol/L; glucose ≥5.6 mmol/L and waist circumference (WC) ≥90th percentile for age and sex or adult cut-off if lower [30, 43]. Amongst those aged between 16 and 19 years old: SBP BP ≥130 or diastolic BP ≥85 mmHg; TG ≥ 1.7 mmol/L; HDL-C < 1.03 mmol/L in males and < 1.29 mmol/L in females; glucose ≥5.6 mmol/L and WC ≥ 94 cm for males and ≥ 80 cm for girls.

Data analysis

Identical analyses were conducted for both the IDF and CR definitions. Subjects' characteristics were described with number and percent for categorical variables and mean and standard deviation for continuous ones. The chi-square test and the independent t-test were used to assess statistically significant differences between groups (MHO vs MUO). We set statistical significance at a two-sided p-value of < 0.05. The associations between MHO status and subjects' characteristics (socio-demographic, anthropometric, dietary, physical activity, sleep, smoking and psychosocial characteristics) were further assessed by creating a logistic regression model with MHO as a dependent variable, and with adjustment for age and sex. Stepwise logistic regression analyses (forward selection) was conducted to determine the independent predictors of MHO. The potential predictors that were entered into the final multivariate regression models included those that were significantly associated with MHO, based on either the IDF or CR definitions, in the age and sex adjusted regression analyses. Moreover, given that available evidence suggests a sleep-gender interaction [25, 44], we tested for a potential interaction between gender and sleep related variables in our study sample. An interaction term was created for gender and number of hours of sleep during weekdays, for gender and number of hours of sleep during week-ends, and for gender and frequency of daytime napping. The interaction terms were entered separately into the logistic regression models, and the interaction was assessed for both models (Model-IDF definition and Model-CR definition). Whenever significant interaction was found, results were reported for both genders separately. Results were reported as odds ratio (OR), and 95% confidence interval (95% CI). We performed all data management and analyses using the Statistical Analysis Software (Version 9.1; 2004).

Results

Of the study sample, 62.6% were boys and 37.4% were girls. The age of the study participants ranged between 10 and 19 years, with a mean of 15.9 years (±1.9) in boys and 15.6 years (±1.8) in girls. The large majority of the students participating in the study were of Saudi nationality (84.9%) (data not shown).

As shown in Tables 1, 219 subjects out of 1047 (20.9%, 95% confidence interval (CI): 18.4–23.4) were categorized as MHO based on the IDF definition and 249 out of 1047 (23.8%, 95% CI: 21.2–26.4) were categorized as MHO based on the CR definition. The results showed

that 12.8% of the participants were classified as being MHO based on both definitions (IDF and CR), while 68.1% were categorized as MUO by both categorizations (data not shown).

Gender disparities were noted in the proportions of MHO and MUO, according to both definitions (Table 1). Significant differences in age were observed with the IDF definition only, whereby subjects with MHO were younger. Across both the IDF and CR categories, the MHO group was significantly shorter, lighter, and less obese (lower BMI values and lower BMI z scores) than their MUO peers (Table 1). WC (cm) was significantly

Table 1 Socio-demographic, anthropometric and cardiometabolic status amongst adolescents ($n = 1047$) in KSA by MUO or MHO status

	IDF			CR		
	MUO ($n = 828$)	MHO ($n = 219$)	p-value	MUO ($n = 798$)	MHO ($n = 249$)	p-value
Socio-demographic						
Age (years)	15.88 ± 1.85	15.41 ± 1.86	0.0008	15.77 ± 1.85	15.81 ± 1.91	0.81
Gender						
Males	534 (64.5)	121 (55.3)	0.01	520 (65.2)	135 (54.2)	0.002
Females	294 (35.5)	98 (44.8)		278 (34.8)	114 (45.8)	
Father's level of education						
Elementary or less	145 (19.7)	35 (18)	0.84	128 (18.1)	52 (23.2)	0.17
Intermediate-high school	331 (45)	91 (46.7)		330 (46.7)	92 (41.1)	
University or higher	259 (35.2)	69 (35.4)		248 (35.1)	80 (35.7)	
Mother's level of education						
Elementary or less	251 (33.7)	57 (28.9)	0.45	235 (32.8)	73 (32.2)	0.82
Intermediate- high school	291 (39)	81 (41.1)		285 (39.8)	87 (38.3)	
University or higher	204 (27.4)	59 (30)		196 (27.4)	67 (29.5)	
Anthropometric						
Height (cm)	162.78 ± 10.43	158.08 ± 11.42	< 0.0001	162.2 ± 10.97	160.5 ± 10.2	0.03
Weight (kg)	88.45 ± 17.4	77.11 ± 14.27	< 0.0001	86.94 ± 17.63	83.31 ± 16.4	0.004
BMI (kg/m^2)	33.28 ± 5.43	30.76 ± 4.25	< 0.0001	32.93 ± 5.44	32.19 ± 4.79	0.04
BMI Z score	2.82 ± 0.75	2.5 ± 0.57	< 0.0001	2.78 ± 0.74	2.67 ± 0.66	0.02
WC (cm)	93.32 ± 18.78	80.97 ± 16.84	< 0.0001	91.08 ± 19.55	89.65 ± 17.37	0.27
Elevated WC	447 (54.0)	0 (0.0)	< 0.0001	357 (44.7)	90 (36.1)	0.02
Cardiometabolic						
SBP (mm Hg)	127.66 ± 11.96	118.05 ± 7.8	< 0.0001	128.6 ± 11.32	116.19 ± 8.08	< 0.0001
DBP (mm Hg)	72.84 ± 10.85	67.75 ± 8.7	< 0.0001	73.37 ± 10.88	66.64 ± 7.9	< 0.0001
TC (mmol/L)	4.35 ± 0.78	4.24 ± 0.62	0.04	4.36 ± 0.77	4.2 ± 0.66	0.001
HDL-C (mmol/L)	1.13 ± 0.23	1.29 ± 0.2	< 0.0001	1.13 ± 0.24	1.27 ± 0.19	< 0.0001
LDL-C (mmol/L)	2.79 ± 0.7	2.63 ± 0.6	0.001	2.8 ± 0.69	2.63 ± 0.64	0.0007
TG (mmol/L)	1.26 ± 0.76	0.87 ± 0.29	< 0.0001	1.3 ± 0.76	0.79 ± 0.21	< 0.0001
Glucose (mmol/L)	4.62 ± 0.96	4.41 ± 0.67	0.0003	4.63 ± 0.97	4.4 ± 0.67	< 0.0001

Numbers are presented as Mean ± SD or as proportions, n(%)
Abbreviations: BMI: Body mass index; cm: Centimeters; CR: Cardiovascular risks; DBP: Diastolic blood pressure; HDL-C: High density lipoprotein-cholesterol; IDF: International Diabetes Federation; kg: Kilograms; kg/m^2: Kilograms per squared meters; KSA: Kingdom of Saudi Arabia; LDL-C: Low density lipoprotein-cholesterol; MHO: Metabolically healthy obesity; mm Hg: Millimeters of mercury; mmol/L:Millimoles per liter; MUO: Metabolically unhealthy obesity; SBP: Systolic blood pressure; SD: Standard deviation; TC: Total cholesterol; TG: Triglycerides; WC: Waist circumference

lower amongst MHO subjects based on the IDF defin-ition. Similarly, the proportion of subjects with elevated WC was significantly lower amongst MHO subjects, based on the CR categorization. As expected, cardiomet-abolic risk factors were in the less healthy direction in the MUO group.

Table 2 shows the dietary and lifestyle characteristics of the study population. In approximately 60% of the study subjects, the daily frequency of fruits' consumption was nil, while another equal proportion reported no con-sumption of milk. Similarly, 60% of the study subjects reported an intake of two or more soft drinks per day. Around half of the adolescents reported irregular break-fast consumption, no intake of vegetables, no exercise at school, and inadequate sleep on week days as well as week-ends. More than 80% of the study population re-ported screen time exceeding 2 h per day. There were no significant differences between the MHO and MUO groups in dietary and lifestyle characteristics, except for the weekly frequency of day napping, which was found to be significantly higher in the MHO group based on the CR definition. Psychosocial variables were also inves-tigated amongst the study subjects (Additional file 1: Table S1). There were no significant differences in any of the psychosocial variables between MHO and MUO groups, according to both definitions.

The predictors of MHO status, after adjustment for age and sex, are shown in Table 3. Across both definitions, fe-male gender was associated with higher odds of MHO (OR = 1.43, 95% CI: 1.06–1.94 based on IDF; OR = 1.59, 95% CI: 1.19–2.12 based on CR). Age was significantly in-versely associated with MHO, based on the IDF categorization (OR = 0.88; 95% CI: 0.81–0.95). Compared to the lowest level of fathers' education (elementary or less), an intermediate or high-school educational level was associated with lower odds of MHO based on the CR def-inition, and the association was close to significance (OR = 0.68, 95% CI: 0.46–1.02). Across both definitions, there was a significant inverse association between MHO, weight, BMI and BMI-z score, with the latter being the strongest anthropometric predictor of MHO. There was also a negative association between WC (cm) and MHO based on the IDF definition, while elevated WC was asso-ciated with lower odds of MHO based on the CR categorization. The daily frequencies of vegetable and soft drink consumption were associated with lower odds of MHO, based on the CR and IDF definitions, respectively. Meeting the sleep recommendations during weekdays as well as the weekly frequency of day napping, were posi-tively associated with MHO. Across both definitions, there was no association between MHO and any of the psycho-social variables under investigation (data not shown).

Stepwise logistic regression was carried out to deter-mine the independent predictors of MHO (Table 4). The model included the variables that were significantly asso-ciated with MHO (for either definition) after age and sex adjustment. As such, the final model included age, gen-der, BMI (kg/m^2), WC (cm), father's level of education, frequency of vegetable consumption per day, frequency of soft drinks' consumption per day, sleep hours per night, and daytime napping. It is important to note that, since the final model included both age and sex, we se-lected BMI (kg/m^2) instead of BMI-z score, given that the latter already adjusts for inter-individual differences in age and sex. In addition, since significant interactions were found between gender, the number of sleep hours during week-days, and the frequency of napping, ana-lyses were performed for boys and girls separately as well as for the total study population. Based on the IDF definition, BMI and WC were the only significant inde-pendent predictors of MHO in the overall sample. Based on the CR categorization, the significant independent predictors of MHO included female gender, BMI and the weekly frequency of day napping. Gender-disparities in MHO predictors were noted. MHO defined·as per the IDF criteria was associated with BMI and WC in both genders, but in boys, the predictors also included the weekly frequency of consuming 2 vegetables per day (in comparison with a reference intake of 0/day). The weekly frequency of day napping as well as meeting the sleep recommendations during week-days also reached borderline significance in boys, but not in girls. Based on the CR categorization, the significant independent pre-dictors of MHO included BMI and the frequency of soft drink consumption in girls, and father's level of educa-tion in boys.

Discussion

This study is the first to investigate MHO amongst ado-lescents in the Eastern Mediterranean Region. The study showed that approximately one in five obese adolescents in KSA was identified as metabolically healthy, despite being obese. In agreement with previous reports [12, 21, 45–53], subjects with MHO were significantly younger, less obese, had smaller waist circumference and were more likely to be females. In addition, sleep habits and vegetable intake were found to be significantly associated with MHO in the study population, particularly in boys. Interestingly, the factors that predicted MHO varied de-pending on the definition that was used to identify sub-jects as MHO or MUO.

The study findings showed that the prevalence of MHO amongst obese adolescents in KSA (20.9–23.8%) falls within the range reported in the literature (3.9–49.3%) [12, 22, 45–56]. Caution must however be exerted when comparing prevalence estimates of MHO given that vari-ous studies may have adopted different definitions and that some studies included both overweight and obese

Table 2 Dietary and lifestyle characteristics amongst adolescents (n = 1047) in KSA by MUO or MHO status

	IDF			CR		
	MUO (n = 828)	MHO (n = 219)	p-value	MUO (n = 798)	MHO (n = 249)	p-value
Dietary habits						
Regular breakfast consumption during the past month						
No	360 (44)	104 (48.2)	0.27	353 (44.7)	111 (45.1)	0.92
Yes	459 (56)	112 (51.9)		436 (55.3)	135 (54.9)	
Frequency of snacks consumption/d						
0	444 (54.1)	124 (57.4)	0.39	437 (55.3)	131 (53.3)	0.5
1	220 (26.8)	48 (22.2)		207 (26.2)	61 (24.8)	
≥ 2	157 (19.1)	44 (20.4)		147 (18.6)	54 (22)	
Frequency of fruits consumption/d						
0	503 (61.1)	134 (61.5)	0.51	475 (59.9)	162 (65.3)	0.31
1	125 (15.2)	27 (12.4)		119 (15)	33 (13.3)	
≥ 2	195 (23.7)	57 (26.2)		199 (25.1)	53 (21.4)	
Frequency of vegetables consumption/d						
0	385 (46.8)	100 (46.1)	0.59	357 (45)	128 (51.8)	0.14
1	266 (32.3)	65 (30)		263 (33.2)	68 (27.5)	
≥ 2	172 (20.9)	52 (24)		173 (21.8)	51 (20.7)	
Frequency of soft drinks consumption/d						
≤ 1	320 (38.8)	95 (44.2)	0.15	317 (39.9)	98 (40.0)	0.98
≥ 2	504 (61.2)	120 (55.8)		477 (60.1)	147 (60.0)	
Frequency of energy drinks consumption/d						
0	657 (79.8)	170 (78.3)	0.63	629 (79.2)	198 (80.5)	0.67
≥ 1	166 (20.2)	47 (21.7)		165 (20.8)	48 (19.5)	
Frequency of milk consumption/d						
0	468 (57.3)	129 (60.3)	0.73	449 (57.1)	148 (60.4)	0.66
1	223 (27.3)	54 (25.2)		215 (27.4)	62 (25.3)	
≥ 2	126 (15.4)	31 (14.5)		122 (15.5)	35 (14.3)	
Frequency of fast food consumption/week	2.03 ± 1.94	1.87 ± 1.78	0.29	2.03 ± 1.95	1.9 ± 1.76	0.36
Physical Activity and sedentary						
Exercise in school						
No	486 (59.7)	130 (60.8)	0.78	464 (59)	152 (62.8)	0.29
Yes	328 (40.3)	84 (39.3)		322 (41)	90 (37.2)	
Frequency of exercise for at least 30 mn during the past week	1.76 ± 2.34	1.64 ± 2.3	0.51	1.8 ± 2.36	1.52 ± 2.2	0.11
Screen time						
≤ 2 h/d	132 (18.7)	37 (19.5)	0.81	126 (18.5)	43 (20)	0.63
> 2 h/d	573 (81.3)	153 (80.5)		554 (81.5)	172 (80)	
Sleep						
Number of hours of sleep per night, during week days						
Adequate	325 (40.3)	100 (46.3)	0.11	312 (40.1)	113 (46.5)	0.07
Inadequate	481 (59.7)	116 (53.7)		467 (60)	130 (53.5)	
Number of hours of sleep per night, during weekends						

Table 2 Dietary and lifestyle characteristics amongst adolescents (n = 1047) in KSA by MUO or MHO status *(Continued)*

	IDF			CR		
Adequate	334 (48.1)	92 (50.8)	0.52	323 (48.4)	103 (49.5)	0.78
Inadequate	360 (51.9)	89 (49.2)		344 (51.6)	105 (50.5)	
Number of days went to sleep during the day in the past week	3.79 ± 2.86	3.86 ± 2.95	0.73	3.69 ± 2.89	4.14 ± 2.83	0.03
Smoking						
Smoking cigarettes during the past month						
No	746 (91.2)	196 (91.2)	0.99	715 (91)	227 (91.9)	0.65
Yes	72 (8.8)	19 (8.8)		71 (9)	20 (8.1)	
Smoking Shisha during the past month						
No	755 (92.4)	200 (93.5)	0.6	726 (92.6)	229 (92.7)	0.95
Yes	62 (7.6)	14 (6.5)		58 (7.4)	18 (7.3)	

Screen time was assessed based on the time spent watching television, using the internet, chatting and playing videogames
Adequate sleep defined as a minimum of 9 h for 10–12 year old adolescents and as a minimum of 8 h for those aged13 years or older [82]
Abbreviations: CR: Cardiovascular risks; d: Day; IDF: International Diabetes Federation; KSA: Kingdom of Saudi Arabia; MHO: Metabolically healthy obesity; mn: Minutes; MUO: Metabolically unhealthy obesity

subjects when assessing MHO. In certain studies, the definition of MHO was based on the presence of insulin resistance as estimated by Homeostasis Model Assessment (HOMA) [12, 21, 22, 48, 50], or as the presence of less than 2 cardiometabolic risk factors [21, 45–47, 54], while in others, including the present study, MHO was identified based on the absence of any cardiometabolic risk factor [12, 22, 48, 49, 51–53, 55, 56]. In addition, the criteria adopted to define individual cardiometabolic abnormalities were often discrepant between studies, and included those proposed by the IDF, the National Cholesterol Education Program (NCEP), the modified Adult treatment Panel III (ATPIII), as well as other ethnic specific criteria. Based on the CR definition proposed by Prince et al. (2014) [12], the prevalence of MHO obtained in this study (23.8%) was lower than the one reported amongst 8–17 year old overweight and obese Canadian children (MHO: 31.5%) and amongst obese German children (mean age: 11.6 ± 2.8 years) (MHO: 49.3%) [51]. The younger age of the children participating in these studies and the fact that both overweight and obese children were included in the study by Prince et al. (2014) [12] may explain the higher proportion of MHO in these studies, compared to our results. Based on the IDF definition, the prevalence of MHO obtained in this study (20.9%) was similar to the one reported amongst obese children and adolescents (10–18 years old) in Belgium (18.6%) [22], and lower than the estimate reported amongst obese youth aged 8–18 years in Austria (30.7%) [55]. Importantly, the results of this study highlighted poor agreement between definitions in classifying subjects as MHO, whereby only 12.8% of the participants were classified as MHO based on both the IDF and CR definitions. Poor agreement between various MHO definitions has also been described by other studies [12, 48], underscoring the need for a

harmonized definition for the identification of MHO in clinical as well as research settings.

It remains important to note that, at the time of this study, the MHO subjects were healthier than their MUO peers based on measures of traditional cardiometabolic health risk, but it is unknown whether this discrepancy would remain stable over time or whether it may be extrapolated to other health domains (such as musculoskeletal, respiratory) or whether the inclusion of other indicators of cardiovascular health (e.g., apo B, inflammatory markers, insulin resistance) would impact the MHO prevalence estimates obtained in this study [12]. It has been debated that MHO may not be a stable phenotype and there are unanswered questions on whether it represents a transient phenotype, changing with age, from childhood into adulthood [57]. However, based on the Bogalusa Heart Study, where 1098 individuals had participated both as children (5–17 years) and as adults (24–43 years), Li et al. (2012) showed that MHO children had favorable cardiometabolic profiles and carotid intima media thickness (CIMT) in adulthood compared with MUO children, thus providing evidence that the MHO phenotype starts in childhood and continues into adulthood [58].

In this study, and in concordance with other reports, there were differences in how MHO related to adiposity, socio-demographic and lifestyle predictors, depending on the classification used to define MHO. First, WC was significantly associated with MHO, based on both the IDF and CR definitions, independently of age and sex, thus highlighting the importance of measuring WC in clinical settings. However, in the fully adjusted model, WC remained an independent predictor of MHO based on the IDF definition only, and not the CR definition. Similar results were obtained by other studies that have

Table 3 Association of socio-demographic, anthropometric, dietary and lifestyle characteristics with MHO after age and sex adjustment

	IDF-MHO		CR-MHO	
	OR (95% CI)*	p-value	OR (95% CI)*	p-value
Socio-demographic				
Age (years)	0.88 (0.81–0.95)	0.001	1.02 (0.94–1.10)	0.65
Gender				
Males	reference		reference	
Females	1.43 (1.06–1.94)	0.02	1.59 (1.19–2.12)	0.002
Father's level of education				
Elementary or less	reference		reference	
Intermediate or high school	1.13 (0.73–1.76)	0.58	0.68 (0.46–1.02)	0.06
University or higher	1.07 (0.68–1.70)	0.76	0.83 (0.55–1.25)	0.37
Mother's level of education				
Elementary or less	reference		reference	
Intermediate or high school	1.18 (0.80–1.73)	0.4	0.99 (0.69–1.42)	0.95
University or higher	1.23 (0.82–1.87)	0.32	1.14 (0.77–1.68)	0.5
Anthropometric				
Weight (Kg)	0.95 (0.94–0.96)	< 0.0001	0.99 (0.98–1.00)	0.01
BMI (Kg/m^2)	0.87 (0.83–0.91)	< 0.0001	0.96 (0.93–1.00)	0.03
BMI Z score	0.36 (0.26–0.51)	< 0.0001	0.78 (0.62–0.98)	0.03
WC (cm)	0.97 (0.96–0.98)	< 0.0001	1.00 (0.99–1.01)	0.74
Elevated WC	NA		0.74 (0.55–1.00)	0.05
Dietary Habits				
Regular breakfast consumption in the past month				
No	reference		reference	
Yes	0.90 (0.66–1.23)	0.51	1.09 (0.81–1.47)	0.55
Frequency of snacks consumption/d				
≥ 3	reference		reference	
2	0.77 (0.49–1.22)	0.27	0.79 (0.52–1.21)	0.28
≤ 1	1.01 (0.68–1.50)	0.96	0.81 (0.56–1.17)	0.27
Frequency of fruits consumption/d				
0	reference		reference	
1	0.78 (0.49–1.25)	0.3	0.83 (0.54–1.27)	0.38
≥ 2	1.04 (0.73–1.49)	0.81	0.81 (0.57–1.15)	0.24
Frequency of vegetables consumption/d				
0	reference		reference	
1	0.89 (0.63–1.27)	0.54	0.70 (0.50–0.98)	0.04
≥ 2	1.12 (0.76–1.65)	0.56	0.83 (0.57–1.20)	0.32
Frequency of soft drinks consumption/d				
≥ 2	reference		reference	
≤ 1	0.73 (0.54–1.00)	0.05	0.94 (0.70–1.26)	0.66
Frequency of power drinks consumption/d				
≥ 1	reference		reference	
0	0.86 (0.60–1.25)	0.43	1.04 (0.72–1.49)	0.84
Frequency of milk drinks consumption/d				

Table 3 Association of socio-demographic, anthropometric, dietary and lifestyle characteristics with MHO after age and sex adjustment *(Continued)*

	IDF-MHO		CR-MHO	
0	reference		reference	
1	0.85 (0.59–1.21)	0.36	0.88 (0.63–1.24)	0.48
≥ 2	0.87 (0.56–1.35)	0.53	0.91 (0.60–1.39)	0.67
Frequency of fast food consumption/week	0.97 (0.90–1.06)	0.50	0.98 (0.91–1.06)	0.58
Physical Activity and Sedentarity				
Exercise in school				
No	reference		reference	
Yes	1.19 (0.81–1.74)	0.37	1.13 (0.79–1.61)	0.51
Screen Time				
> 2 h/day	reference		reference	
≤ 2 h/day	1.01 (0.67–1.52)	0.96	1.08 (0.73–1.59)	0.71
Frequency of exercise for at least 30 mn in the past week	0.98 (0.91–1.04)	0.45	0.96 (0.90–1.02)	0.21
Sleep				
Number of sleep hrs per night, during week days				
Inadequate	reference		reference	
Adequate	1.31 (0.97–1.78)	0.08	1.34 (1.00–1.80)	0.05
Number of sleep hrs per night, during weekends				
Inadequate	reference		reference	
Adequate	1.10 (0.79–1.53)	0.57	1.03 (0.75–1.41)	0.86
Number of days went to sleep during the day in the past week	1.02 (0.97–1.08)	0.44	1.05 (1.00–1.11)	0.05
Smoking				
Smoking cigarette during the past month				
Yes	reference		reference	
No	0.75 (0.43–1.30)	0.3	1.00 (0.59–1.71)	0.99
Smoking shisha during the past month				
Yes	reference		reference	
No	0.88 (0.47–1.63)	0.68	0.88 (0.50–1.55)	0.66

*Analyses were adjusted for age and sex except for BMI Z score since this variable already adjusts for inter-individual differences in age and sex
Abbreviations: BMI: Body mass index; CI: Confidence interval; cm: Centimeters; CR: Cardiovascular risks; d: Day; hrs: Hours; IDF: International Diabetes Federation; kg: Kilograms; kg/m^2: Kilograms per squared meters; MHO: Metabolically healthy obesity; mn: Minutes; OR: Odds ratio; WC: Waist circumference

adopted the CR definition. For instance, Prince et al. (2014) has shown that WC was no longer significantly related with MHO in Canadian children, after adjustment for lifestyle factors [12]. In addition, the results of this study showed that, based on both definitions, BMI-z score was the strongest predictor of MHO amongst adolescents in KSA, and that, after adjustment for dietary and lifestyle factors, BMI was more strongly associated with MHO, compared to WC. These results are in agreement with those reported by a longitudinal study amongst adolescents, where BMI and its changes over time were more strongly related to cardiovascular factors compared with WC [51]. It is important to acknowledge that WC may not always be reflective of visceral fat as it is not able to differentiate between subcutaneous fat in the abdominal area and visceral fat accumulation [59].

Taken together, these findings suggest that the screening of an obese adolescent may include WC as a proxy of abdominal obesity [60, 61], in conjunction with BMI which may be able to better predict metabolic health in this age group. It has in fact been argued that BMI is one of the most consistent determinants of MHO in adolescents [12, 52, 56] and that MHO status may not be really found at higher levels of obesity [21].

In this study, we found an association between the frequency of consumption of vegetables and MHO amongst boys, but not girls. Gender-based differences in the association of diet composition with MHO have been previously reported amongst adults [44] but no studies have examined these differences in children and adolescents. Such gender-based disparities may reflect differences in physiology or in the reporting of dietary

Table 4 Independent associations of socio-demographic, anthropometric, and lifestyle characteristics with MHO status

Model-IDF definition*	OR (95%CI)	p-value
Among All		
BMI (kg/m^2)	0.89 (0.84–0.93)	< 0.0001
WC (cm)	0.97 (0.96–0.98)	< 0.0001
Model-CR definition*		
Female Gender	1.76 (1.29–2.41)	0.0004
BMI (kg/m^2)	0.97 (0.94–1.00)	0.06
Number of days went to sleep during the day in the past week	1.06 (1.00–1.12)	0.04
Among Boys		
Model-IDF definition*		
BMI (kg/m^2)	0.91 (0.85–0.96)	0.001
WC (cm)	0.97 (0.96–0.99)	< 0.0001
Frequency of vegetable consumption/d, ≥2/day	1.77 (1.07–2.91)	0.02
Number of sleep hours during week days, adequate	1.51 (0.99–2.35)	0.07
Number of days went to sleep during the day in the past week	1.07 (0.99–1.16)	0.08
Model-CR definition*		
Father's level of education, intermediate-high school	0.60 (0.39–0.92)	0.02
Among Girls		
Model-IDF definition*		
BMI (kg/m^2)	0.84 (0.77–0.92)	0.0001
WC (cm)	0.97 (0.96–0.99)	0.0005
Model-CR definition*		
BMI (kg/m^2)	0.95 (0.89–1.00)	0.06
Frequency of soft drinks consumption/d, ≤1/day	0.49 (0.30–0.81)	0.006

*For each definition of MHO, the variables included in the model were: age (by unit increase of 1 year), gender (reference: male), BMI (by unit increase of 1 kg/m^2), waist circumference (by unit increase of 1 cm), father's level of education (reference: lowest), frequency of vegetables' consumption per day (reference: 0), Frequency of soft drinks' consumption per day (reference: ≥2), Number of sleep hours per night, during week days (reference: < 9 h for 6–12 years old; < 8 h for those aged 13 years and above), number of days went to sleep during the day (by unit increase of 1 day). Since the model included age and gender as variables, we included BMI in the regression model instead of BMI-zcore, given that the latter already adjusts for inter-individual differences in age and sex
Abbreviations: BMI: Body mass index; CI: Confidence interval; cm: Centimeters; CR: Cardiovascular risks; hrs: Hours; IDF: International Diabetes Federation; kg/m^2: Kilograms per squared meters; MHO: Metabolically healthy obesity; OR: Odds ratio; WC: Waist circumference

intakes between sexes. The combination of phytochemicals, antioxidants, and dietary fiber brought by a diet rich in vegetables may decrease oxidative stress, mitigate the inflammatory response, improve insulin sensitivity and decrease cardio-metabolic risk, which may explain our study findings [62]. It is worth noting that some studies have reported a positive association of MHO with the intake of milk and fruits, and an inverse association with the consumption of soft drinks [47, 50, 54], while other studies found no association between MHO and food groups' intakes [12, 48]. Surprisingly, our results showed that, in girls, a lower intake of soft drinks was associated with lower odds of MHO. This may be due to the fact that adolescent girls, and particularly those with high adiposity, tend to under-report their intakes of energy-dense, nutrient-poor foods [63–65]. It is important to note that the questionnaire adopted in this study was qualitative in nature, and did not obtain quantitative information on portions or serving sizes usually

consumed. In addition, the questionnaire did not allow for the estimation of energy and macronutrient intakes, and hence differences between MHO and MUO groups in this respect, could not be investigated.

Based on the CR definition, the results showed that meeting the recommended number of sleep hours per night was associated with higher odds of MHO in the total sample, after adjustment for age and sex. This sleep indicator was also associated with MHO in boys, based on the IDF definition. These findings are in line with those reported by Li et al. (2015) amongst Chinese children and adolescents, where MHO subjects had significantly longer sleep hours, and with those reported by Spruyt et al. (2010), where shorter sleep durations among children in the United States (US) were strongly associated with adverse metabolic outcomes such as higher plasma levels of insulin, low density lipoprotein (LDL) and high sensitivity C-reactive protein [50, 66]. Interestingly, the results of our study have also shown that the weekly frequency of day napping was an independent positive predictor of MHO status, particularly in boys. Studies on the association between day napping and metabolic health are scarce. In adults, longer napping durations (> 60–90 mn) were associated with higher risk of Metabolic syndrome and incidence of coronary heart disease, while this association was not observed for shorter nap durations (< 30–60 mn) [67–69]. In high school students, afternoon or evening naps, as assessed by actigraphy, were associated with higher levels of interleukin 6, while this association was not found for morning naps [70]. The same study has reported that diary-reported napping was not associated with any inflammatory marker. In addition, although some studies have suggested that daytime naps may be associated with reduced nocturnal sleep and with increased food craving amongst adolescents [71], others have found no association between daytime sleep and increased risk of adiposity in children and adolescents [72, 73]. It has been proposed that nighttime sleep and naps serve different physiological functions. Naps may in fact reduce daytime psychosocial stress and cortisol levels, which may, at least partly explain the observed associations in our study [72, 74, 75].

It is of interest that, in our study, sleep indicators were associated with MHO in boys only, and not in girls. Gender-based differences in the association between sleep and metabolic health have been previously described amongst adults [25], but few studies have tackled this association in adolescents. In a nationally representative survey of 7–15 year old children and adolescents, short sleep duration was associated with elevated waist circumference, and this association was observed amongst boys only [76]. In a study conducted on children and adolescents aged 6–20 years, short sleep duration was associated with lower resting energy expenditure in boys and with higher leptin levels in girls [77, 78]. These results suggest a possible gender difference in the impact of sleep duration on hormonal and physiologic parameters during childhood and adolescence [78]. Alternatively, the gender-based disparities in the association between sleep and MHO may reflect differences in lifestyle-related factors. In fact, the widespread use of videogames and technology among teenage boys, may delay the onset of sleep, possibly introducing daytime napping as well [79]. Consequently, this group is at higher risk of disruption of the normal circadian rhythmicity related to sleep and the hormonal systems involved in metabolic regulation [79]. Taken together, our findings highlight the need for the integration of sleep in the development of effective prevention, treatment, and intervention programs targeting adolescent obesity and related metabolic abnormalities [76, 80]. The inclusion of sleep questions in health assessments can provide a clear picture of whether the adolescent has good or poor sleeping habits

and help in planning for lifestyle and behavior modification interventions when needed [80].

In the present study, there was no association between physical activity, sedentary behavior, and MHO amongst adolescents. The link between physical activity and MHO status in youth is not well understood, since only few studies have examined this association. Prince et al. (2014) [12] showed that higher physical activity was independently associated with MHO amongst Canadian children, while Camhi et al. (2013), Heinzle et al. (2015) and Senechayl et al. (2013) reported no associations between physical activity, screen time and MHO amongst US and Canadian adolescents [21, 46, 52]. The lack of association between MHO and physical activity in the present study may be due to the low prevalence of physical activity amongst obese adolescents in KSA whereby the frequency of engaging in physical activity for at least 30 min was less than 2 times per week in this population group. Alternatively, other factors such as cardiorespiratory or musculoskeletal fitness, which may offer additional insight as to why some obese adolescents experience metabolic abnormalities while others do not [45, 52], were not assessed in this study.

The strengths of this study included the large sample and the national representativeness of the study population. Anthropometric measurements were obtained using standardized protocols rather than being self-reported. The findings of this study should however be interpreted in light of the following limitations. First, the study instrument was self-administered which may be associated with recall bias, and a high cognitive burden [81]. However, the questionnaire underwent several rounds of expert review and was pilot-tested for clarity, appropriate wording and comprehension amongst the target respondent group, i.e. adolescents in KSA. Second, pubertal stage and the levels of sex hormones, which may affect the cardiometabolic profile, were not assessed in this study [22, 48, 50, 51]. In addition, direct measures of adiposity, such as fat mass, percent body fat and visceral fat, which may play a crucial role in the pathogenesis of metabolic abnormalities, were not obtained. It is also important to note that physical activity and dietary assessment were not investigated using objective measurements, but were self-reported based on questions that were formulated in congruence with those included in the Youth Risk Behavior Survey [33] and the Global School-based Student Health Survey [28, 34], with cultural adaptation. It is worth noting that, although the questionnaire inquired about the frequency of daytime sleeping, it did not allow for the assessment of nap duration or its timing during the day. In addition, the questionnaire used in the Jeeluna study did not inquire about the age of onset of obesity, and thus did not allow us to examine the association between obesity duration and MHO/MUO status in the study sample. Furthermore, those who consented to blood withdrawal and provided blood samples represented 58.3% of the originally surveyed population. A comparison between those who provided blood samples and those who did not, showed that socio-economic characteristics did not differ significantly between the groups. However, the group that provided blood was older (15.9 ± 1.83 vs. 15.69 ± 1.84 years), heavier (BMI: 22.77 ± 5.92 vs. 22.36 ± 6.06 kg/m^2), and included more girls compared to boys (50.9% girls vs. 49.1% boys) ($p < 0.05$). Such differences could have resulted in an underestimation of MHO in the study sample, given that BMI has been repetitively shown to be inversely associated with MHO in youth. Despite the above, these differences in age, BMI and gender are less likely to have affected the association between dietary, anthropometric and sleep indicators, as identified in this study. Lastly, the cross-sectional nature of this study does not allow for causality inference. There is a need for longitudinal studies to further confirm the role of adiposity, dietary, psychosocial, socio-demographic and lifestyle- related factors in modulating metabolic profiles in obese youth.

Conclusion
In a national survey conducted in KSA, this study showed that approximately one out of five adolescents had a favorable metabolic profile, despite being obese. The increasing rate of pediatric obesity underscores the importance of distinguishing MHO and MUO, to optimize the delivery of health services for obesity management in a manner that is both efficient and effective [50]. This study has importantly identified anthropometric factors as predictors of MHO and suggested gender-based differences in the association between diet, sleep and MHO in adolescents. The poor agreement between the two MHO definitions adopted in this study (IDF and CR) and the fact that the use of different definitions yielded different predictors highlight the need for harmonized definitions for the identification of MHO in adolescence. Taken together, the study's findings provide additional insights into the heterogeneity of obesity, while also having possible impact on intervention strategies aimed at improving metabolic heath in obese adolescents in a region that harbors one of the highest burdens of pediatric obesity worldwide.

Abbreviations
ATPIII: Adult Treatment Panel III; BMI: Body Mass Index; BP: Blood pressure; CDC: Center for Disease Control and Prevention; CI: Confidence interval; CIMT: Carotid intima media thickness; cm: Centimeters; CR: Cardiovascular risk; CVD: Cardiovascular diseases; d: Day; DBP: Diastolic blood pressure; EMR: Eastern Mediterranean Region; GCC: Gulf Cooperation Council; HDL-

C: High density lipoprotein-cholesterol; HOMA: Homeostasis Model Assessment; hrs: Hours; IDF: International Diabetes Federation; IRB: Institutional review board; KAIMRC: King Abdullah International Medical Research Center; kg: Kilograms; kg/m^2: Kilograms per squared meters; KSA: Kingdom of Saudi-Arabia; LDL-C: Low density lipoprotein-cholesterol; MHO: Metabolically healthy obesity; mm Hg: Millimeters of mercury; mmol/L: Millimoles per liter; mn: Minutes; MOE: Ministry of Education; MUO: Metabolically unhealthy obese; NCD: Non-communicable diseases; NCEP: National Cholesterol Education Program; OR: Odd ratio; SBP: Systolic blood pressure; TC: Total cholesterol; TG: Triglycerides; US: United States; WC: Waist circumference; WHO: World Health Organization

Acknowledgements
We would like to thank Dr. Waleed Tamimi from the Department of Pathology and Laboratory Medicine at King Abdulaziz Medical City for providing the technical laboratory related information.

Funding
This work was supported by King Abdullah International Medical Research Center (Protocol RC08–092).

Authors' contribution
LN contributed to the conceptualization of the study objectives and methodology, write up of the paper and the interpretation of the data. HT conducted data analyses and contributed to data interpretation and the write up of the manuscript. AM contributed to data analysis and data interpretation; FSA led and supervised the implementation of the Jeeluna survey in KSA, obtained funding, contributed to data interpretation, and critically reviewed the manuscript. LN and HT contributed equally to this manuscript. All authors have contributed to, read and approved the final manuscript.

Competing interests
The authors declare that they have no competing interests.

Author details
[1]Department of Nutrition and Food Science, Faculty of Agricultural and Food Sciences, American University of Beirut, P.O. Box 11-0236, Riad El Solh, Beirut, Lebanon. [2]Clinical Research Institute, Biostatistics Unit, American University of Beirut Medical Center, Riad El Solh, Beirut, Lebanon. [3]Department of Pediatrics and Adolescent Medicine, AlDara Hospital and Medical Center, P.O. Box 1105, Riyadh 11431, Saudi Arabia. [4]Department of Population, Family, and Reproductive Health, Bloomberg School of Public Health, Johns Hopkins University, Baltimore, MD, USA.

References
1. Hossain P, Kawar B, El Nahas M. Obesity and diabetes in the developing world—a growing challenge. N Engl J Med. 2007;356:213–5.
2. Food and Nutrition Administration/Ministry of Health Kuwait. Kuwait National Surveillance System (KNSS). Annu Rep. 2013:2014.
3. Rootwelt MS, Christine, Beinnes Fosse K, Tuffaha A, Said H, Sandridge A, Janahi I, Greer W, Hedin L. Qatar' s Youth Is Putting On Weight: The Increase In Obesity Between 2003 And 2009. In Qatar Foundation Annual Research Conference. 2014: HBSP1130.
4. Wang Y, Lobstein T. Worldwide trends in childhood overweight and obesity. Pediatr Obes. 2006;1:11–25.
5. Black RE, Victora CG, Walker SP, Bhutta ZA, Christian P, De Onis M, Ezzati M, Grantham-McGregor S, Katz J, Martorell R. Maternal and child undernutrition and overweight in low-income and middle-income countries. Lancet. 2013; 382:427–51.
6. Nasreddine L, Ouaijan K, Mansour M, Adra N, Sinno D, Hwalla N. Metabolic syndrome and insulin resistance in obese prepubertal children in Lebanon: a primary health concern. Ann Nutr Metab. 2010;57:135–42.

7. Weiss R, Dziura J, Burgert TS, Tamborlane WV, Taksali SE, Yeckel CW, Allen K, Lopes M, Savoye M, Morrison J. Obesity and the metabolic syndrome in children and adolescents. N Engl J Med. 2004;350:2362–74.
8. Ebbeling CB, Pawlak DB, Ludwig DS. Childhood obesity: public-health crisis, common sense cure. Lancet. 2002;360:473–82.
9. Krebs NF, Jacobson MS. Prevention of pediatric overweight and obesity. Pediatrics. 2003;112:424–30.
10. Bonora E, Kiechl S, Willeit J, Oberhollenzer F, Egger G, Targher G, Alberiche M, Bonadonna RC, Muggeo M. Prevalence of insulin resistance in metabolic disorders: the Bruneck study. Diabetes. 1998;47:1643–9.
11. Ferrannini E, Natali A, Bell P, Cavallo-Perin P, Lalic N, Mingrone G. Insulin resistance and hypersecretion in obesity. European Group for the Study of insulin resistance (EGIR). J Clin Invest. 1997;100:1166–73.
12. Prince RL, Kuk JL, Ambler KA, Dhaliwal J, Ball GD. Predictors of metabolically healthy obesity in children. Diabetes Care. 2014;37:1462–8.
13. Hinnouho G-M, Czernichow S, Dugravot A, Batty GD, Kivimaki M, Singh-Manoux A. Metabolically healthy obesity and risk of mortality. Diabetes Care. 2013;36:2294–300.
14. Lassale C, Tzoulaki I, Moons KG, Sweeting M, Boer J, Johnson L, Huerta JM, Agnoli C, Freisling H, Weiderpass E. Separate and combined associations of obesity and metabolic health with coronary heart disease: a pan-European case-cohort analysis. Eur Heart J. 2017;39:397–406.
15. Lee H-J, Choi E-K, Lee S-H, Kim Y-J, Han K-D, Oh S. Risk of ischemic stroke in metabolically healthy obesity: a nationwide population-based study. PLoS One. 2018;13:e0195210.
16. Zheng R, Zhou D, Zhu Y. The long-term prognosis of cardiovascular disease and all-cause mortality for metabolically healthy obesity: a systematic review and meta-analysis. J Epidemiol Community Health. 2016jech-2015-206948.
17. Bell JA, Kivimaki M, Hamer M. Metabolically healthy obesity and risk of incident type 2 diabetes: a meta-analysis of prospective cohort studies. Obes Rev. 2014;15:504–15.
18. Johnson ST, Kuk JL, Mackenzie KA, Huang TT, Rosychuk RJ, Ball GD. Metabolic risk varies according to waist circumference measurement site in overweight boys and girls. J Pediatr. 2010;156:247–52. e1.
19. Sims EA. Are there persons who are obese, but metabolically healthy? Metabolism. 2001;50:1499–504.
20. Huang TT-K, Sun SS, Daniels SR. Understanding the nature of metabolic syndrome components in children and what they can and cannot do to predict adult disease. J Pediatr. 2009;155:e13.
21. Heinzle S, Ball G, Kuk J. Variations in the prevalence and predictors of prevalent metabolically healthy obesity in adolescents. Pediatr Obes. 2016;11:425–33.
22. Bervoets L, Massa G. Classification and clinical characterization of metabolically "healthy" obese children and adolescents. J Pediatr Endocrinol Metab. 2016;29:553–60.
23. Coleman K, Austin BT, Brach C, Wagner EH. Evidence on the chronic care model in the new millennium. Health Aff. 2009;28:75–85.
24. Camhi SM, Crouter SE, Hayman LL, Must A, Lichtenstein AH. Lifestyle behaviors in metabolically healthy and unhealthy overweight and obese women: a preliminary study. PLoS One. 2015;10:e0138548.
25. Hankinson AL, Daviglus ML, Horn LV, Chan Q, Brown I, Holmes E, Elliott P, Stamler J. Diet composition and activity level of at risk and metabolically healthy obese American adults. Obesity. 2013;21:637–43.
26. Matta J, Nasreddine L, Jomaa L, Hwalla N, Mehio Sibai A, Czernichow S, Itani L, Naja F. Metabolically healthy overweight and obesity is associated with higher adherence to a traditional dietary pattern: a cross-sectional study among adults in Lebanon. Nutrients. 2016;8:432.
27. Mehio Sibai A, Nasreddine L, Mokdad AH, Adra N, Tabet M, Hwalla N. Nutrition transition and cardiovascular disease risk factors in Middle East and North Africa countries: reviewing the evidence. Ann Nutr Metab. 2010; 57:193–203.
28. AlBuhairan FS, Tamim H, Al Dubayee M, AlDhukair S, Al Shehri S, Tamimi W, El Bcheraoui C, Magzoub ME, De Vries N, Al Al. Time for an adolescent health surveillance system in Saudi Arabia: findings from "Jeeluna". J Adolesc Health. 2015;57:263–9.
29. El-Hazmi MA, Warsy AS. A comparative study of prevalence of overweight and obesity in children in different provinces of Saudi Arabia. J Trop Pediatr. 2002;48:172–7.
30. International Diabetes Federation. The IDF consensus definition of the metabolic syndrome in children and adolescents. 2006. https://www.idf.org/e-library/consensus-statements/61-idf-consensus-definition-of-metabolic-syndrome-in-children-and-adolescents. Accessed 5 Sept 2011.
31. Onis Md, Onyango AW, Borghi E, Siyam A, Nishida C, Siekmann J. Development of a WHO growth reference for school-aged children and adolescents. Bull World Health Organ. 2007;85:660–7.
32. Kuczmarski RJ, Ogden CL, Guo SS, Grummer-Strawn LM, Flegal KM, Mei Z, Wei R, Curtin LR, Roche AF, Johnson CL. CDC growth charts for the United States: methods and development. Vital Health Stat. 2000;11:20021–190.
33. Kann L, Kinchen S, Shanklin SL, Flint KH, Hawkins J, Harris WA, Lowry R, Olsen EOM, McManus T, Chyen D. Youth risk behavior surveillance—United States. 2013;2014
34. World Health Organization. Global school-based student health survey (GSHS). WHO CHP. 2009.
35. Center for Disease Control and Prevention-World Health Organization: Global School-Based Student Health Survey. Jordan GSHS Report. 2004.
36. AlBuhairan F. Jeeluna study: national assessment of the health needs of adolescents in Saudi Arabia. Riyadh: King Adbullah International Medical Research Center, ISBN: 978–603–90316-1-1.2016.
37. Malak MZ. Patterns of health-risk behaviors among Jordanian adolescent students. Health. 2015;7:58.
38. Lee RD, Nieman DC. Nutritional Assessment. 4th ed. New York: McGraw–Hill; 2007.
39. Marfell-Jones MJ, Stewart A, De Ridder J. International standards for anthropometric assessment. 2012.
40. Pediatrics AAo. National high blood pressure education program working group on high blood pressure in children and adolescents. Pediatrics 2004;114:iv-iv.
41. Cook S, Weitzman M, Auinger P, Nguyen M, Dietz WH. Prevalence of a metabolic syndrome phenotype in adolescents: findings from the third National Health and nutrition examination survey, 1988-1994. Arch Pediatr Adolesc Med. 2003;157:821–7.
42. Lee S, Bacha F, Gungor N, Arslanian S. Comparison of different definitions of pediatric metabolic syndrome: relation to abdominal adiposity, insulin resistance, adiponectin, and inflammatory biomarkers. J Pediatr. 2008;152:177–84. e3.
43. Fernández JR, Redden DT, Pietrobelli A, Allison DB. Waist circumference percentiles in nationally representative samples of African-American, European-American, and Mexican-American children and adolescents. J Pediatr. 2004;145:439–44.
44. Slagter SN, Corpeleijn E, Van Der Klauw MM, Sijtsma A, Swart-Busscher LG, Perenboom CW, De Vries JH, Feskens EJ, Wolffenbuttel BH, Kromhout D. Dietary patterns and physical activity in the metabolically (un) healthy obese: the Dutch lifelines cohort study. Nutr J. 2018;17:18.
45. Cadenas-Sanchez C, Ruiz JR, Labayen I, Huybrechts I, Manios Y, González-Gross M, Breidenassel C, Kafatos A, De Henauw S, Vanhelst J. Prevalence of metabolically healthy but overweight/obese phenotype and its association with sedentary time, physical activity, and fitness. J Adolesc Health. 2017;
46. Camhi SM, Waring ME, Sisson SB, Hayman LL, Must A. Physical activity and screen time in metabolically healthy obese phenotypes in adolescents and adults. J Obes. 2013;2013
47. Chun S, Lee S, Son H-J, Noh H-M, Oh H-Y, Jang HB, Lee H-J, Kang J-H, Song H-J, Paek Y-J. Clinical characteristics and metabolic health status of obese Korean children and adolescents. Korean J Fam Med. 2015;36:233–8.
48. Ding W, Yan Y, Zhang M, Cheng H, Zhao X, Hou D, Mi J. Hypertension outcomes in metabolically unhealthy normal-weight and metabolically healthy obese children and adolescents. J Hum Hypertens. 2015;29:548.
49. Elmaogullari S, Demirel F, Hatipoglu N. Risk factors that affect metabolic health status in obese children. J Pediatr Endocrinol Metab. 2017;30:49–55.
50. Li L, Yin J, Cheng H, Wang Y, Gao S, Li M, Grant SF, Li C, Mi J, Li M. Identification of genetic and environmental factors predicting metabolically healthy obesity in children: data from the BCAMS study. J Clin Endocrinol Metab. 2016;101:1816–25.
51. Reinehr T, Wolters B, Knop C, Lass N, Holl RW. Strong effect of pubertal status on metabolic health in obese children: a longitudinal study. J Clin Endocrinol Metab. 2014;100:301–8.
52. Sénéchal M, Wicklow B, Wittmeier K, Hay J, MacIntosh AC, Eskicioglu P, Venugopal N, McGavock JM. Cardiorespiratory fitness and adiposity in metabolically healthy overweight and obese youth. Pediatrics. 2013;132:e85–92.
53. Vukovic R, Milenkovic T, Mitrovic K, Todorovic S, Plavsic L, Vukovic A, Zdravkovic D. Preserved insulin sensitivity predicts metabolically healthy obese phenotype in children and adolescents. Eur J Pediatr. 2015;174:1649–55.
54. Camhi SM, Evans EW, Hayman LL, Lichtenstein AH, Must A. Healthy eating index and metabolically healthy obesity in US adolescents and adults. Prev Med. 2015;77:23–7.

55. Mangge H, Zelzer S, Puerstner P, Schnedl WJ, Reeves G, Postolache TT, Weghuber D. Uric acid best predicts metabolically unhealthy obesity with increased cardiovascular risk in youth and adults. Obesity. 2013;21

56. Weghuber D, Zelzer S, Stelzer I, Paulmichl K, Kammerhofer D, Schnedl W, Molnar D, Mangge H. High risk vs."metabolically healthy" phenotype in juvenile obesity–neck subcutaneous adipose tissue and serum uric acid are clinically relevant. Exp Clin Endocrinol Diabetes. 2013;121:384–90.

57. Phillips CM. Metabolically healthy obesity across the life course: epidemiology, determinants, and implications. Ann N Y Acad Sci. 2017;1391:85–100.

58. Li S, Chen W, Srinivasan SR, Xu J, Berenson GS. Relation of childhood obesity/cardiometabolic phenotypes to adult cardiometabolic profile: the Bogalusa heart study. Am J Epidemiol. 2012;176:S142–S9.

59. Eloi JC, Epifanio M, de Gonçalves MM, Pellicioli A, Vieira PFG, Dias HB, Bruscato N, Soder RB, Santana JCB, Mouzaki M. Quantification of abdominal fat in obese and healthy adolescents using 3 tesla magnetic resonance imaging and free software for image analysis. PLoS One. 2017;12:e0167625.

60. Hatipoglu N, Mazicioglu MM, Poyrazoglu S, Borlu A, Horoz D, Kurtoglu S. Waist circumference percentiles among Turkish children under the age of 6 years. Eur J Pediatr. 2013;172:59–69.

61. McCarthy HD, Ellis SM, Cole TJ. Central overweight and obesity in British youth aged 11–16 years: cross sectional surveys of waist circumference. BMJ. 2003;326:624.

62. Esmaillzadeh A, Kimiagar M, Mehrabi Y, Azadbakht L, Hu FB, Willett WC. Fruit and vegetable intakes, C-reactive protein, and the metabolic syndrome. Am J Clin Nutr. 2006;84:1489–97.

63. Collins C, Watson J, Burrows T. Measuring dietary intake in children and adolescents in the context of overweight and obesity. Int J Obes. 2010;34:1103.

64. Collins CE, Dewar DL, Schumacher TL, Finn T, Morgan PJ, Lubans DR. 12 month changes in dietary intake of adolescent girls attending schools in low-income communities following the NEAT girls cluster randomized controlled trial. Appetite. 2014;73:147–55.

65. Moore LL, Singer MR, Qureshi MM, Bradlee ML, Daniels SR. Food group intake and micronutrient adequacy in adolescent girls. Nutrients. 2012;4: 1692–708.

66. Spruyt K, Molfese DL, Gozal D. Sleep duration, sleep regularity, body weight, and metabolic homeostasis in school-aged children. Pediatrics. 2011;127: e345–e52.

67. Yamada T, Hara K, Shojima N, Yamauchi T, Kadowaki T. Daytime napping and the risk of cardiovascular disease and all-cause mortality: a prospective study and dose-response meta-analysis. Sleep. 2015;38:1945–53.

68. Yang L, Xu Z, He M, Yang H, Li X, Min X, Zhang C, Xu C, Angileri F, Légaré S. Sleep duration and midday napping with 5-year incidence and reversion of metabolic syndrome in middle-aged and older Chinese. Sleep. 2016;39:1911–8.

69. Yang L, Yang H, He M, Pan A, Li X, Min X, Zhang C, Xu C, Zhu X, Yuan J. Longer sleep duration and midday napping are associated with a higher risk of CHD incidence in middle-aged and older Chinese: the Dongfeng-Tongji cohort study. Sleep. 2016;39:645–52.

70. Jakubowski KP, Hall MH, Marsland AL, Matthews KA. Is daytime napping associated with inflammation in adolescents? Health Psychol. 2016;35:1298.

71. Landis AM, Parker KP, Dunbar SB. Sleep, hunger, satiety, food cravings, and caloric intake in adolescents. J Nurs Scholarship. 2009;41:115–23.

72. Bell JF, Zimmerman FJ. Shortened nighttime sleep duration in early life and subsequent childhood obesity. Arch Pediatr Adolesc Med. 2010;164:840–5.

73. Tikotzky L, De Marcas G, HAR-TOOV J, Dollberg S, BAR-HAIM Y, Sadeh A. Sleep and physical growth in infants during the first 6 months. J Sleep Res. 2010;19:103–10.

74. Pervanidou P, Chrousos GP. Stress and obesity/metabolic syndrome in childhood and adolescence. Pediatr Obes. 2011;6:21–8.

75. Ward TM, Gay C, Alkon A, Anders TF, Lee KA. Nocturnal sleep and daytime nap behaviors in relation to salivary cortisol levels and temperament in preschool-age children attending child care. Biol Res Nurs. 2008;9:244–53.

76. Eisenmann JC, Ekkekakis P, Holmes M. Sleep duration and overweight among Australian children and adolescents. Acta Paediatr. 2006;95:956–63.

77. Hitze B, Bosy-Westphal A, Bielfeldt F, Settler U, Plachta-Danielzik S, Pfeuffer M, Schrezenmeir J, Mönig H, Müller M. Determinants and impact of sleep duration in children and adolescents: data of the Kiel obesity prevention study. Eur J Clin Nutr. 2009;63:739.

78. Van Cauter E, Knutson KL. Sleep and the epidemic of obesity in children and adults. Eur J Endocrinol. 2008;159:S59–66.

79. Klingenberg L, Chaput J-P, Holmbäck U, Visby T, Jennum P, Nikolic M, Astrup A, Sjödin A. Acute sleep restriction reduces insulin sensitivity in adolescent boys. Sleep. 2013;36:1085–90.

80. Chaput J-P, Dutil C. Lack of sleep as a contributor to obesity in adolescents: impacts on eating and activity behaviors. Int J Behav Nutr Phys Act. 2016;13:103.

81. Bowling A. Mode of questionnaire administration can have serious effects on data quality. J Public Health. 2005;27:281–91.

82. Feinberg I. Recommended sleep durations for children and adolescents: the dearth of empirical evidence. 2013.

10

Serum and urine FGF23 and IGFBP-7 for the prediction of acute kidney injury in critically ill children

Zhenjiang Bai[1†], Fang Fang[2†], Zhong Xu[1], Chunjiu Lu[3], Xueqin Wang[3], Jiao Chen[1], Jian Pan[2], Jian Wang[2] and Yanhong Li[2,3*]

Abstract

Background: Fibroblast growth factor 23 (FGF23) and insulin-like growth factor binding protein 7 (IGFBP-7) are suggested to be biomarkers for predicting acute kidney injury (AKI). We compared them with proposed AKI biomarker of cystatin C (CysC), and aimed (1) to examine whether concentrations of these biomarkers vary with age, body weight, illness severity assessed by pediatric risk of mortality III score, and kidney function assessed by estimated glomerular filtration rate (eGFR), (2) to determine the association between these biomarkers and AKI, and (3) to evaluate whether these biomarkers could serve as early independent predictors of AKI in critically ill children.

Methods: This prospective single center study included 144 critically ill patients admitted to the pediatric intensive care unit (PICU) regardless of diagnosis. Serum and spot urine samples were collected during the first 24 h after PICU admission. AKI was diagnosed based on the AKI network (AKIN) criteria.

Results: Twenty-one patients developed AKI within 120 h of sample collection, including 11 with severe AKI defined as AKIN stages 2 and 3. Serum FGF23 levels were independently associated with eGFR after adjustment in a multivariate linear analysis ($P < 0.001$). Urinary IGFBP-7 (Adjusted OR = 2.94 per 1000 ng/mg increase, $P = 0.035$), serum CysC (Adjusted OR = 5.28, $P = 0.005$), and urinary CysC (Adjusted OR = 1.13 per 1000 ng/mg increase, $P = 0.022$) remained significantly associated with severe AKI after adjustment for body weight and illness severity, respectively. Urinary IGFBP-7 level was predictive of severe AKI and achieved the AUC of 0.79 ($P = 0.001$), but was not better than serum (AUC = 0.89, $P < 0.001$) and urinary (AUC = 0.88, $P < 0.001$) CysC in predicting severe AKI.

Conclusions: Serum FGF23 levels were inversely related to measures of eGFR. In contrast to serum and urinary FGF23 which are not associated with AKI in a general and heterogeneous PICU population, an increased urinary IGFBP-7 level was independently associated with the increased risk of severe AKI diagnosed within the next 5 days after sampling, but not superior to serum or urinary CysC in predicting severe AKI in critically ill children.

Keywords: Acute kidney injury, Critically ill children, Cystatin C, Fibroblast growth factor 23, Insulin-like growth factor binding protein 7, Pediatric risk of mortality III score

* Correspondence: liyanhong@suda.edu.cn
†Zhenjiang Bai and Fang Fang contributed equally to this work.
²Institute of Pediatric Research, Children's Hospital of Soochow University, Suzhou, JiangSu province, China
³Department of nephrology, Institute of pediatric research, Children's Hospital of Soochow University, Suzhou, JiangSu province, China
Full list of author information is available at the end of the article

Background

Critically ill children are at a high risk of developing acute kidney injury (AKI), which is an independent risk factor associated with high mortality and morbidity [1–4]. Research in AKI has focused on identifying biomarkers for early diagnosis, which is crucial to initiate effective therapies [5–10]. Although potential biomarkers for predicting AKI have been identified during the last decade, strong evidence is still lacking to confirm that early biomarkers of AKI have beneficial effects on the clinical outcomes in a general intensive care unit (ICU) population, which leads to attempts to identify novel biomarkers that can predict the development of AKI at an earlier stage [5, 7, 11, 12]. Two of the emerging biomarkers of AKI are fibroblast growth factor 23 (FGF23) [13–19] and insulin-like growth factor binding protein 7 (IGFBP-7) [20–24].

FGF23, a circulating 26-kDa peptide produced by osteocytes, plays an important role in regulating phosphate and vitamin D homeostasis as a phosphate-regulating hormone [13]. Although it has been studied less extensively in AKI, a number of previous studies revealed that plasma FGF23 levels rise rapidly during AKI, suggesting that plasma FGF23 has the potential to diagnose AKI [15–19]. In adult patients undergoing cardiac surgery [18] or in children undergoing cardiopulmonary bypass [19], plasma FGF23 was significantly higher and independently associated with adverse outcomes [18]. So far, two studies of FGF23 with small sample size have been carried out in adult ICU patients [14, 15]. Elevated level of FGF23 was reported in a cohort of 12 ICU patients with AKI compared with 8 control ICU patients without AKI [14]. Subsequently, a prospective observational study of 60 hospitalized adult patients, including 27 from ICU, showed that FGF23 level is elevated and associated with greater risk of death or need for renal replacement therapy [15]. Analysis of larger cohorts is necessary to see if these findings can be replicated in general ICU patients, and whether these findings can apply to critically ill children remains unclear.

IGFBP-7, also known as IGFBP-related protein 1 (IGFBP-rP1), is an additional member of the IGFBP family and involved with the phenomenon of G1 cell-cycle arrest [24]. Renal tubular cells can enter a short period of G1 cell-cycle arrest during the very early phases of cell injury, representing an early response to renal injury [25]. Indeed, urinary IGFBP-7 was identified by proteomics as an early prognostic marker of AKI severity [20]. IGFBP-7 and tissue inhibitor of metalloproteinases-2 (TIMP-2) were further validated in a large multicenter of ICU patients as a predictor of AKI defined by risk, injury, failure, loss, end-stage renal disease (RIFLE) criteria, suggesting that the urinary concentration of IGFBP7 multiplied by TIMP-2 is a novel prognostic urinary biomarker of AKI [23, 24]. However, whether IGFBP-7 alone is a new candidate predictive biomarker of AKI remains to be validated. Serum IGFBP-7 was reported to be associated with insulin resistance and diabetes [26] that may have direct renal effects, resulting in glomerular hyperfiltration and renal damage [27]. However, whether serum IGFBP-7 correlates with renal function, and whether there is a relationship between the serum IGFBP-7 concentration and urinary IGFBP-7 excretion remain elucidated.

In the present study, we assessed concentrations of both FGF23 and IGFBP-7 in serum and urine, and compared them with proposed biomarkers of AKI, serum and urinary cystatin C (CysC). We aimed (1) to examine whether concentrations of these biomarkers vary with age, body weight, and illness severity as assessed by the pediatric risk of mortality III (PRISM III) score, as well as with kidney function as assessed by estimated glomerular filtration rate (eGFR) in critically ill children, (2) to determine the association between these biomarkers and AKI, and (3) to evaluate whether serum and urinary FGF23 and IGFBP-7 could serve as early predictors of AKI, independently of potential confounders, in critically ill children.

Methods

Cohorts, setting, and data collection

All patients who were admitted to the pediatric ICU (PICU) regardless of diagnosis in the university-affiliated tertiary children hospital from May to August 2012 were considered for inclusion in the prospective study. The criteria for PICU admission in our hospital were adopted from guidelines for developing admission and discharge policies for the PICU, as described previously [28, 29], including both medical and surgical patients and age between 1 month and 16 years. The exclusion criteria were the presence of congenital abnormality of the kidney, discharge from PICU before sampling, and unexpected discharge from the PICU or withdrawal of therapy. The Institutional Review Board of the Children's Hospital of Soochow University approved the study. Informed parental written consent was obtained at enrollment of each patient, and all clinical investigations were conducted according to the principles expressed in the Declaration of Helsinki.

Assessment of illness severity

The PRISM III score, based on age-related physiological parameters collected in the first 24 h after PICU admission, was used as a measure to assess illness severity of critically ill children [30].

Diagnosis of AKI

The diagnosis of AKI developed within 120 h of sample collection was based on the serum creatinine (Cr) level defined by the AKI network (AKIN) criteria [1, 31] without urine output criteria. For patients with elevated serum Cr ≥ 106.1 μmol/L at PICU admission, the lowest Cr value during hospitalization was considered as the baseline Cr, in accordance with previous studies [32, 33]. Severity of AKI was characterized by the AKIN criteria. AKIN stage 1 was defined as mild AKI, and AKIN stages 2 and 3 were defined as severe AKI.

Measurement of serum and urinary FGF23 and IGFBP-7

Non-fasting venous blood and spot urine were collected during the first 24 h after PICU admission and immediately aliquoted and stored at − 80 °C. Serum and urine were first centrifuged at 1500×g at 4 °C for 15 min and the supernatants were used for the measurement. The FGF23 level was quantified by the human enzyme-linked immunosorbent assay (ELISA) kit (SEA746Hu, Cloud-Clone Corp, USA), according to the manufacturer's protocol. The minimum detectable level of FGF23 was < 6.7 pg/mL, and the coefficient of variation of intra-assay and inter-assay were less than 10 and 12% respectively, corresponding to that reported by the manufacturer. The FGF23 levels were detectable in all serum samples and in 118 (81.9%) urinary samples. For those samples with undetectable FGF23 levels (18.1%), the FGF23 value was assumed to have a concentration at 6.7 pg/mL equivalent to the detection limit of the assay to facilitate the calculation for urinary FGF23/urinary Cr ratios.

The human IGFBP-rp1/IGFBP-7 ELISA kit (DY1334–05, R&D Systems, USA) was used for the measurement. The samples were diluted 20-fold to 100-fold in Reagent Diluent to ensure that the enzymatic reaction was maintained within the linear range. The coefficient of variation of intra-assay and inter-assay were less than 10%. The level of IGFBP-7 was detectable in all samples.

Measurement of serum and urinary CysC and Cr

The levels of CysC and Cr from the aliquoted samples were measured on an automatic biochemical analyzer (Hitachi 7600, Japan), as described previously [6]. The CysC level was measured using latex enhanced immuno-turbidimetry assay, and the detection limit for CysC was 0.01 mg/L. The coefficient of variation of intra-assay and inter-assay were ≤ 10%. The CysC levels were detectable in all serum samples and in 131 (91.0%) urinary samples. Urinary CysC values for those with undetectable CysC levels were assumed to have the concentration at 0.01 mg/L equivalent to the detection limit of the assay for calculation of the urinary CysC/urinary Cr ratio. The serum and urinary Cr levels were measured automatically using the sarcosine oxidase method on the automatic biochemical analyzer.

Estimated glomerular filtration rate

Estimated GFR was calculated according to the following formula published by Bouvet et al. [34]: eGFR (ml/min) $= 63.2 \times [1.2/\text{serum CysC (mg/L)}]^{0.56} \times [1.09/\text{serum Cr (mg/dL)}]^{0.35} \times [\text{weight (kg)}/45]^{0.3} \times [\text{age (years)}/14]^{0.4}$. The results of Cr and CysC were obtained from the aliquoted serum samples.

Statistical analysis

Data analyses were performed using SPSS statistical software. We first checked assumptions of normality and homogeneity of variance. The Mann-Whitney U test was used to analyze differences between two groups, and the Kruskal-Wallis H test was used to analyze differences among three groups. The chi-square test or Fisher's exact test were used to compare differences in categorical variables among groups. Spearman's analysis was performed to examine correlations. Univariate and multivariate linear analyses were used to analyze the association of variables with eGFR. The data for continuous variables were log-transformed to meet the assumptions of homogeneity of variances. Univariate and multivariate logistic regression analyses were used to calculate odds ratio (OR) to assess the association of biomarkers with AKI, and to identify independent variables associated with AKI. Model fit was assessed by the Hosmer-Lemeshow goodness-of-fit test with $P > 0.05$, suggesting the absence of a biased fit. The area under-the-receiver-operating-characteristic curve (AUC) was calculated to assess the predictive strength, and the nonparametric method of Delong was performed to compare differences between AUCs. Optimal cut-off points to maximize both sensitivity and specificity were determined using Sigma Plot 10.0 software.

Results
Patient characteristics

The study involved 144 critically ill children. Of a total of 179 children were admitted to the PICU during the study period, 35 were excluded: 2 died and 5 were discharged from PICU before sampling, 3 had withdrawal of therapy, and 25 had a failure in collecting blood and urine samples during the first 24 h after PICU admission. The leading cause of PICU admission in the cohort was neurologic diseases (33.3%), followed by respiratory diseases (30.6%). Twenty-four (16.7%) patients were diagnosed with sepsis.

Of the 144 patients, 21 (14.6%) developed AKI within 120 h of sample collection. Ten patients fulfilled the AKIN criteria stage 1 defined as mild AKI: 5 on the first, 3 on the second, 1 on the third, and 1 on the fifth day after PICU admission. Eleven patients fulfilled the criteria of AKIN stages 2 and 3 defined as severe AKI, including 6 patients developed AKIN stage 2: 5 on the first and 1 on the third day after admission; and 5 patients developed AKIN stage 3: 2 on the first, 2 on the second, and 1 on the fourth day after admission.

A comparison of the demographic and clinical characteristics and outcomes among patients with non-AKI, mild AKI, and severe AKI is displayed in Table 1.

Correlation of serum and urinary biomarkers with age, body weight, gender, sepsis, and illness severity

Spearman's correlation analyses of biomarkers with age, body weight, gender, sepsis, and PRISM III score are displayed in Table 2. Multivariate linear regression analyses, including variables of age, body weight, gender, sepsis, and PRISM III score, were further performed. Serum levels of FGF23 ($P = 0.010$) and CysC ($P = 0.003$) remained independently associated with age. In addition, when we grouped the patients into two age categories: ≤3 years ($n = 102$) and > 3 years ($n = 42$), the negative correlation between age and serum FGF23 levels was

only significant in patients aged ≤3 years ($r = -0.590$, $P < 0.001$), but not in patients aged > 3 years ($r = 0.064$, $P = 0.682$). Moreover, the correlation of sepsis with serum FGF23 ($P = 0.068$), urinary IGFBP-7 ($P = 0.350$), and urinary CysC ($P = 0.391$), however, did not remain significant after adjustment for age, body weight and illness severity in a multivariate analysis.

Association of serum and urinary biomarkers with eGFR

Univariate and multivariate linear analyses were used to analyze the association of biomarkers with kidney function as assessed by eGFR. Serum levels of FGF23 ($P < 0.001$), IGFBP-7 ($P = 0.003$), and CysC ($P < 0.001$) and urinary levels of FGF23 ($P = 0.001$) and CysC ($P = 0.022$) were associated with eGFR in the univariate linear regression analysis in Table 3. To identify whether these biomarkers were independently associated with eGFR, the multivariate linear analysis was further conducted. The association of eGFR with serum FGF23 ($P = 0.040$) and

Table 1 Demographic and clinical characteristics grouped according to AKI status

Variable	Non-AKI	Mild AKI	Severe AKI	P
	($n = 123$)	($n = 10$)	($n = 11$)	
Age, months	12 [4–48]	30.5 [11.25–98]	59 [4–98]	0.049[&]
Body weight, kg	10 [6.5–14]	14 [8.75–26.25]	20 [6.5–30]*	0.024[&]
Male, n	70 (56.9)	5 (50.0)	7 (63.6)	0.819
PRISM III score	3 [0.25–6.75]	7.5 [4.25–10.5]*	17 [8–20]*[#]	< 0.001
Arterial pH[a]	7.409 [7.363–7.468]	7.461 [7.392–7.481]	7.400 [7.203–7.497]	0.297
Blood bicarbonate[a], mmol/L	20.0 [17.6–22.2]	17.1 [15.5–20.0]*	17.1 [8.1–19.6]*	0.020[φ]
Serum albumin[a], g/L	41.7 [38.5–44.4]	40.2 [34.9–46.9]	35.3 [26.7–43.8]*	0.026[φ]
Serum creatinine[a], μmol/L	24.6 [19.5–31.8]	44.3 [26.9–72.1]*	86.4 [77.3–140.0]*[#]	< 0.001[φ]
Blood urea nitrogen[a], μmol/L	3.30 [2.54–4.40]	6.34 [3.41–8.53]*	7.00 [5.84–13.44]*	< 0.001[φ]
Serum sodium[a], μmol/L	134.6 [132.3–136.6]	135.8 [133.2–140.3]	132.8 [130.3–133.7]*[#]	0.008[ζ]
Serum potassium[a], μmol/L	4.02 [3.57–4.56]	4.31 [3.77–4.47]	4.32 [3.83–5.60]	0.157
MODS[b], n	3 (2.4)	2 (20.0)*	6 (54.5)[*]	< 0.001[φ]
Shock/DIC[b], n	11 (8.9)	2 (20.0)	5 (45.5)[*]	< 0.001[ζ]
MV[c], n	45 (36.6)	6 (60.0)	10 (90.9)[*]	0.001[ζ]
Duration of MV[c], hours	0 [0–44]	35 [0–123.5]	115 [12–134][*]	0.001[ζ]
Prolonged MV (> 48 h)[c], n	26 (21.1)	4 (40.0)	8 (72.7)[*]	0.002[φ]
Antibiotics[c], n	116 (94.3)	10 (100)	11 (100)	0.322
Inotrope[c], n	23 (18.7)	1 (10.0)	8 (72.7)*[#]	0.001[φ]
Furosemide[c], n	31 (25.2)	3 (30.0)	11 (100)*[#]	0.032[φ]
Steroids[c], n	45 (36.6)	3 (30.0)	5 (45.5)	0.757
PICU LOS, hours	66 [36–141]	77.5 [38.25–256]	152 [118–181]*	0.032[ζ]
Death, n	5 (4.1)	1 (10.0)	2 (18.2)	0.093

Values are median [interquartile range]. Numbers in parentheses denote percentages
AKI network stage 1 was defined as mild AKI, and AKIN stages 2 and 3 were defined as severe AKI. *AKI* acute kidney injury, *DIC* disseminated intravascular coagulation, *LOS* length of stay, *MODS* multiple organ dysfunction syndrome, *MV* mechanical ventilation, *PICU* pediatric intensive care unit, *PRISM III* pediatric risk of mortality III
[a]The first available laboratory results during the first 24 h after PICU admission. [b]Developed during PICU stay. [c]Administration during PICU stay
*$P < 0.05$, compared with non-AKI; [#]$P < 0.05$, compared with mild AKI. [&]$P > 0.05$, after adjustment for PRISM III score. [ζ]$P > 0.05$, [φ]$P < 0.05$, after adjustment for body weight and PRISM III score

Table 2 Correlation of biomarkers with age, body weight, gender, sepsis, and illness severity

Variable	Statistics	sFGF23 pg/mL	sIGFBP-7 ng/mL	sCysC mg/L	uFGF23 pg/mg uCr	uIGFBP-7 ng/mg uCr	uCysC ng/mg uCr
Age, months	r	−0.608	− 0.274	− 0.369	− 0.209	0.049	− 0.114
	P	< 0.001*	0.001	< 0.001*	0.012	0.556	0.175
Body weight, kg	r	−0.598	− 0.253	− 0.346	−0.233	0.066	−0.102
	P	< 0.001	0.002	< 0.001	0.005	0.433	0.224
Gender	Z	−0.051	−0.682	−0.077	−1.271	− 0.020	−0.444
	P	0.959	0.495	0.939	0.204	0.984	0.657
Sepsis	Z	−2.144	−1.812	−.901	− 1.614	−2.037	−2.589
	P	0.032	0.070	0.368	0.107	0.042	0.010
PRISM III score	r	−0.002	0.093	0.084	0.054	0.327	0.253
	P	0.981	0.269	0.317	0.524	< 0.001*	0.002*

PRISM III pediatric risk of mortality III, r = Spearman's correlation coefficient; Z: The Mann-Whitney U test
*$P < 0.05$, multivariate linear regression analysis, including variables of age, body weight, gender, and PRISM III score. Continuous variables were log-transformed in multivariate analysis

urinary CysC (P = 0.001) remained significant in the multivariate analysis after adjustment for age and body weight, as shown in Table 3.

Association of serum and urinary biomarkers with severe AKI

Comparisons of serum and urinary levels of FGF23, IGFBP-7, and CysC among patients with non-AKI, mild AKI, and severe AKI are shown in Table 4 and Fig. 1. Since there was no significant difference in serum and urinary levels of FGF23, IGFBP-7, and CysC between patients with mild AKI and without AKI (P > 0.05), univariate and multivariate logistic analyses were used to analyze the association of biomarkers with severe AKI in Table 5.

The association of serum CysC (P = 0.005), urinary IGFBP-7 (P = 0.035), and urinary CysC (P = 0.022) with severe AKI remained significant after controlling for body weight and illness severity as assessed by PRISM III score (Table 5).

Ability of serum and urinary biomarkers to predict severe AKI

The predictive ability of serum and urinary CysC and urinary IGFBP-7 levels for severe AKI is shown in Table 6. Serum CysC displayed the highest AUC of 0.89 (P < 0.001), which was similar to the result obtained based on the PRISM III score (AUC = 0.92, P < 0.001), for predicting severe AKI in critically ill children, followed by urinary CysC (AUC = 0.88, P < 0.001).

Table 3 Association of variables with eGFR

Variable	Univariate regression		Multivariate regression	
	B coefficient (SE)	P	B coefficient (SE)	P
Age, months	0.524 (0.025)	< 0.001		
Body weight, kg	1.129 (0.067)	< 0.001		
Gender	−0.063 (0.062)	0.317		
PRISM III score	0.000 (0.006)	0.959		
MV	−0.033 (0.063)	0.595		
Duration of MV, hours	0.000 (0.000)	0.302		
sFGF23, pg/mL	−0.842 (0.108)	< 0.001	−0.156 (0.075)[a]	0.040
sIGFBP-7, ng/mL	−0.657(0.214)	0.003	−0.111 (0.113)[a]	0.327
sCysC, mg/L	−1.062 (0.113)	< 0.001	−0.702 (0.048)[a]	< 0.001
uFGF23, pg/mg uCr	−0.169 (0.051)	0.001	−0.050 (0.027)[a]	0.061
uIGFBP-7, ng/mg uCr	−0.013 (0.065)	0.843		
uCysC, ng/mg uCr	−0.097 (0.042)	0.022	−0.067 (0.020)[a]	0.001

eGFR estimated glomerular filtration rate, *MV* mechanical ventilation, *PRISM III* pediatric risk of mortality III. eGFR was calculated based on age, body weight, and serum levels of creatinine and cystatin C
[a]After adjustment for age and body weight. All continuous variables were log-transformed

Table 4 Serum and urinary FGF23, IGFBP-7 and CysC levels grouped according to AKI status

Biomarker	Non-AKI	Mild AKI	Severe AKI	P
	(n = 123)	(n = 10)	(n = 11)	
sFGF23, pg/mL	79.33 [49.88–115.84]	59.97 [50.25–81.57]	92.33 [49.98–107.50]	0.372
sIGFBP-7, ng/mL	107.92 [87.47–125.02]	108.17 [83.65–135.71]	125.26 [103.07–148.35]	0.255
sCysC, mg/L	0.60 [0.47–0.78]	0.73 [0.54–0.96]	1.10 [1.06–1.72]*#	< 0.001
uFGF23, pg/mg uCr	74.40 [39.20–225.8]	47.14 [28.82–130.6]	172.93 [114.37–448.25]*#	0.033
uIGFBP-7, ng/mg uCr	291.57 [135.60–539.04]	244.33 [87.51–478.73]	653.50 [301.94–2072.06]*#	0.005
uCysC, ng/mg uCr	183.17 [94.62–494.96]	122.38 [80.27–332.97]	6559.79 [1224.42–30,414.64]*#	< 0.001

Values are median [interquartile range]
AKI network stage 1 was defined as mild AKI, and AKIN stages 2 and 3 were defined as severe AKI
*$P < 0.05$, compared with non-AKI; #$P < 0.05$, compared with mild AKI

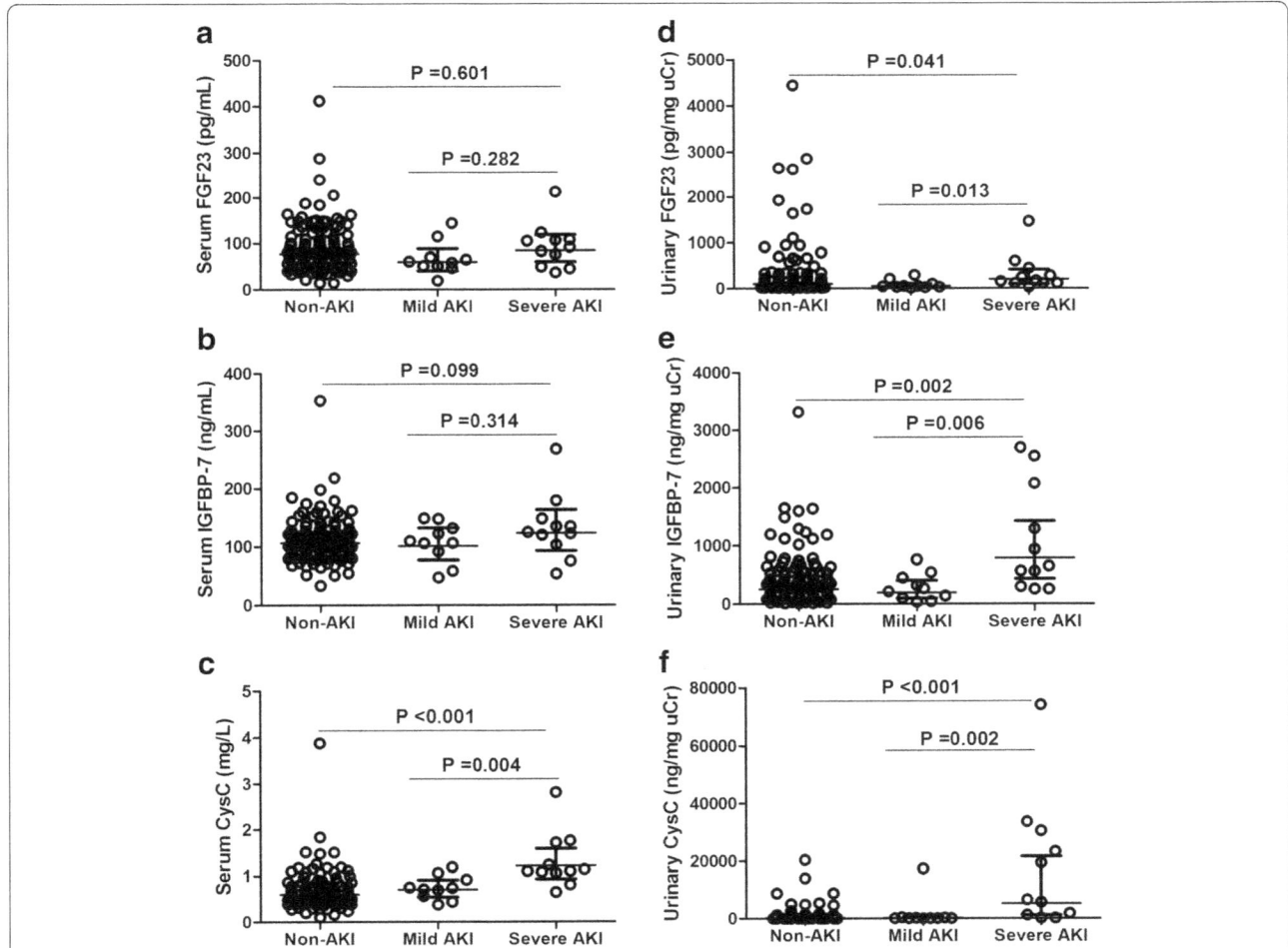

Fig. 1 Comparison of the levels of biomarkers among critically ill children with non-AKI, mild AKI, and severe AKI. **a** serum level of FGF23, **b** serum level of IGFBP-7; **c** serum level of CysC, **d** urinary level of FGF23, **e** urinary level of IGFBP-7, **f** urinary level of CysC. AKI network stage 1 was defined as mild AKI. AKI network stages 2 and 3 were defined as severe AKI. Each circle represents an individual patient; the horizontal lines indicate geometric means with 95% confidence interval. Probability values: the Mann-Whitney U test. The P value for comparison between non-AKI (n = 123) and severe AKI (n = 11), and for comparison between mild (n = 10) and severe (n = 11) AKI

Table 5 Association of variables with severe AKI

Variable	OR	95% CI	P	AOR	95% CI	P
Age, months	1.01	1.00–1.03	0.026	1.01[d]	0.99–1.02	0.567
Body weight, kg	1.09	1.03–1.16	0.003	1.03[d]	0.96–1.12	0.428
Gender	0.74	0.21–2.65	0.642			
PRISM III score	1.36	1.18–1.55	< 0.001	1.32[e]	1.15–1.53	<0.001
MV	16.08	2.00–129.36	0.009	5.03[f]	0.50–50.56	0.170
Duration of MV, hours	1.00	1.00–1.00	0.494			
Sepsis	3.23	0.87–12.05	0.081			
eGFR, mL/min	0.98	0.96–1.01	0.138			
sFGF23, pg/mL	1.00	0.99–1.01	0.730			
sIGFBP-7, ng/mL	1.01	0.99–1.02	0.096			
sCysC, mg/L	6.67	1.84–24.18	0.004	5.28[f, g]	1.64–16.99	0.005
uFGF23, pg/mg uCr	1.15[a]	0.47–2.82	0.761			
uIGFBP-7, ng/mg uCr	4.37[b]	1.82–10.49	0.001	2.94[b, f, g]	1.08–8.01	0.035
uCysC, ng/mg uCr	1.21[c]	1.10–1.34	< 0.001	1.13[c, f, g]	1.02–1.25	0.022

AKI, acute kidney injury; AOR, Adjusted OR; CI, confidence interval; eGFR, estimated glomerular filtration rate; MV, mechanical ventilation; OR, odds ratio; PRISM III, pediatric risk of mortality III
Severe AKI was defined as AKI network stages 2 and 3
[a]Odds ratio represents the increase in risk per 1000 pg/mg increase in uFGF23/uCr. [b]Odds ratio represents the increase in risk per 1000 ng/mg increase in uIGFBP-7/uCr. [c]Odds ratio represents the increase in risk per 1000 ng/mg increase in uCysC/uCr
[d]After adjustment for PRISM III score. [e]After adjustment for age and body weight. [f]After adjustment for body weight and PRISM III score. [g]P < 0.05, after adjustment for body weight, sepsis, and PRISM III score

Urinary IGFBP-7 level was predictive of severe AKI and achieved the AUC of 0.79 (P = 0.001), but was not better than serum CysC and urinary CysC, in predicting severe AKI. However, the difference between the two AUCs of either urinary IGFBP-7 (AUC = 0.79) and serum CysC (AUC = 0.89) (P = 0.103) or urinary IGFBP-7 and urinary CysC (AUC = 0.88) (P = 0.225) did not reach statistically significant. In addition, combining urinary IGFBP-7 with serum and urinary CysC improved the predictive performance, which was superior to urinary IGFBP-7 alone (P = 0.029), but not significantly better than serum CysC alone (P = 0.689). ROC curves for the ability of serum CysC, urinary IGFBP-7, urinary CysC, and PRISM III score to predict severe AKI in critically ill children are shown in Fig. 2.

Discussion

Our results demonstrated that serum FGF23 level was inversely related to measures of eGFR, and an increased urinary level of IGFBP-7 was associated with the increased risk of severe AKI diagnosed within the next 5 days after sampling. However, urinary IGFBP-7 was not superior to serum or urinary CysC in predicting severe AKI in critically ill children.

Previous findings indicate that variables, such as age, gender, and illness severity, may interfere with CysC and other traditional renal biomarkers [6, 35]. We found that both serum CysC and FGF23 levels were independently associated with age. Serum CysC concentration has been reported to be gradually declined with increasing age in younger children less than 3 years old, which reflects

Table 6 Predictive characteristics of biomarkers for severe AKI

Variable	AUC	95% CI	P	Optimal cut-off value	Sensitivity (%)	Specificity (%)
PRISM III score	0.92	0.84–0.99	< 0.001	7.5	90.9	77.4
sCysC, mg/L	0.89	0.82–0.97	< 0.001	0.81	90.9	78.2
uCysC, ng/mg uCr	0.88	0.76–0.99	< 0.001	1145.0	81.8	86.5
uIGFBP-7, ng/mg uCr	0.79	0.66–0.92	0.001	563.4	72.7	79.0
uIGFBP-7, combined with sCysC	0.89	0.79–0.99	< 0.001			
uIGFBP-7, combined with uCysC	0.88	0.79–0.98	< 0.001			
uIGFBP-7, combined with sCysC and uCysC	0.90	0.81–1.00	< 0.001			

Severe AKI was defined as AKI network stages 2 and 3
AKI acute kidney injury, AUC the area under the ROC curve, CI confidence interval, PRISM III pediatric risk of mortality III

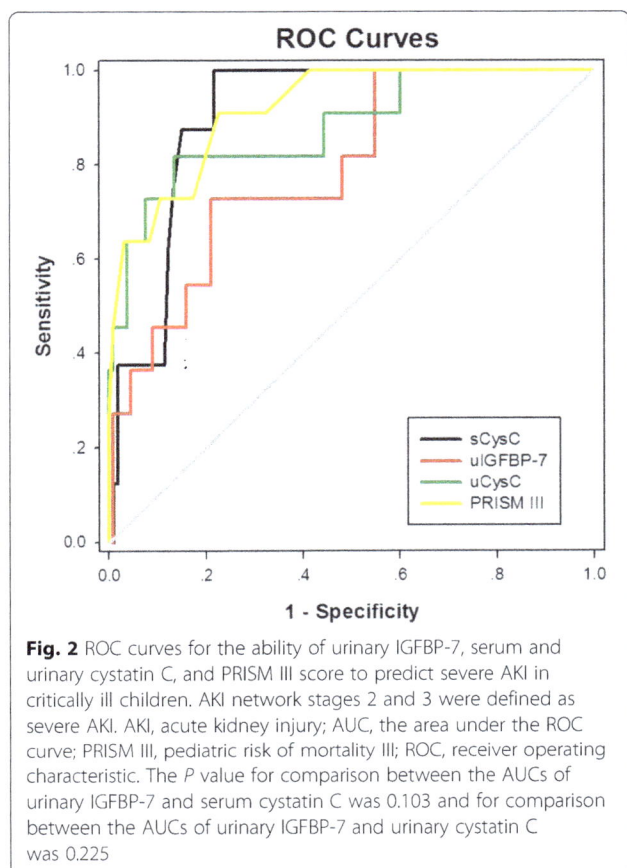

Fig. 2 ROC curves for the ability of urinary IGFBP-7, serum and urinary cystatin C, and PRISM III score to predict severe AKI in critically ill children. AKI network stages 2 and 3 were defined as severe AKI. AKI, acute kidney injury; AUC, the area under the ROC curve; PRISM III, pediatric risk of mortality III; ROC, receiver operating characteristic. The *P* value for comparison between the AUCs of urinary IGFBP-7 and serum cystatin C was 0.103 and for comparison between the AUCs of urinary IGFBP-7 and urinary cystatin C was 0.225

renal maturation [35]. Similarly, the decreased serum FGF23 level with increasing age during the first 3 years of age as seen in the present study may also reflect renal maturation. This result is consistent with a previous finding that FGF23 concentration was elevated at birth and higher than reported in adults [36]. Moreover, the FGF23 is a circulating peptide produced by osteocytes. Previous studies have shown that there is a relationship between FGF23 and bone formation [37, 38], suggesting that the negative correlation between serum FGF23 level and age might be related to osteogenesis and skeletal maturation. However, the decreased serum FGF23 level with increasing age was only seen in younger children less than 3 years old. Data on 1,25-dihydroxyvitamin D and parathyroid hormone (PTH) levels were not available in the study, and thus the association between FGF23 and PTH could not be studied. Further studies are necessary to identify whether the association of serum FGF23 with age is in relation to osteogenesis and skeletal maturation.

Significant correlations between biomarkers and measures of kidney function assessed by eGFR were identified in the present study. Previous studies have suggested that eGFR based on both serum Cr and CysC levels is more accurate than equations based on either [34, 39]. Therefore,

we calculated eGFR based on both serum Cr and CysC, and demonstrated that the association of eGFR with serum FGF23 levels persisted even after adjustment for age and body weight, indicating that serum FGF23 levels have an inverse relationship to kidney function. This result is in line with a previous study conducted in adult patients with preserved renal function, where higher plasma FGF23 concentration was associated with lower estimated GFR [40]. Our data highlight the need to determine whether serum FGF23 is a potential marker for monitoring kidney dysfunction in critically ill children in large multicenter studies.

To our knowledge, this study is the first to examine the relationships between serum and urinary IGFBP-7 and FGF23 levels with AKI in critically ill children. Of note, our observation of FGF23 levels in critically ill children with AKI is not consistent with previous research [16, 18, 19], and furthermore FGF23 levels in both urine and serum are not useful for the prediction of AKI in critically ill children. The most likely explanation for this discrepancy between our data and previous data could be that we evaluated the predictive accuracy of FGF23 in a general and heterogeneous PICU population rather than in a specific clinical setting, such as in patients undergone cardiac surgery [16, 18, 19] or in randomly selected ICU patients [14, 15]. Given the heterogeneity and dynamic nature of AKI, the predictive performance is dependent strongly on the underlying conditions. The poor results derived from a mixed heterogeneous PICU might be related to the low specificity of FGF23 for AKI. Indeed, upregulation of FGF23 was reported in patients with hypertension, advanced diabetic nephropathy, and cardiovascular disease [41] or in patients with end stage liver disease [42]. Our data support the concept that the usefulness of biomarkers should be addressed differently for different clinical settings [7]. In addition, the level of FGF23 was substantially influenced by age and body weight, which might be considered as disadvantages in the clinical utility of FGF23 as an AKI biomarker in PICU population. The age did not remain significantly associated with severe AKI after adjustment for illness severity in the present study, suggesting that the positive correlation of age with AKI might be due to the higher prevalence of severe underlying diseases in older children, rather than due to a direct effect of age.

One of our major findings was a significant association of urinary IGFBP-7 with severe AKI in critically ill children, which is in line with the previous report from Aregger et al. [20], where urinary IGFBP-7 was identified by proteomics as an early prognostic marker of AKI severity. We verified the use of urinary IGFBP-7 and evaluated the impact of urinary IGFBP-7 on predicting severe AKI in a general PICU population, independent of the severity of illness. It is well accepted that a desirable biomarker should be characterized by a high accuracy and unaffected by potential confounders. The odds ratio for urinary IGFBP-7 to predict severe AKI occurrence remained significant after adjustment for body weight and severity of illness, as assessed by PRISM III score, demonstrating that urinary IGFBP-7 was independently associated with increased risk for severe AKI in critically ill children.

Our study provides the first evidence of a significant association of urinary IGFBP-7 with severe AKI in critically ill children; however, urinaryIGFBP-7 level is not superior to serum or urinary CysC in predicting severe AKI. Since multiple pathways are involved in the development and progression of AKI, a single biomarker may be unlikely to provide the required predictive accuracy in general PICU population, and a panel of biomarkers for accurately predicting AKI might be necessary. Nevertheless, despite the biological diversity, the combination of urinary IGFBP-7 and serum or urinary CysC did not substantially improve the prediction of severe AKI in critically ill children.

The ROC curve analysis in the present study showed that serum CysC appeared to play a greater role in predicting severe AKI, which is in agreement with previous studies where serum CysC has been reported to be associated with an increased risk of AKI in various pediatric cohorts [8, 9]. Notably, although two studies have shown that serum CysC is an early and accurate biomarker for AKI in general critically ill children [8, 9], we are the first to demonstrate that serum CysC was independently associated with AKI, even after adjustment for body weight and illness severity as assessed by PRISM III score. Our results strongly indicate that serum CysC could serve as an independent biomarker to predict severe AKI in critically ill children.

This present study has some limitations. Firstly, we utilized elevated serum Cr levels as a reference standard to define AKI. Although serum Cr remains a widely used marker for evaluating kidney function in PICU, its disadvantage has been well discussed and recognized. Secondly, although the use of urine output criteria for AKI diagnosis has not been well validated [43], it has been suggested that patients meeting both serum Cr and urine output criteria for AKI have worse outcomes compared with patients who manifest AKI predominantly by one criterion [44]. The diagnosis and staging of AKI based only on serum Cr without urine output criteria may have under estimated incidence and grade of AKI. Thirdly, previous studies have indicated that AKI incidence is best estimated by choosing the lowest Cr value within the first week in the ICU as baseline Cr, suggesting that any reasonable estimate based on Cr measures is likely to be better than an estimate that takes into account only age, gender, and race [32]. However, the use of the lowest Cr value during hospitalization as the

baseline Cr for patients with elevated serum Cr (≥106.1 μmol/L) at PICU admission has not been validated in critically ill children. Fourthly, the lack of serial measurements of these biomarkers during PICU stay might reduce the likelihood of observing the difference between AKI and non-AKI groups. Fifthly, although the urinary levels of IGFBP-7 and CysC were affected by sepsis; urinary IGFBP-7 and CysC were independently associated with increased risk for severe AKI, even after adjustment for the presence of sepsis. The present study was not powered to specifically detect differences in these biomarkers between septic children with versus without AKI. Finally, the relatively small sample size limited the power to perform logistic regression between these biomarkers and mortality.

Conclusions

Our results have shown that serum FGF23 levels are inversely related to measures of eGFR, irrespective of illness severity, suggesting that the elevated serum FGF23 level may reflect a decline in kidney function independently. In contrast to serum and urinary FGF23 which are not associated with AKI in a general and heterogeneous PICU population, an increased urinary level of IGFBP-7 was independently associated with increased risk of severe AKI diagnosed within the next 5 days after sampling. However, urinary IGFBP-7 was not superior to serum or urinary CysC in predicting severe AKI in critically ill children. Further investigation is needed to explore the role of FGF23 and IGFBP-7 for prediction of AKI in various pediatric cohorts.

Abbreviations
AKI: Acute kidney injury; AKIN: AKI network; AOR: Adjusted odds ratio; CI: Confidence interval; Cr: Creatinine; CysC: Cystatin C; eGFR: Estimated glomerular filtration rate; FGF23: Fibroblast growth factor 23; IGFBP-7: Insulin-like growth factor binding protein 7; IQR: Interquartile range; LOS: Length of stay; MV: Mechanical ventilation; OR: Odds ratio; PICU: Pediatric intensive care unit; PRISM III score: Pediatric risk of mortality III; PTH: Parathyroid hormone

Acknowledgements
We thank the staff in biochemistry laboratory for technical assistance.

Funding
This work was supported by grants from the National Natural Science Foundation of China (81370773, 81741054, 81571551, and 81501840), JiangSu province's science and technology support Program (Social Development BE2016675), Natural Science Foundation of Jiangsu province (BK20171217, BK20151206), Key talent of women's and children's health of JiangSu province (FRC201738), SuZhou clinical key disease diagnosis and treatment technology foundation (LCZX201611). The funders had no role in study design, data collection, preparation of the manuscript, and decision to publish.

Authors' contributions
ZB was responsible for collecting data and samples, participated in data analysis. FF participated in data analysis and helped to draft the manuscript.

ZX participated in collecting data and samples. CL carried out the human enzyme-linked immunosorbent assay (ELISA) and participated in data collection. XW carried out ELISA and participated in data collection. JC participated in data analysis. JP participated in data analysis and interpretation. JW participated in the design of the study and coordination. YL had primary responsibility for study design, performing the experiments, data analysis, interpretation of data, and writing of the manuscript. All authors read and approved the final manuscript.

Competing interests
The authors declare that they have no competing interests.

Author details
[1]Pediatric Intensive Care Unit, Children's Hospital of Soochow University, Suzhou, JiangSu province, China. [2]Institute of Pediatric Research, Children's Hospital of Soochow University, Suzhou, JiangSu province, China. [3]Department of nephrology, Institute of pediatric research, Children's Hospital of Soochow University, Suzhou, JiangSu province, China.

References
1. Singbartl K, Kellum JA. AKI in the ICU: definition, epidemiology, risk stratification, and outcomes. Kidney Int. 2012;81:819–25.
2. Alkandari O, Eddington KA, Hyder A, Gauvin F, Ducruet T, Gottesman R, et al. Acute kidney injury is an independent risk factor for pediatric intensive care unit mortality, longer length of stay and prolonged mechanical ventilation in critically ill children: a two-center retrospective cohort study. Crit Care. 2011;15:R146.
3. Sanchez-Pinto LN, Goldstein SL, Schneider JB, Khemani RG. Association between progression and improvement of acute kidney injury and mortality in critically ill children. Pediatr Crit Care Med. 2015;16:703–10.
4. Volpon LC, Sugo EK, Consulin JC, Tavares TL, Aragon DC, Carlotti AP. Epidemiology and outcome of acute kidney injury according to pediatric risk, injury, failure, loss, end-stage renal disease and kidney disease: Improving Global Outcomes Criteria in Critically Ill Children-A Prospective Study. Pediatr Crit Care Med. 2016;17:e229–38.
5. Coca SG, Yalavarthy R, Concato J, Parikh CR. Biomarkers for the diagnosis and risk stratification of acute kidney injury: a systematic review. Kidney Int. 2008;73:1008–16.
6. Li Y, Fu C, Zhou X, Xiao Z, Zhu X, Jin M, et al. Urine interleukin-18 and cystatin-C as biomarkers of acute kidney injury in critically ill neonates. Pediatr Nephrol. 2012;27:851–60.
7. Vanmassenhove J, Vanholder R, Nagler E, Van Biesen W. Urinary and serum biomarkers for the diagnosis of acute kidney injury: an in-depth review of the literature. Nephrol Dial Transplant. 2013;28:254–73.
8. Ataei N, Bazargani B, Ameli S, Madani A, Javadilarijani F, Moghtaderi M, et al. Early detection of acute kidney injury by serum cystatin C in critically ill children. Pediatr Nephrol. 2014;29:133–8.
9. Volpon LC, Sugo EK, Carlotti AP. Diagnostic and prognostic value of serum cystatin C in critically ill children with acute kidney injury. Pediatr Crit Care Med. 2015;16:e125–31.
10. Sellmer A, Bech BH, Bjerre JV, Schmidt MR, Hjortdal VE, Esberg G, et al. Urinary neutrophil gelatinase-associated Lipocalin in the evaluation of patent ductus arteriosus and AKI in very preterm neonates: a cohort study. BMC Pediatr. 2017;17:7.
11. Ronco C. Acute kidney injury: from clinical to molecular diagnosis. Crit Care. 2016;20:201.
12. Lameire NH, Vanholder RC, Van Biesen WA. How to use biomarkers efficiently in acute kidney injury. Kidney Int. 2011;79:1047–50.
13. Kovesdy CP, Quarles LD. FGF23 from bench to bedside. Am J Physiol Renal Physiol. 2016;310:F1168–74.
14. Zhang M, Hsu R, Hsu CY, Kordesch K, Nicasio E, Cortez A, et al. FGF-23 and PTH levels in patients with acute kidney injury: a cross-sectional case series study. Ann Intensive Care. 2011;1:21.
15. Leaf DE, Wolf M, Waikar SS, Chase H, Christov M, Cremers S, et al. FGF-23 levels in patients with AKI and risk of adverse outcomes. Clin J Am Soc Nephrol. 2012;7:1217–23.
16. Christov M, Waikar SS, Pereira RC, Havasi A, Leaf DE, Goltzman D, et al. Plasma FGF23 levels increase rapidly after acute kidney injury. Kidney Int. 2013;84:776–85.
17. Neyra JA, Moe OW, Hu MC. Fibroblast growth factor 23 and acute kidney injury. Pediatr Nephrol. 2015;30:1909–18.
18. Leaf DE, Christov M, Juppner H, Siew E, Ikizler TA, Bian A, et al. Fibroblast growth factor 23 levels are elevated and associated with severe acute kidney injury and death following cardiac surgery. Kidney Int. 2016;89:939–48.
19. Ali FN, Hassinger A, Price H, Langman CB. Preoperative plasma FGF23 levels predict acute kidney injury in children: results of a pilot study. Pediatr Nephrol. 2013;28:959–62.
20. Aregger F, Uehlinger DE, Witowski J, Brunisholz RA, Hunziker P, Frey FJ, et al. Identification of IGFBP-7 by urinary proteomics as a novel prognostic marker in early acute kidney injury. Kidney Int. 2014;85:909–19.
21. Konvalinka A. Urine proteomics for acute kidney injury prognosis: another player and the long road ahead. Kidney Int. 2014;85:735–8.
22. Lameire N, Vanmassenhove J, Van Biesen W, Vanholder R. The cell cycle biomarkers: promising research, but do not oversell them. Clin Kidney J. 2016;9:353–8.
23. Wetz AJ, Richardt EM, Wand S, Kunze N, Schotola H, Quintel M, et al. Quantification of urinary TIMP-2 and IGFBP-7: an adequate diagnostic test to predict acute kidney injury after cardiac surgery? Crit Care. 2015;19:3.
24. Kashani K, Al-Khafaji A, Ardiles T, Artigas A, Bagshaw SM, Bell M, et al. Discovery and validation of cell cycle arrest biomarkers in human acute kidney injury. Crit Care. 2013;17:R25.
25. Price PM, Safirstein RL, Megyesi J. The cell cycle and acute kidney injury. Kidney Int. 2009;76:604–13.
26. Liu Y, Wu M, Ling J, Cai L, Zhang D, Gu HF, et al. Serum IGFBP7 levels associate with insulin resistance and the risk of metabolic syndrome in a Chinese population. Sci Rep. 2015;5:10227.
27. Tucker BJ, Anderson CM, Thies RS, Collins RC, Blantz RC. Glomerular hemodynamic alterations during acute hyperinsulinemia in normal and diabetic rats. Kidney Int. 1992;42:1160–8.
28. Guidelines for developing admission and discharge policies for the pediatric intensive care unit. American Academy of Pediatrics. Committee on hospital care and section of critical care. Society of Critical Care Medicine. Pediatric section admission criteria task force. Pediatrics. 1999;103:840–2.
29. Bai Z, Zhu X, Li M, Hua J, Li Y, Pan J, et al. Effectiveness of predicting in-hospital mortality in critically ill children by assessing blood lactate levels at admission. BMC Pediatr. 2014;14:83.
30. Pollack MM, Patel KM, Ruttimann UE. PRISM III: an updated pediatric risk of mortality score. Crit Care Med. 1996;24:743–52.
31. Mehta RL, Kellum JA, Shah SV, Molitoris BA, Ronco C, Warnock DG, et al. Acute kidney injury network: report of an initiative to improve outcomes in acute kidney injury. Crit Care. 2007;11:R31.
32. Pickering JW, Endre ZH. Back-calculating baseline creatinine with MDRD misclassifies acute kidney injury in the intensive care unit. Clin J Am Soc Nephrol. 2010;5:1165–73.
33. Li Y, Wang J, Bai Z, Chen J, Wang X, Pan J, et al. Early fluid overload is associated with acute kidney injury and PICU mortality in critically ill children. Eur J Pediatr. 2016;175:39–48.
34. Bouvet Y, Bouissou F, Coulais Y, Seronie-Vivien S, Tafani M, Decramer S, et al. GFR is better estimated by considering both serum cystatin C and creatinine levels. Pediatr Nephrol. 2006;21:1299–306.
35. Finney H, Newman DJ, Thakkar H, Fell JM, Price CP. Reference ranges for plasma cystatin C and creatinine measurements in premature infants, neonates, and older children. Arch Dis Child. 2000;82:71–5.
36. Fatani T, Binjab A, Weiler H, Sharma A, Rodd C. Persistent elevation of fibroblast growth factor 23 concentrations in healthy appropriate-for-gestational-age preterm infants. J Pediatr Endocrinol Metab. 2015;28:825–32.
37. Lima F, El-Husseini A, Monier-Faugere MC, David V, Mawad H, Quarles D, et al. FGF-23 serum levels and bone histomorphometric results in adult patients with chronic kidney disease on dialysis. Clin Nephrol. 2014;82:287–95.
38. Samadfam R, Richard C, Nguyen-Yamamoto L, Bolivar I, Goltzman D. Bone formation regulates circulating concentrations of fibroblast growth factor 23. Endocrinology. 2009;150:4835–45.

39. Deng F, Finer G, Haymond S, Brooks E, Langman CB. Applicability of estimating glomerular filtration rate equations in pediatric patients: comparison with a measured glomerular filtration rate by iohexol clearance. Transl Res. 2015;165:437–45.

40. Dhayat NA, Ackermann D, Pruijm M, Ponte B, Ehret G, Guessous I, et al. Fibroblast growth factor 23 and markers of mineral metabolism in individuals with preserved renal function. Kidney Int. 2016;90:648–57.

41. Scialla JJ, Wolf M. Roles of phosphate and fibroblast growth factor 23 in cardiovascular disease. Nat Rev Nephrol. 2014;10:268–78.

42. Prie D, Forand A, Francoz C, Elie C, Cohen I, Courbebaisse M, et al. Plasma fibroblast growth factor 23 concentration is increased and predicts mortality in patients on the liver-transplant waiting list. PLoS One. 2013;8:e66182.

43. Md Ralib A, Pickering JW, Shaw GM, Endre ZH. The urine output definition of acute kidney injury is too liberal. Crit Care. 2013;17:R112.

44. Kellum JA. Diagnostic criteria for acute kidney injury: Present and Future. Crit Care Clin. 2015;31:621–32.

11

DTwP-HB-Hib: antibody persistence after a primary series, immune response and safety after a booster dose in children 18–24 months old

Hartono Gunardi[1*], Kusnandi Rusmil[2], Eddy Fadlyana[2], Soedjatmiko[1], Meita Dhamayanti[2], Rini Sekartini[1], Rodman Tarigan[2], Hindra Irawan Satari[1], Bernie Endyarni Medise[1], Rini Mulia Sari[3], Novilia Sjafri Bachtiar[3], Cissy B. Kartasasmita[2] and Sri Rezeki S. Hadinegoro[1]

Abstract

Background: The new combination of DTwP-HB-Hib vaccines has been developed in Indonesia following World Health Organization (WHO) recommendation and integrated into national immunization program. The aims of the study were to measure 1) antibody persistence 12–18 months after a primary series, 2) immune response and safety after a booster dose of DTwP-HB-Hib.

Methods: This was a multi-center, open-labeled, prospective, interventional study. Subjects who had received complete primary dose of DTwP-HB-Hib vaccine from the previous phase III trial were recruited in this trial. Subjects were given one dose of DTwP-HB-Hib (Pentabio®) booster at age 18–24 months old. Diphtheria, tetanus, pertussis, hepatitis B, *Hemophilus influenza* type B antibodies were measured before and after booster to determine antibody persistence and immune response. Vaccine adverse events were assessed immediately and monitored until 28 days after the booster recorded with parent's diary cards.

Results: There were 396 subjects who completed the study. Increased proportion of seroprotected subjects from pre-booster to post-booster were noted in all vaccine antigens: 74.5 to 99.7% for diphtheria; 100 to 100% for tetanus; 40.4 to 95.5% for pertussis; 90.2 to 99.5% for hepatitis B; and 97.7 to 100% for Hib. Common systemic adverse events (AEs) were irritability (23.7–25%) and fever (39.9–45.2%). Local AEs such as redness, swelling, and induration were significantly less common in the thigh group (7.7, 11.3, and 7.1%) than in the deltoid group (28.9, 30.7, and 25%) ($P < 0.001$). Most AEs were mild and resolved spontaneously within three-day follow-up period.

Conclusions: Booster of DTwP-HB-Hib vaccine at age 18–24 months is required to achieve and maintain optimal protective antibody. The vaccine is safe and immunogenic to be used for booster vaccination.

Keywords: Booster dose, DTwP-HB-Hib vaccine, Immunogenicity, Safety, Children

* Correspondence: hartono@ikafkui.net
[1]Department of Child Health, Faculty of Medicine, Universitas Indonesia/Dr. Cipto Mangunkusumo Hospital, Jl. Diponegoro No 71, Jakarta 10430, Indonesia
Full list of author information is available at the end of the article

Background

Infections related with vaccine-preventable diseases including hepatitis B, diphtheria, pertussis, and *Haemophilus influenzae* type B (Hib) were accounted for high morbidity and mortality among children younger than 5 years of age in many underdeveloped countries [1–4]. In accordance with the Expanded Program on Immunization (EPI) recommendation, the Indonesian National Immunization schedule comprises primary vaccination with 3 doses of DTwP-HB-Hib at 2, 3, and 4 months, followed by a booster dose at age 18–24 months. DTwP-HB-Hib is a new vaccine produced by Bio Farma, Indonesia, combining diphtheria toxoid and tetanus toxoid, inactive pertussis bacteria, hepatitis B surface antigen, and Hib [5]. Combination vaccine reduces number of injections, number of visits to healthcare or hospital, cost, discomfort; these ultimately increase parental compliance and improve immunization coverage rates [6, 7].

In India, DTwP-HB-Hib pentavalent vaccine trial showed low reactogenicity, minimal adverse events (AEs), and high level of seroprotective rates [8, 9]. A randomized trial in Latin American children has also shown that primary and booster vaccination with a DTwP-HB-Hib combination vaccine showed good seroprotection rate and good persistence of antibodies against all vaccine antigens. The vaccine was also well-tolerated as primary and booster doses [10]. However, immunogenicity and safety of DTwP-HB-Hib combined vaccine has not been well understood in Indonesia, especially as a booster dose vaccination.

This study was a follow-up of the previous phase III study [11]. The objectives of this study were to measure antibody persistence after three primary doses at age 2,4,6 months old, to asses immune response, and to ensure safety of a booster dose of DTwP-HB-Hib vaccine.

Methods

Study design and population

This open-labeled, prospective, interventional and multicenter trial was conducted from March to October 2014 in Bandung (Group A) and Jakarta (Group B), Indonesia. The main criteria of subjects were children aged 18–24 months who had received hepatitis B birth dose and three primary doses of DTwP-HB-Hib vaccine from the previous Phase III trial recruited from three primary health centers in Bandung (Group A) and three primary health centers in Jakarta (Group B) [11].

Exclusion criteria in this trial were mild, moderate or severe illness, especially infectious diseases or fever (axillary temperature ≥ 37.5°C on day 0); history of allergy to any components of the vaccines; history of uncontrolled coagulopathy or blood disorders contraindicated intramuscular injection; history of acquired immunodeficiency (including HIV infection); received a treatment likely to alter immune response in the previous 4 weeks (e.g. intravenous

immunoglobulin, blood-derived products or long-term corticosteroid therapy (> 2 weeks); receiving other vaccines within 1 month prior to trial enrollment; any abnormalities or chronic diseases determined by investigators that might interfere the trial objectives; and children with history of either diphtheria, tetanus, pertussis, Hib, and hepatitis B infection.

All subjects were recruited following written form of informed consent authorized by parents or legal representative after the explanation of the trial, potential risks, and his/her obligations. The study protocol had been approved by the Quality Assurance Division of Bio Farma, the Institutional Ethics Committee, and Indonesian Regulatory Authorities. This trial was conducted in accordance with ICH Good Clinical Practice guidelines and local regulatory requirement.

Study procedure

There were two visit in the study. At the first visit, blood sample from the subjects aged 18–24 months (12–18 months after the last dose of three primary doses) were obtained for pre-booster antibody titer. Then each subject was given one dose (0.5 mL) of DTwP-HB-Hib vaccine as a booster, intra-muscularly into the middle-third anterolateral region of the thigh or the deltoid muscle with a 23G, 25 mm needle. Anterolateral thigh muscle was the preferred site but the deltoid muscle could also serve as site of injection if pediatrician considered the muscle mass was adequate.

After the booster vaccination, all parents were given a diary to record information for any local and systemic adverse events (AEs) until 28 days after the vaccination. Collection of any local or systems AEs within 3 days after immunization were conducted by a nurse or designated person by home visit or phone call.

At the second visit (28 days after the booster vaccination), blood samples were acquired from the subjects to measure post-booster antibody. Subjects' diary were then reviewed for any notes in local and systemic AEs.

Study vaccine

DTwP-HB-Hib vaccine (Pentabio®, batch number 5010613, with expired date: June 2015) used in this study were manufactured by Bio Farma, Bandung, Indonesia. Each 0.5 mL dose of vaccine contained ≥30 IU of purified diphtheria toxoid, ≥60 IU of purified tetanus toxoid, ≥4 IU of inactivated *Bordetella pertussis*, 10 μg hepatitis B surface antigen (HBsAg, recombinant), 10 μg Hib in the form of polyribosil-ribitol-phosphate (PRP) conjugated to tetanus toxoid, 1.5 μg aluminium phosphate, 4.5 mg sodium chloride, and 0.025 mg thimerosal. Vaccines were stored in the refrigerator at temperature + 2° to + 8°C (as standart protocol) at the clinical trial centers to assure quality.

Blood sampling and antibody measurement

For each subject, 4 mL of blood was drawn in vacutainer tubes and then coded. After clotted at room temperature in 30 min to 2 h, each speciment was centrifuged at 3000 rpm for 15 min and the sera stored in cryotubes within 24 h after sampling. Sera of the coded samples were stored at – 20 C.

Serology antibody testing was started after the samples had been blinded. The blinding code and list were prepared by the statistician and witnessed by the investigators.

Serology assays, except for anti-HBs, were conducted in Immunology Laboratory of Product Evaluation Department of Bio Farma by technicians who were blinded to samples' visit. Test for anti-HBs was conducted in Prodia Laboratory which had been assessed by Quality Assurance of Bio Farma and had been certificated by ISO 9001 and National Accreditation Committee. Tetanus and diphtheria antibody were measured by validated ELISA. Pertussis antibody was measured by microagglutination method. Antibody to hepatitis B surface antigen (anti-HBs) was measured by Chemiluminescent Microparticle Immunoassay (CMIA) AUSAB reagent kit by Abbott. Antibody to PRP was measured by using Improved Phipps ELISA; a competitive ELISA was used for measuring the levels of serum antibody to *Haemophilus influenzae* type B. All antibody assays were validated previously.

Measures

This study measured antibody persistence after three doses of primary vaccinations and immune response after a single booster dose at 18–24 months of age. Antibody persistence is defined as having antibody level above the protective threshold for each given vaccination after primary doses. Immune response after booster was expressed in three parameters: (1) seroprotection (antibody level above the basic protective threshold), (2) seroconversion (conversion of seronegative to seropositive), and (3) four-times increase of antibody level [12, 13]. Primary outcome was the short-term or basic protective antibody, defined as: diphtheria antibody ≥ 0.01 IU/mL, tetanus antibody ≥ 0.01 IU/mL, pertussis antibody $\geq 1/40$, hepatitis B antibody ≥ 10 mIU/mL, and Hib antibody titer (PRP) ≥ 0.15 µg/mL. Secondary outcome was long-term or full protective antibody, defined as diphtheria antibody ≥ 0.1 IU/mL, tetanus antibody ≥ 0.1 IU/mL, pertussis antibody $\geq 1/80$, and Hib antibody titer (PRP) ≥ 1 µg/mL [14–18].

Safety assessment

Immediate local and systemic AEs 30 min after vaccination were observed and recorded at the health centers. A digital thermometer, a plastic measuring scale, and a diary card were provided for the parents to measure and record axillary temperature and the size of redness and swelling, respectively. Appearance, duration, and intensity

of any local or systemic adverse events (indicated as 1 [mild], 2 [moderate], or 3 [severe]) were recorded at home. Local reactions were defined as the presence of local pain, redness, induration, or swelling at the injection site; the systemic events were defined as the occurrence of fever (axillary temperature $\geq 38.0°C$), irritability, or both. Local and systemic AEs were recorded in two interval of time: (1) within 30 min to 72 h and (2) 72 h – 28 days after vaccination.

Vaccine AEs were retrieved by interviewing the parents and assessing the diary card during the follow-up visit.

Statistical analysis

The vaccine immunogenicity and safety were analyzed using intention-to-treat (ITT) and per-protocol (PP) analyses. Immunogenicity analysis was done regarding response to each vaccine antigen pre- and post-booster. Seroprotection, increase in antibody level, and seroconversion were calculated for each vaccine antigen. AEs were analyzed using Chi-square test with at least p value < 0.05 considered to be statistically significant.

Results

There were 399 subjects enrolled at the first visit. These subjects were subsequently divided into two groups: of 238 children in Group A (Bandung); and 161 children in Group B (Jakarta) (Fig. 1). One subject in Group B was lost to follow-up because the child moved to another province, and there were two subjects were withdrawn from the study. After these drop-outs, the total of the subjects were 396 subjects (238 subjects in Group A and 158 subjects in Group B). All subjects were of Indonesian race, with their demographic and baseline characteristics of presented in Table 1.

Diphtheria antibody

The protective level of diphtheria antibody was 74.5% prior the booster immunization, and 99.7% after booster. As many as 87.1% subjects had increment in their antibody titer ≥ 4 times, and all of seronegative subjects experienced seroconversion after the administration of booster dose. The Geometric Mean Titer (GMT) of the diphtheria antibody increased 9.4 times (0.054 to 0.508) after booster (Table 2).

Tetanus antibody

Subjects who had the protective level of tetanus antibody were 100%, before and after the booster. However, there was an increment of GMT 20.6 times, from 0.187 to 3.853 after the booster. The proportion of subjects with 4-times increased in antibody titer was 91.7% (Table 2).

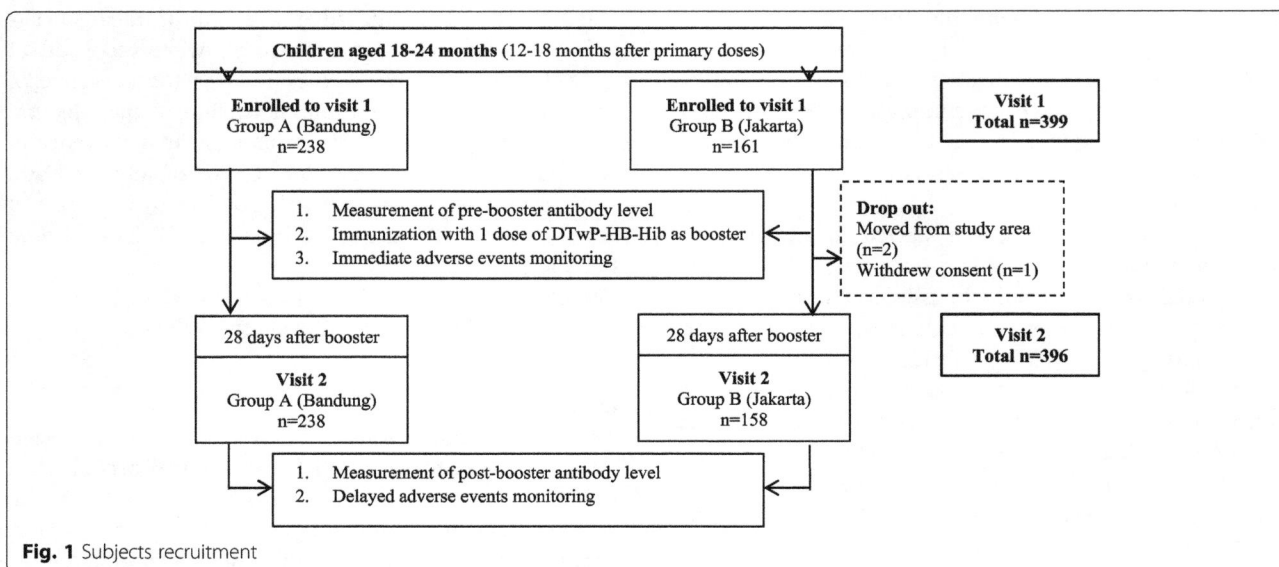

Fig. 1 Subjects recruitment

Pertussis antibody

The subjects with pertussis micro-agglutination level ≥ 1/40 were 40.4% before booster and this number was increased to 95.5% after the booster. There were 90.9% of the subjects whose antibody titer was increased four times from the baseline, and increased of the GMT by 22.8 times, from 28.086 to 639.145, after the booster (Table 2).

Hepatitis B antibody

Prior the booster, the proportion of subjects with protective hepatitis B antibody were 90.2, and 99.5% after booster. As many as 97.2% subjects had four times increment in their antibody titer and 94.9% subjects had seroconversion to seropositive. The GMT of hepatitis B antibody increased 65.6 times from 85.27 to 5591.13 after booster (Table 2).

Haemophilus influenza B

The proportion of subjects with protective level of Hib antibody was 97.7% before booster and 100% after booster. As many as 82.3% subject had 4-times increment in antibody titer, and all subjects who previously were seronegative had converted to seropositive after the booster.

Table 1 Demographic characteristics of subjects

Description	Group A (N = 238)	Group B (N = 161)	Total
Gender			
Male (n)	112	69	181 (45.4%)
Female (n)	126	92	218 (45.4%)
Age (months)			
Mean ± SD	19 ± 0.8	20 ± 0.9	20 ± 1.0
Min-max	18–22	19–24	18–24

Overall, the GMT of Hib antibody increased 20.7 times, from 3.399 to 70.226 after booster (Table 2).

Local adverse events 30 min after booster vaccination

Local AEs were reported in 17.3% subjects in the deltoid group and 14.9% subjects in the thigh group within 30 min after vaccination. The pain was reported in 10.8% subjects in the deltoid group and in 8.3% subjects in the thigh group. All of the symptoms were slightly less common in the thigh than in the deltoid group, but not statistically significant ($P = 0.515$).

Systemic adverse events 30 min after booster vaccination

The most common AE was irritability, which was found in 11.7% subjects of the deltoid group and 6.5% of the thigh group.

Local adverse events > 30 min to 72 h after booster vaccination

Local AEs were reported in 51.3% subjects of the deltoid group and 41.7% of the thigh group within 30 min to 72 h following booster vaccination. All of the symptoms were less common in the thigh group than in the deltoid group. Pain was reported in 43.4% subjects in the deltoid group and 38.1% subjects in the thigh group. Local AEs such as redness, swelling, and induration were found significantly less common in the thigh group (7.7, 11.3, 7.1%), compared to the deltoid group (28.9, 30.7, 25%) ($P < 0.001$) (Fig. 2).

Systemic adverse events > 30 min to 72 h after booster vaccination

There were 42.1% subjects in the deltoid group and 51.2% subjects in the thigh group who had systemic

Table 2 Summary of pre-booster and post-booster antibody level of tested antibodies[*]

Antibody	$N = 396$	Subjects (%)	95% CI	GMT(Range)
Diphtheria				
Pre-booster titer (IU/mL)				0.054 (0.047–0.061)
Anti-D ≥ 0.01[a]	295	74.5		
Anti-D ≥ 0.1[b]	81	20.5	16.8–24.7	
Post-booster titer (IU/mL)				0.508 (0.446–0.580)
Anti-D ≥ 0.01[a]	394	99.7		
Anti-D ≥ 0.1[b]	344	87.1	83.4–90.0	
Increased antibody titer[c]	345	87.1		
Seroconversion [d]	98/98	100		
Tetanus				
Pre-booster titer (IU/mL)				0.187 (0.169–0.206)
Anti-tetanus ≥0.01 [a]	396	100		
Anti-tetanus ≥0.1 [b]	286	72.2	67.4–76.2	
Post-booster titer (IU/mL)				3.853 (3.531–4.205)
Anti-tetanus ≥0.01 [a]	396	100		
Anti-tetanus ≥0.1 [b]	394	95.5	98.2–99.9	
Increased antibody titer[c]	363	91.7		
Pertussis				
Pre-booster titer				28.086 (24.791–31.812)
≥ 1/40[a]	160	40.4	35.7–45.3	
≥ 1/80[b]	99	25.0	21.0–29.5	
Post-booster titer				639.145 (550.807–741.651)
≥ 1/40[a]	378	95.5	92.9–97.1	
≥ 1/80[b]	367	92.7	89.7–94.9	
Increased antibody titer[c]	360	90.9		
Hepatitis B				
Pre-booster titer (mIU/mL)				85.27 (74.199–98.016)
Anti-HBs ≥10	357	90.2	86.8–92.7	
Post-booster titer (mIU/mL)				5591.13 (4761.02–6564.47)
Anti-HBs ≥10	394	99.5	97.8–98.7	
Increased antibody titer[c]	385	97.2		
Seroconversion[d]	37/39	94.9		
PRP-T (Hib)				
Pre-booster titer (µg/mL)				3.399 (3.006–3.844)
Anti-Hib ≥0.15[a]	387	97.7		
Anti-Hib ≥1.0[b]	343	86.6	82.9–89.6	
Post-booster titer (µg/mL)				70.226 (61.249–80.501)
Anti-Hib ≥0.15[a]	396	100		
Anti-Hib ≥1.0[b]	394	99.5	98.2–99.9	
Increased antibody titer[c]	326	82.3		
Seroconversion[d]	9/9	100		

[*]Based on per-protocol analysis
[a]Short-term protection, [b]Long-term protection, [c]Increased antibody titer ≥4 times from the pre-booster level, [d]Transition from seronegative to seropositive

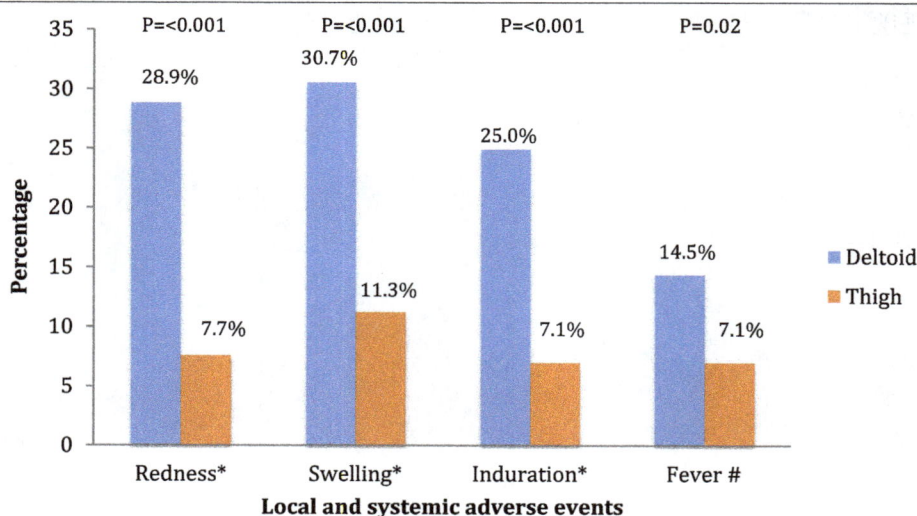

Fig. 2 Local and systemic adverse events
*local and systemic adverse events 30 minutes – 72 hours, #Systemic adverse events 72 hours – 28 days, No significant differences in AEs for pain, irritability, and others between deltoid and thigh group

adverse events in > 30 min to 72 h after vaccination. The most common systemic AE was irritability (39.9% in deltoid group and 45.2% in thigh group), with the second most common systemic AE was fever (23.7% in deltoid group and 25% in thigh group). Both occurred slightly less common in the deltoid groups.

Local adverse events > 72 h to 28 days after booster vaccination

No local reaction occurred within 72 h to 28 days after the booster vaccination, except 3 subjects with induration in deltoid group.

Systemic adverse events > 72 h to 28 days after booster vaccination

There were 23.2% subjects in the deltoid group and 16.1% subjects in the thigh group who were reported to have systemic adverse events within 72 h to 28 days after vaccination. The most common symptom reported was fever (14.5% in the deltoid group vs. 7.1% in the thigh group), which statistically more significant to be found in the deltoid group ($P = 0.02$, Fig. 2). All of the other symptoms (irritability and others) were found to be slightly less common in the thigh group than in the deltoid group, but not statistically significant.

Local and systemic reaction intensity

Most of the adverse events that were reported were mild and resolved spontaneously within the 72 h follow-up period. There was one report of acute diarrhea as a serious AE from Group B, which was classified as unrelated. The subject was recovered after several days of hospitalization. There was no other vaccine-related serious AE reported.

Discussion

This study has demonstrated good immunogenicity and tolerability of the new combined DTwP-HB-Hib (Pentabio®) vaccine as a booster dose in children age 18–24 months old. Although the persistence of antibody following the primary doses were quite good for each vaccine antigen, there were some degrees of waning immunity during 18–24 months of age, especially diphtheria and pertussis. This justified the necessity for a booster dose in children age 18–24 months.

In a previous study, 1 month after the third dose of DTwP-HB-Hib (Pentabio®) as primary vaccination, most of the children (84–100%) had protective antibody level [11]. In this study, the antibodies prior booster vaccinations were low in subjects with protective antibody of diphtheria and pertussis (74.5 and 40.4%, respectively). After the booster, the seroprotection had increased to 99.7 and 95.5% for diphtheria and pertussis, respectively. Another DTPw-HB-Hib vaccine trial in El Salvador finds the seroconversion of B. pertussis after a booster dose was 94.4%. In addition, a trial in Latin America finds at least 99.1% had the seroprotective level of antibodies against diphtheria, tetanus and hepatitis B [10, 19].

Currently, there is no international standard definition determined for the seroprotection for B. pertussis. A study in France used the ratio 1: 80 as cut-off, but in it was stated that the cut-off might had been too high as a cut-off [20]. We used the 1/40 as cut-off, only 40.4% of our subjects had the seroprotection before the booster doses. However, this proportion had increased greatly to 95.5% after one dose of booster. The 1/40 cut-off was also used in the pertussis outbreak in a university in Japan [21]. In this study, the protective titer was found in 92.7% subjects for the long-term protection of using the 1/80 cut-off.

The persistent protective antibody after three primary doses in children aged 18–24 months was 90.2% for hepatitis B, and 97.7% for Hib. After primary immunization, anti-HBs concentrations wane quite rapidly within the first year and more slowly thereafter. Even with the waning immunity, the immune memory to hepatitis B continues to persist over a longer period. Protective antibody had risen to 99.5 and 100%; and following the booster dose, seroconversion occurred in 94.9 and 100% subjects to hepatitis B and Hib, respectively, indicating effective priming and induction of the immune memory [22].

The long-term protection of tetanus from our earlier study was 72.2% 1 month after primary DTP-HB-Hib vaccination [11], then decreased to 72.2% at 18–24 months of age. After the booster, the long-term protection had increased to 95.5% with the GMT level of 3.85 IU/mL, which will provide 3–5 years of protection [23].

DTwP-HB-Hib vaccine was found to be highly immunogenic in our booster vaccination study. One month following the booster vaccination of this vaccine, our study finds at least 95.5% of the study subjects reached protective levels of antibodies (seroprotected) against the antigens employed in the vaccine. Another report of DTwP-HB-Hib (Quinvaxem®) immunogenicity showed 99.4% seroprotection at 1-month after booster dose [24]. Other previous studies of similar pentavalent vaccine in Latin America and Costa Rica showed that it could induce both persisting immunity and boostable memory, therefore provided an efficient and reliable way of implementing this vaccine to the routine program [25, 26].

In this study, no serious adverse events were considered related to vaccine or procedure. This study has demonstrated that the occurrence of local AEs such as redness, swelling and induration within 30 min – 72 h, and fever as systemic AE in 72 h – 28 days were significantly less common in the thigh group than in the deltoid group. This findings are similar to a previous study conducted in Vaccine Safety Datalink population that included 1.4 million of children in the USA, which finds injection in thigh was associated with significantly lower risk of local reaction to DTaP vaccination among children 1–2 years of age. This finding supports the current recommendation for thigh as intramuscular site injection in this age group [27].

The three doses of primary immunization and a booster dose of DTwP-HB-Hib were all immunogenic and well-tolerated by the study subjects. DTwP-HB-Hib vaccine is a suitable for immunization program in developing countries. [9, 11, 19, 25, 26].

Limitation of study
There were only 399 (69.4%) out of 575 subjects were recruited. A total of 396 subjects who completed the DTwP-HB-Hib primary immunization were analyzed.

The reason for this limitation was due to unpredictable heavy flood in the study area, which caused so many subjects moved to other areas. Regardless the limitation, this was the first study of immunogenicity and safety of DTwP-HB-Hib booster in Indonesian children.

Conclusions
The new combination of DTwP-HB-Hib vaccines (Pentabio) as a booster at age 18–24 months is necessary to achieve and maintain optimal protective antibody. The vaccine is safe and immunogenic to be used for booster vaccination.

Abbreviations
DTwP: Diphtheria tetanus whole-cell pertussis; GMT: Geometric mean titer; HB: Hepatitis B; HBsAg: Hepatitis B surface antigen; Hib: *Haemophilus influenza* type b; PRP: Polyribosil-ribitol-phosphate

Acknowledgments
PT Bio Farma was the funding stakeholder of this study. The authors would like to thank all of the children and parents who participated in this study, head of Bandung District Health Office, Jakarta Province Health Office, head and staff of Garuda, Ibrahim Adjie, Puter Primary Health Center in Bandung; head and staff of Jatinegara, Mampang, and Tebet Primary Health Center in Jakarta for their supports. We would also like to express our appreciation for the tremendous support of Indonesian National AEFI Committee as auditor of SAEs in this study. We also thank Mr. Hadyana Sukandar for his statistical work in this study, and Dr. Natharina Yolanda for her invaluable editorial assistance.

Funding
This study was funded by PT Bio Farma, number 06815/DIR/XII/2013 (Bandung site) and 06818/DIR/XII/2013 (Jakarta site).

Authors' contributions
KR was a national principal investigator and principal investigator in Bandung city. HG was the principal investigator in Jakarta city. KR, HG, EF, RMS, and NSB conceived the study and its design. HG, KR, EF, and S wrote and review the manuscript. MD and RT reviewed the design, recruited the subjects and conducted the study in Bandung city. S, RS, BEM and HIS reviewed the design, recruited the subjects and conducted the study in Jakarta city. SRH was the medical advisor of Jakarta site and reviewed the study and manuscript. CBK was the medical advisor of Bandung site and reviewed the study and manuscript. All authors read and approved the final manuscript.

Competing interests
Hartono Gunardi, Kusnandi Rusmil, Eddy Fadlyana, Soedjatmiko, Meita Dhamayanti, Rini Sekartini, Rodman Tarigan, Hindra Irawan Satari, Bernie Endyarni Medise, Cissy B Kartasasmita, Sri Rezeki S Hadinegoro, received grant support through their institutions. Rini Mulia Sari and Novilia Sjafri Bachtiar were employees of PT Bio Farma at the time of the conduct of this study and manuscript preparation.

Author details
[1]Department of Child Health, Faculty of Medicine, Universitas Indonesia/Dr. Cipto Mangunkusumo Hospital, Jl. Diponegoro No 71, Jakarta 10430, Indonesia. [2]Department of Child Health, Faculty of Medicine, Padjadjaran University/Dr. Hasan Sadikin Hospital, Jl. Pasteur No 38, Bandung 40161, Indonesia. [3]PT Bio Farma, Jl. Pasteur No 28, Bandung, Jawa Barat, Indonesia.

References
1. CDC. Haemophilus influenzae type B. In: Hamborsky J, Kroger A, Wolfe S, editors. Epidemiology and prevention of vaccine-preventable diseases. 13th ed. Washington D.C.: Public Health Foundation; 2015. p. 119–34.

2. Pertussis CDC. In: Hamborsky J, Kroger A, Wolfe S, editors. Epidemiology and prevention of vaccine-preventable diseases. 13th ed. Washington D.C.: Public Health Foundation; 2015. p. 261–78.

3. CDC. Hepatitis B. In: Hamborsky J, Kroger A, Wolfe S, editors. Epidemiology and prevention of vaccine-preventable diseases. 13th ed. Washington D.C.: Public Health Foundation; 2015. p. 149–74.

4. CDC. Diphtheria. In: Hamborsky J, Kroger A, Wolfe S, editors. Epidemiology and prevention of vaccine-preventable diseases. 13th ed. Washington D.C.: Public Health Foundation; 2015. p. 107–18.

5. Rusmil K, Fadlyana E, Bachtiar NS. Safety and immunogenicity of the DTP/HB/Hib combination vaccine: phase I study. Paed Indones. 2013;53:309–14.

6. Decker MD. Principles of pediatric combination vaccines and practical issues related to use in clinical practice. Pediatr Infect Dis J. 2001;20(11 Suppl):S10–8.

7. Marshall GS, Happe LE, Lunacsek OE, Szymanski MD, Woods CR, Zahn M, et al. Use of combination vaccines is associated with improved coverage rates. Pediatr Infect Dis J. 2007;26:496–500.

8. Gandhi DJ, Dhaded SM, Ravi MD, Dubey AP, Kundu R, Lalwani SK, et al. Safety, immune lot-to-lot consistency and non-inferiority of a fully liquid pentavalent DTwp-HepB-Hib vaccine in healthy Indian toddlers and infants. Hum Vaccin Imunother. 2016;12:946–54.

9. Sharma H, Yadav S, Lalwani S, Gupta V, Kapre S, Jadhav S, et al. A phase III randomized, controlled study to assess the immunogenicity and tolerability of DTPw-HBV-Hib, a liquid pentavalent vaccine in Indian infants. Vaccine. 2011;29:2359–64.

10. Espinoza F, Tregnaghi M, Gentile A, Abarca K, Casellas J, Collard A, et al. Primary and booster vaccination in Latin American children with a DTPw-HBV/Hib combination: a randomized controlled trial. BMC Infect Dis. 2010;10:297.

11. Rusmil K, Gunardi H, Fadlyana E, Soedjatmiko, Dhamayanti M, Sekartini R, et al. The immunogenicity, safety, and consistency of an Indonesia combined DTP-HB-Hib vaccine in expanded program on immunization schedule. BMC Pediatr. 2015;15:219.

12. Gold R, Barreto L, Ferro S, Thippawong J, Guasparini R, Meekison W, Russell M, et al. Safety and immunogenicity of a fully liquid vaccine containing five-component pertussis-diphtheria-tetanus-inactivated poliomyelitis-*Haemophilus influenzae* type b conjugate vaccines administered at two, four, six and 18 months of age. Can J Infect Dis Med Microbiol. 2007;18(4):241–8.

13. Nauta J. Statistics in clinical vaccine trials. New York: Springer; 2011. p. 28.

14. WHO. The immunological basis for immunization series. Module 2 diphtheria. Geneva: WHO; 2009. p. 4–19.

15. Borrow R, Balmer P, Roper MH. The immunological basis for immunization series. Module 3, tetanus. Geneva: WHO; 2006. p. 2–24.

16. WHO. The immunological basis for immunization series. Module 22 hepatitis B. Geneva: WHO; 2011. p. 2–15.

17. WHO. The immunological basis for immunization series. Module 4: pertussis update; 2009. p. 26–36.

18. WHO. Recommendations for the production and control of Haemophilus influenza type b conjugate vaccine. Technical Report Series 897 Annex 1. Geneva 2000;57–59.

19. Suarez E, Asturias EJ, Hilbert AK, Herzog C, Aeberhard U, Spyr C. A fully liquid DTPw-HepB-Hib combination vaccine for booster vaccination of toddlers in El Salvador. Rev Panam Salud Publica 2010;27:117–124.

20. Relyveld E, Oato NH, Guerin N, Coursaget P, Huet M, Gupta RK. Determination of circulating antibodies directed to pertussis toxin and of agglutinogens in children vaccinated with either the whole cell or component pertussis vaccine in France, Japan and Senegal. Vaccine. 1991;9:843–50.

21. Kamano H, Mori T, Maeta H, Taminato T, Ishida T, Kishimoto N, et al. Analysis of Bordetella pertussis agglutinin titers during an outbreak of pertussis at a university in Japan. Jpn J Infect Dis. 2010;63:108–12.

22. Marshall H, McIntyre P, Roberton D, Dinan L, Hardt K. Primary and booster immunization with a diphtheria, tetanus, acellular pertussis, hepatitis B (DTPa-HBV) and Haemophilus influenzae type b (Hib) vaccine administered separately or together is safe and immunogenic. Int J Infect Dis. 2010;14:e41–9.

23. World Health Organization (WHO). Tetanus vaccines: WHO position paper. February 2017. Wkly Epidemiol Rec. 2017;92:53–76.

24. Schmid DA, Macura-Biegun A, Rauscher M. Development and introduction of a ready-to-use pediatric pentavalent vaccine to meet and sustain the needs of developing countries–Quinvaxem(R): the first 5 years. Vaccine. 2012;30:6241–8.

25. Tregnaghi M, Lopez P, Rocha C, Rivera L, David MP, Ruttimann R, et al. A new DTPw-HB/Hib combination vaccine for primary and booster vaccination of infants in Latin America. Rev Panam Salud Publica. 2006;19:179–88.

26. Faingezicht I, Avila-Aguerro ML, Cervantes Y, Fourneau M, Clemens SA. Primary and booster vaccination with DTPw/HB/Hib pentavalent vaccine in Costa Rican children who had received a birth dose of hepatitis B vaccine. Rev Panam Salud Publica. 2002;12:247–57.

27. Jackson LA, Peterson D, Nelson JC, Marcy SM, Naleway AL, Nordin JD, et al. Vaccination site and risk of local adverse events in children 1 through 6 years of age. Pediatrics. 2013;131:283–9.

12

The paediatric version of Wisconsin gait scale, adaptation for children with hemiplegic cerebral palsy

Agnieszka Guzik[1]*[ID], Mariusz Drużbicki[1], Andrzej Kwolek[1], Grzegorz Przysada[1], Katarzyna Bazarnik-Mucha[1], Magdalena Szczepanik[1], Andżelina Wolan-Nieroda[1] and Marek Sobolewski[2]

Abstract

Background: In clinical practice there is a need for a specific scale enabling detailed and multifactorial assessment of gait in children with spastic hemiplegic cerebral palsy. The practical value of the present study is linked with the attempts to find a new, affordable, easy-to-use tool for gait assessment in children with spastic hemiplegic cerebral palsy. The objective of the study is to evaluate the Wisconsin Gait Scale (WGS) in terms of its inter- and intra-rater reliability in observational assessment of walking in children with hemiplegic cerebral palsy.

Methods: The study was conducted in a group of 34 patients with hemiplegic cerebral palsy. At the first stage, the original version of the ordinal WGS was used. The WGS, consisting of four subscales, evaluates fourteen gait parameters which can be observed during consecutive gait phases. At the second stage, a modification was introduced in the kinematics description of the knee and weight shift, in relation to the original scale. The same video recordings were rescored using the new, paediatric version of the WGS. Three independent examiners performed the assessment twice. Inter and intra-observer reliability of the modified WGS were determined.

Results: The findings show very high inter- and intra-observer reliability of the modified WGS. This was reflected by a lack of systematically oriented differences between the repeated measurements, very high value of Spearman's rank correlation coefficient $0.9 \leq |R| < 1$, very high value of ICC > 0.9, and low value of CV < 2.5% for the specific physical therapists.

Conclusions: The new, ordinal, paediatric version of WGS, proposed by the authors, seems to be useful as an additional tool that can be used in qualitative observational gait assessment of children with spastic hemiplegic cerebral palsy. Practical dimension of the study lies in the fact that it proposes a simple, easy-to-use tool for a global gait assessment in children with spastic hemiplegic cerebral palsy. However, further research is needed to validate the modified WGS by comparing it to other observational scales and objective 3-dimensional spatiotemporal and kinematic gait parameters.

Keywords: Hemiplegic gait, Cerebral palsy, Wisconsin gait scale, Intra-observer reliability, Inter-observer reliability, Scale adaptation

* Correspondence: agnieszkadepa2@wp.pl
[1]Institute of Physiotherapy, University of Rzeszów, Warszawska 26 a, 35-205 Rzeszów, Poland
Full list of author information is available at the end of the article

Background

Development of children with cerebral palsy is determined by the degree of intellectual disability and the associated learning ability which mostly determines participation in society [1, 2]. In functional assessment, mobility is also important [3, 4]. In cerebral palsy gait pattern functions and walking can be impaired. Neuromusculoskeletal impairment may be related to muscle function and control of voluntary movement functions [5].

Walking analysis in children with cerebral palsy is a sensitive tool used in evaluating progress resulting from treatment, enabling accurate assessment of functional performance and providing information necessary for determining goals of therapy [6, 7]. Advanced methods of assessing gait in this group of patients enable in-depth multidimensional analysis, yet they require considerable financial resources and sophisticated non-standard equipment due to which they are often inaccessible. On the other hand, observational gait analysis, an affordable method which can be used easily and quickly, is commonly applied in the clinical practice as a basic tool for evaluating gait abnormalities in children with cerebral palsy [6–8]. In observational gait assessment the examiner performs visual analysis of gait pattern using video recordings and scales describing abnormalities in both temporospatial and kinematic parameters of gait [9]. In the literature there are few studies focusing on tools designed for assessment of children with spastic cerebral palsy, therefore their clinical use cannot be judged based on the existing evidence [6]. Scales enabling assessment of gait in children with cerebral palsy include: Observational Gait Scale [10], Visual Gait Assessment Scale [11], Salford Gait Tool [12], and Edinburgh Visual Gait Scale [13]. However, the first of the above scales is only used for documenting gait changes in children after injections of botulinum toxin A [10], otherwise it does not present good results for all evaluated parameters [7]; the second scale can achieve only reliable sagittal plane assessment of the knee and ankle, yet it is not a reliable tool for assessing sagittal plane hip motion and additionally, it does not attempt to characterise either transverse or coronal plane deviations [11]; similarly the third scale is only sagittal plane observational gait assessment tool [12]; finally, the last scale on the above list is most extensive and detailed, enabling analysis in other planes of motion, yet just like all the others it focuses exclusively on assessing kinematic gait parameters [13]. In the clinical practice there is a need for a simple and practicable tool enabling detailed and multifactorial gait assessment (i.e. taking into account all the planes as well as spatiotemporal and kinematic parameters) and monitoring of rehabilitation outcomes, specifically in children with spastic hemiplegic cerebral palsy.

According to many researchers the Wisconsin Gait Scale (WGS) is a valuable tool which can easily be used in observational analysis, enabling detailed and accurate multidimensional assessment of spatiotemporal and kinematic gait parameters and evaluation of progress achieved in gait re-education by patients with hemiplegia, yet it is designed for adult stroke patients [14–18]. However, gait in children with hemiplegic cerebral palsy is very similar to gait observed in adult individuals with hemiplegia after stroke. It is also characterised by decreased walking speed, longer stance phase and shorter swing phase on unaffected leg, longer gait cycle, short stride, high stride frequency, impaired motor coordination and stability during walking; additionally, there are significant differences in kinematic parameters of the hip, knee, and ankle joints compared to healthy children [19, 20]. This observation provided inspiration for the present study and for the attempt to adapt WGS for children with spastic hemiplegic cerebral palsy. Moreover, it has been suggested by some researchers that psychometric properties of WGS should be analysed in more detail in patients with various neurological disorders other than stroke [21]. The practical value of the present study is linked with the attempts to find a new, affordable, easy-to-use tool for gait assessment in children with spastic hemiplegic cerebral palsy. The main objective of the study is to assess WGS in terms of its inter- and intra-observer reliability in observational gait analysis based on examination of video recording of children with hemiplegic cerebral palsy.

Methods
Participants and setting

The study was carried out in a group of 34 patients with hemiplegic cerebral palsy. It was conducted at University of Rzeszów gait laboratory. Inclusion criteria: hemiplegic cerebral palsy, age 6–18 years, independent gait without assistance of another person (with use of walking aids or AFO orthosis - if necessary). Exclusion criteria: cognitive function deficits impairing the ability to understand and follow instructions, unstable medical condition, differences in the length of extremities exceeding two centimetres, surgical intervention in the area of lower extremities less than 6 months before the study, and botulinum toxin treatment less than 6 months before the study. A total of 56 patients participating in outpatient rehabilitation program at the Regional Hospital No. 2 in Rzeszów in 2014–2016, who met the inclusion criteria, were selected out of 120 patients with a medical history of cerebral palsy. After being contacted by phone, 40 caregivers agreed for their children to participate in the gait analysis, however two children failed to report for the trial, one child gave up during the trial and in three cases complete gait assessment on WGS turned out impossible due to very poor quality of the recording. Finally, WGS based gait analysis was performed for 34 children. Figure 1 shows the flow of the subjects through the study and Table 1 presents the characteristics of the group.

Study protocol

The study protocol this prospective observational study was approved by the local Bioethics Commission of the Medical Faculty (5/2/2017) and was registered with Australian New Zealand Clinical Trials Registry (ACTRN12617000436370). Experimental conditions conformed to the Declaration of Helsinki.

Procedure and measures

At the first stage original version of WGS was used to assess gait in the patients with hemiplegic cerebral palsy. The WGS, consisting of four subscales, evaluates 14 gait parameters which can be observed in the affected leg during consecutive gait stages, i.e. stance, toe off, swing and heel strike phases. Additionally, it accounts for the use of hand held gait aid while walking. The first subscale is designed to assess spatiotemporal gait parameters, while kinematic parameters are evaluated by subscale one, two, three and four. In all the items of the scale subjects can score from 1 to 3 points, except for Item One (1–5 points) and Item Eleven (1–4 points). The total number of points falls between 13.35 and 42, a higher score corresponding to greater gait impairments.

WGS assessment was performed based on video material acquired during trails registered with synchronised system designed for three-dimensional recording (BTS Smart system). For this purpose, two video cameras were located at two different places and simultaneously recorded images in the frontal and sagittal plane. The camera recording the frontal plane view was set in the middle of the delineated route, at a distance of two metres from the path walked by the subject. The camera recording the sagittal plane view was placed in line with the path walked. In the case of each subject, six trials comprising at least three complete gait cycles were recorded. Ultimately, the video material used by the rater for gait assessment provided back and front as well as left and right side view of the patient. The subjects were asked to walk at a comfortable, self-selected speed, and they were allowed to use their own orthopaedic aids.

The video material was analysed and the WGS based gait assessment was performed independently by three physical therapists with expertise in gait disorders associated with hemiplegic cerebral palsy, and familiar with assessment criteria used in WGS. While assessing the video recordings the three physiotherapists were unable to perform complete assessment with the original version of WGS in all the children, and to determine the final score, because in two points of WGS (item 4 - weight shift to the affected side and item 11 - knee flexion from toe off to mid swing) the gait patterns did not match any description. Complete gait assessment

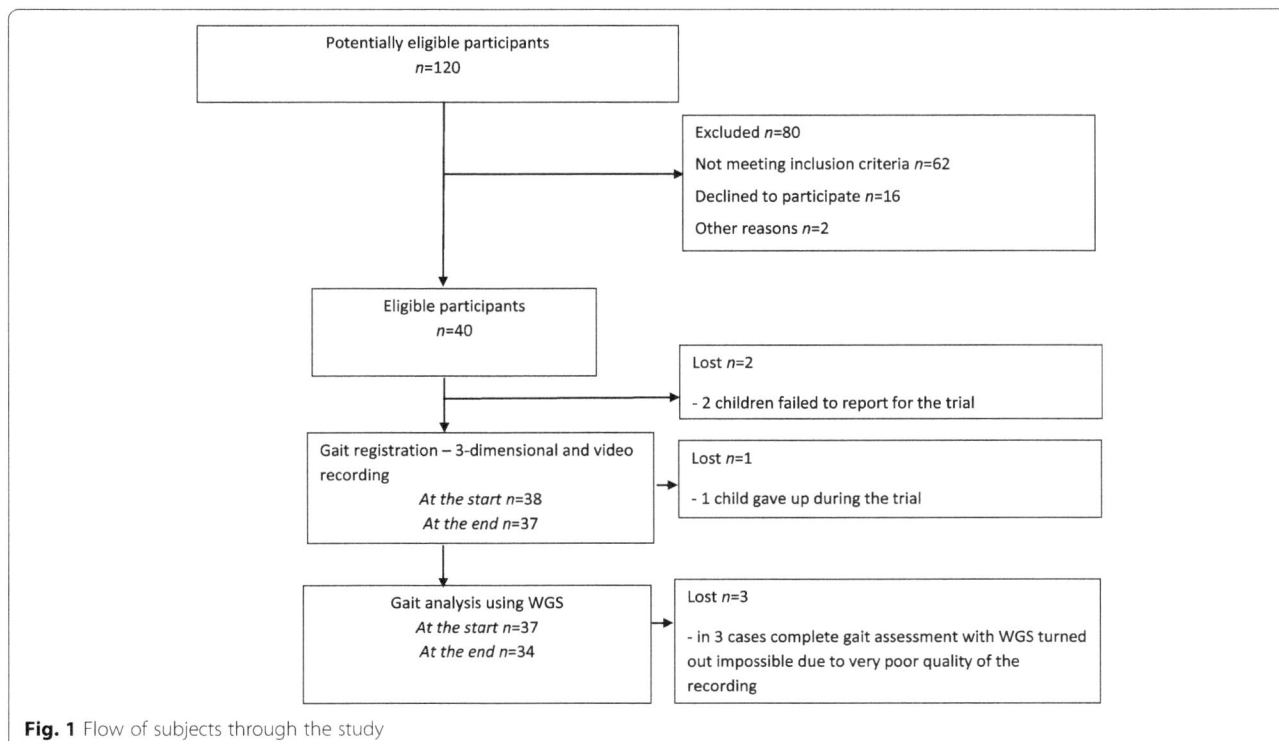

Fig. 1 Flow of subjects through the study

Table 1 Baseline characteristics of individuals with cerebral palsy

	Group ($n = 34$)
Age [years], mean (sd)	10.9 (2.3)
Sex [female/male]	19/15
Paretic limb [right/left]	19/15
Height [cm], mean (sd)	138.9 (11.26)
Weight [kg], mean (sd)	35.9 (8.97)
BMI [kg/m2], mean (sd)	18.79 (4.12)
Comorbidities:	
- epilepsy	3
- insulin dependent diabetes	1
- visual disorder corrected with glasses	5
- auditory limitations	1

sd standard deviation, *BMI* Body Mass Index

Table 2 Comparison of the original and modified Wisconsin Gait Scale in items 4 and 11

Original Wisconsin Gate Scale	Modified Wisconsin Gait Scale
4. Weight Shift to the Affected Side, with or without a gait aid	4. Weight Shift to the weight bearing leg, with or without a gait aid
1 = Full shift	1 = Full shift
2 = Decreased shift: head and trunk crosses midline, but not over the affected foot	2a = Decreased shift: head and trunk crosses midline, but not over the affected foot
3 = Very limited shift: head and trunk does not cross midline, minimal weight shift in the direction of the affected side	2b = Decreased shift: head and trunk crosses midline, but not over the unaffected foot, head and trunk for part of stance phase leaning towards the affected side
	3a = Very limited shift: head and trunk does not cross midline, minimal weight shift in the direction of the affected side
	3b = Very limited shift: head and trunk does not cross midline, minimal weight shift in the direction of the unaffected side, head and trunk during entire stance phase leaning towards the affected side
11. Knee flexion from toe off to mid swing	11. Knee flexion from toe off to mid swing
1 = normal (affected knee flexes equally to unaffected side)	1 = normal (affected knee flexes equally to unaffected side)
2 = some (affected knee flexes, but less than unaffected knee)	2a = some (affected knee flexes, but less than unaffected knee)
3 = minimal (minimal flexion noted in affected knee (hardly visible)	2b = some (affected knee flexes, but more than unaffected knee)
	3a = minimal (minimal flexion noted in affected knee (hardly visible)
	3b = maximal (maximal flexion noted in affected knee (well visible)
4 = none (knee remains in extension throughout swing)	4 = none (knee remains in extension throughout swing)

could not be performed in 16 out of the 34 children in the study group. More specifically in item 4 of WGS some subjects presented with decreased shift or very limited shift but not over the affected foot but over the unaffected foot, because head and trunk for part of the duration of the stance phase or for the entire duration of the stance phase were leaning towards the affected side. Assessment in item 11 of WGS was impossible due to the fact that some patients were found with increased unaffected knee flexion or maximal flexion in affected knee rather than with decreased or minimal flexion in affected knee.

Due to the fact that in the first phase it was impossible to perform complete assessment of gait pattern with WGS, including items 4 and 11, each of these points was discussed in detail and then points 4 and 11 were expanded and a common opinion was specified with regard to the gait patterns observed in the subjects. At the second stage of the study a modified WGS was introduced and the same video recordings were rescored by the same three physiotherapists, after 2 weeks, using the new, modified paediatric version of WGS (Table 2).

Inter-observer reliability of the modified WGS in the assessment of children with hemiplegic cerebral palsy was determined by comparing evaluation results acquired by three examiners independently analysing video recordings. Intra-observer reliability of the modified WGS in the assessment of children with hemiplegic cerebral palsy was determined by comparing evaluation results acquired by three examiners during two assessments carried out by each of them 2 weeks apart (test-retest).

Statistical analysis

The scores were subjected to statistical analyses performed using Statistica 10.0 (StatSoft, Poland). Wilcoxon test was applied to assess test-retest differences independently for each of the physiotherapists as well as the

relevant differences between the specific physiotherapists. Significance of correlations between the results was examined with Spearman's correlation coefficient. Correspondence of test-retest results, for each of the physiotherapists and between the specific physiotherapists, was assessed with intra-class correlation coefficient (ICC) and value of intra-subject coefficient of variation (CV), which is calculated as a quotient of standard deviation and mean value in both measurements and shows relative variation between results obtained in both examinations. In order to determine what difference in two WGS-based measurements could be considered non-accidental, the minimal detectable change (MDC) was calculated. Repeatability of the results was calculated using Bland- Altman method. Statistical significance was assumed for $p < 0.05$.

Sample size

The minimum size of the sample was calculated taking into account the number of children with spastic hemiplegic cerebral palsy treated at the rehabilitation clinic at Regional Hospital No. 2 in Rzeszów in 2014–2016. A fraction size of 0.8 was used, with a maximum error of 5%, a sample size of 30 patients was obtained. The study involved 34 children.

Results

General results

WGS score was determined for each patient six times, i.e. twice by three different physiotherapists. The following table presents the basic descriptive statistics characterizing WGS distribution in the specific series of measurement. The mean level of WGS score in the specific measurement series was very similar – on average differences between them were not higher than 0.5 point. There was also similar level of variation (standard deviation) - Table 3.

Analysis of test vs. re-test

Comparison of results obtained using test-retest method showed no systematically oriented changes between the results determined during the two exams by any of the physiotherapists. Therefore, there are no grounds for claiming that the first examination produced higher or lower results than the second examination. Very low value of standard deviation in the differences between the two exams (for the specific physiotherapists amounting to 0.60; 0.72 and 0.94, respectively) allows a conclusion that deviations between the test-retest results do not exceed a few percent in relation to the outcome value (on average amounting to approx. 19.5 points) – Table 4.

Findings of comparative analysis of the test-retest results are also shown in Table 5, which presents the result of Wilcoxon test, Spearman's rank correlation coefficient with assessment of significance, intra-class correlation coefficient (ICC), and value of intra-subject coefficient of variation (CV) and minimal detectable change (MDC), between the two examinations (test-retest). All the

figures show very good test-retest reliability. The findings show no systematically oriented differences between the two examination (insignificant value of Wilcoxon test), very high correlation between the scores (value of Spearman's rank correlation coefficient $0.9 \leq |R| < 1$), very high ICC, low value of CV (up to 2.5% for the specific physiotherapists) and value of MDC up to 2 points. The Bland- Altman plots for comparison of test-retest results, separately for each physiotherapist are shown in Fig. 2.

Comparison of assessments made by the physiotherapists during the test and the retest

Analysis of consistency between scores determined by the specific physiotherapists during exam 1 (test) and exam 2 (retest) showed no systematically oriented differences between WGS values assigned to the patients by various physiotherapists; *p*-values calculated with Wilcoxon test significantly exceed 0.05 (Table 6).

Another important issue is the fact that correlations between assessments performed by the physiotherapists in exam 1 (test) and exam 2 (retest) were very high (value of Spearman's rank correlation coefficient $0.9 \leq |R| < 1$); only in exam 2 (retest) the correlation Physiotherapist 3 vs. Physiotherapist 2 was $0.7 < |R| < 0.9$. A wider range of statistics related to the paired comparison of assessments performed by the specific physiotherapists is presented in Table 7. The values of all the defined measures and coefficients show very high consistency of the results determined by the physiotherapists. The Bland- Altman plots for paired comparison of the scores between the specific physiotherapists in exam 1 (test) and in exam 2 (retest) are shown in Figs. 3 and 4.

Discussion

Researchers have been looking for an optimal tool designed for systematic assessment of gait in children with spastic hemiplegic cerebral palsy. The inspiration for this study was the fact that whereas classifications taking into account community involvement, activity, hand function as well as secondary conditions in children with cerebral

Table 3 Distribution of WGS in the specific measurement series

WGS	$\bar{x}$	Me	sd	min	max	95% c.i.
Physiotherapist 1 / exam 1	19.58	19.10	3.24	15.35	25.10	(18.45; 20.71)
Physiotherapist 1 / exam 2	19.64	19.10	3.05	15.35	25.10	(18.57; 20.70)
Physiotherapist 2 / exam 1	19.46	19.10	3.17	14.35	25.10	(18.35; 20.56)
Physiotherapist 2 / exam 2	19.75	19.60	3.10	15.10	25.10	(18.67; 20.83)
Physiotherapist 3 / exam 1	19.69	19.10	3.18	14.35	26.10	(18.58; 20.80)
Physiotherapist 3 / exam 2	19.86	20.23	3.26	14.35	26.10	(18.73; 21.00)

$\bar{x}$ – arithmetic mean, *Me* median, *sd* standard deviation, *min* minimum, *max* maximum, 95% c.i. – estimation of mean value in the entire population constructed as 95% confidence intervals

Table 4 Comparison of test-retest results determined independently for each physiotherapist

	$\bar{x}$	Me	sd	min	max	95% c.i.
WGS (Physiotherapist 1)						
test	19.58	19.10	3.24	15.35	25.10	(18.45; 20.71)
re-test	19.64	19.10	3.05	15.35	25.10	(18.57; 20.70)
re-test vs. test ($p = 0.4413$)	0.06	0.00	0.60	− 1.00	2.00	(− 0.15; 0.27)
WGS (Physiotherapist 2)						
test	19.46	19.10	3.17	14.35	25.10	(18.35; 20.56)
re-test	19.75	19.60	3.10	15.10	25.10	(18.67; 20.83)
re-test vs. test ($p = 0.0597$)	0.29	0.00	0.72	−1.00	2.00	(0.04; 0.54)
WGS (Physiotherapist 3)						
test	19.69	19.10	3.18	14.35	26.10	(18.58; 20.80)
re-test	19.86	20.23	3.26	14.35	26.10	(18.73; 21.00)
re-test vs. test ($p = 0.3109$)	0.18	0.00	0.94	−2.00	3.00	(−0.15; 0.50)

$\bar{x}$ – arithmetic mean, *Me* median, *sd* standard deviation, *min* minimum, *max* maximum, 5% c.i. – estimation of mean value in the entire population constructed as 95% confidence intervals, *p* – Wilcoxon test probability values

palsy are widely available in the literature [22–27], there are few scales focused on assessment of the walking pattern in this group of patients [7, 10–13]. Furthermore, there is no specific scale enabling multivariate assessment of both spatiotemporal and kinematic gait parameters designed typically for children with spastic hemiplegic cerebral palsy.

Observation gait scales are an auxiliary tool in the gait analysis of children over 6 years of age, allowing for a basic assessment of the gait pattern [11]. The scales available for assessing walking skills in children with cerebral palsy focus only of examining kinematic gait parameters [10–13]. On the other hand, WGS is a simple, ordinal scale based on observation. The scale does not measure specific spatiotemporal and kinematic parameters, yet it enables a subjective assessment and categorisation of gait patterns into orderly groups, providing however only global description of gait. Thus the scale describes positions of parts of the lower limbs and joints in the gait cycle of the affected and unaffected legs. Descriptions of the walking pattern refer mainly to the symmetry of the gait. The scale is divided into subscales which may correspond to temporal (stance time), spatial (step length, stance width) and kinematic parameters of

Table 5 Comparison of test-retest results, separately for each physiotherapist

Physiotherapist	Comparison of test-retest				
	Wilcoxon test	Rank correlation	ICC	CV	MDC
1	0.4413	0.97 ($p < 0.001$)	0.9821	1.6%	1.20
2	0.0597	0.97 ($p < 0.001$)	0.9701	2.1%	1.52
3	0.3109	0.95 ($p < 0.001$)	0.9575	2.3%	1.82

p – test probability values, *ICC* intraclass correlation coefficient, *CV* intrasubject coefficient of variation, *MDC* minimal detectable change (calculated for 95% confidence level)

hip, knee, ankle and pelvis joints, in the sagittal, transverse, and frontal planes [14–18, 21].

The present study is part of a larger research project where the authors have performed detailed assessment of test-retest reliability and internal consistency of WGS [28], and have examined 3-diemensional gait parameters in relation to WGS-based observational gait assessment in patients with post-stroke hemiparesis [15]. The above studies demonstrated that, in addition to being an easy-to-use tool, WGS can effectively assess walking ability in hemiparetic patients after stroke, and it is characterised by high internal consistency and test-retest reliability. Ultimately, it was also shown that there was a moderate and good level of correspondence between spatiotemporal parameters identified during 3-dimensional gait examination and results of gait assessment based on observational WGS [15, 28]. The acquired results have encouraged the authors to carry out further research to investigate feasibility of WGS based assessment in other groups of neurological patients with hemiplegia. Furthermore, Gor-García-Fogeda and co-authors emphasize the importance of this type of research and recommend more in-depth analysis of psychometric properties of observational gait scales, including WGS, in patients with varied neurological disorders other than stroke [21]. In view of the above, the present study is the first report from research designed as an attempt to adapt WGS scale for children with spastic hemiplegic cerebral palsy.

The present findings show very good intra-observer reliability of the modified WGS (consistency of test-retest results independently for each physiotherapist). This was reflected by a lack of systematically oriented differences between the test-retest measurements (insignificant result in Wilcoxon test), very high value of Spearman's rank correlation coefficient $0.9 \leq |R| < 1$, very

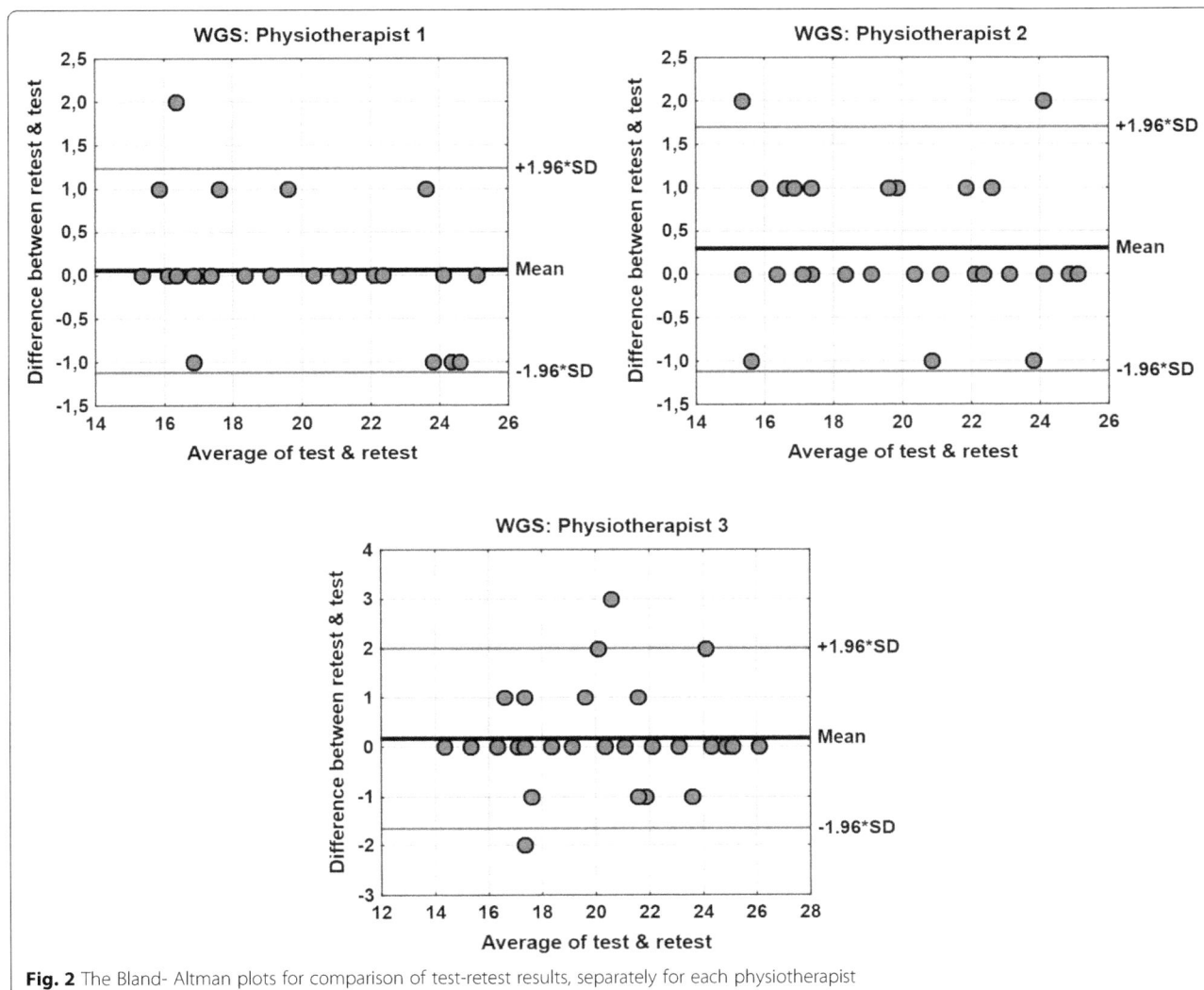

Fig. 2 The Bland- Altman plots for comparison of test-retest results, separately for each physiotherapist

high value of ICC > 0.9, and low value of CV < 2.5% for the specific physical therapists. It was also shown there was very good inter-observer reliability of the modified WGS (consistency of results between the specific physiotherapists in the first exam and in the second exam).

This was also reflected by a lack of systematically oriented differences between WGS scores assigned to the patients by the different physiotherapists (insignificant result in Wilcoxon test), very high value of Spearman's rank correlation coefficient. Furthermore, the

Table 6 Paired comparison of the scores determined by the specific physiotherapists in exam 1 (test) and exam 2 (retest)

	$\bar{x}$	Me	sd	min	max	95% c.i.
WGS (total) exam 1 (test)						
Physiotherapist 2 vs. Physiotherapist 1 (p = 0.4446)	−0.12	0.00	0.81	−2.00	2.00	(−0.40; 0.16)
Physiotherapist 3 vs. Physiotherapist 2 (p = 0.2575)	0.23	0.00	1.15	−3.00	3.00	(−0.17; 0.63)
Physiotherapist 3 vs. Physiotherapist 1 (p = 0.3078)	0.11	0.00	0.58	−1.00	1.00	(−0.09; 0.31)
WGS (total) exam 2 (retest)						
Physiotherapist 2 vs. Physiotherapist 1 (p = 0.6529)	0.12	0.00	0.91	−1.00	3.00	(−0.20; 0.44)
Physiotherapist 3 vs. Physiotherapist 2 (p = 0.6292)	0.11	0.00	1.32	−4.00	2.00	(−0.35; 0.57)
Physiotherapist 3 vs. Physiotherapist 1 (p = 0.1702)	0.23	0.00	1.08	−3.00	2.00	(−0.15; 0.60)

$\bar{x}$ – arithmetic mean, Me median, sd standard deviation, min minimum, max maximum, 5% c.i. – estimation of mean value in the entire population constructed as 95% confidence intervals, p – Wilcoxon test probability values

Table 7 Paired comparison of the scores between the specific physiotherapists in exam 1 (test) and in exam 2 (retest)

	Wilcoxon test	Rank correlation	ICC	CV	MDC
Physiotherapist	Exam 1 (test)				
2 vs. 1	0.4446	0.96 ($p < 0.001$)	0.9685	2.1%	1.59
3 vs. 2	0.2575	0.92 ($p < 0.001$)	0.9335	3.1%	2.26
3 vs. 1	0.3078	0.98 ($p < 0.001$)	0.9835	1.6%	1.15
Physiotherapist	Exam 2 (re-test)				
2 vs. 1	0.6529	0.94 ($p < 0.001$)	0.9564	2.4%	1.77
3 vs. 2	0.6292	0.88 ($p < 0.001$)	0.9162	3.5%	2.49
3 vs. 1	0.1702	0.91 ($p < 0.001$)	0.9410	2.9%	2.05

p – test probability values, *ICC* intraclass correlation coefficient, *CV* intra-subject coefficient of variation, *MDC* minimal detectable change (calculated for 95% confidence level)

determined values of ICC and CV also reflect very high consistency of the results between the physiotherapists.

Evaluation of intra and inter-rater reliability has been in focus of numerous studies related to available scales enabling assessment of gait in children with cerebral palsy. For example, Araújo and co-authors examined intra- and inter-rater reliability of the Observational Gait Scale (OGS) for children with spastic cerebral palsy. In accordance with the study design, the OGS was applied in the process of rating 23 videos of children with spastic diplegia and hemiplegic cerebral palsy. The assessment was performed in two sessions, by four physical therapists, who had been trained on the use of the OGS and instructed about the significance of all the items of the scale. In order to avoid memory bias the second evaluation was performed 2 weeks after the first one. Each rater was provided with a CD containing the OGS file as well as video material presenting frontal and sagittal plane view of each subject examined. The authors

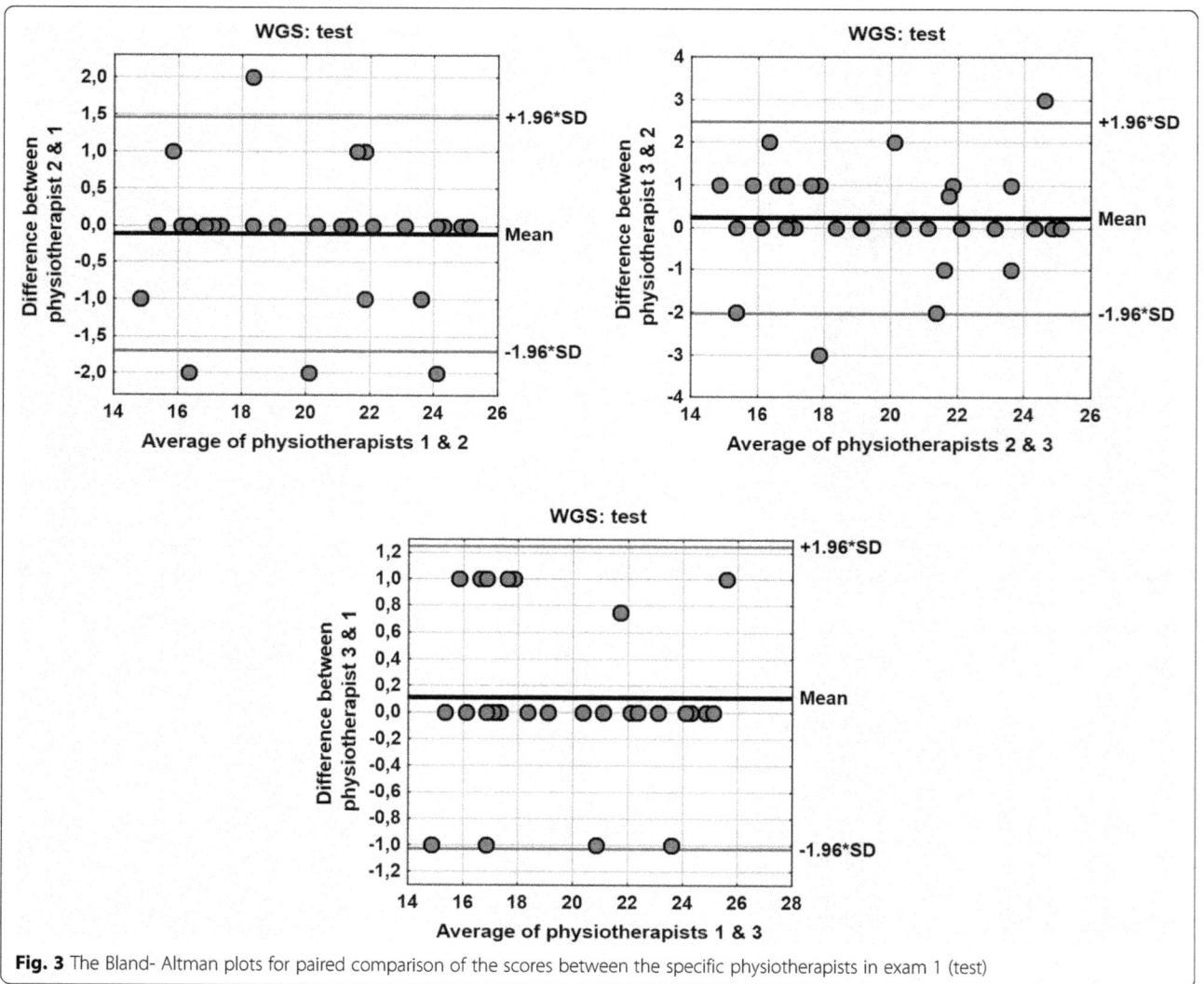

Fig. 3 The Bland- Altman plots for paired comparison of the scores between the specific physiotherapists in exam 1 (test)

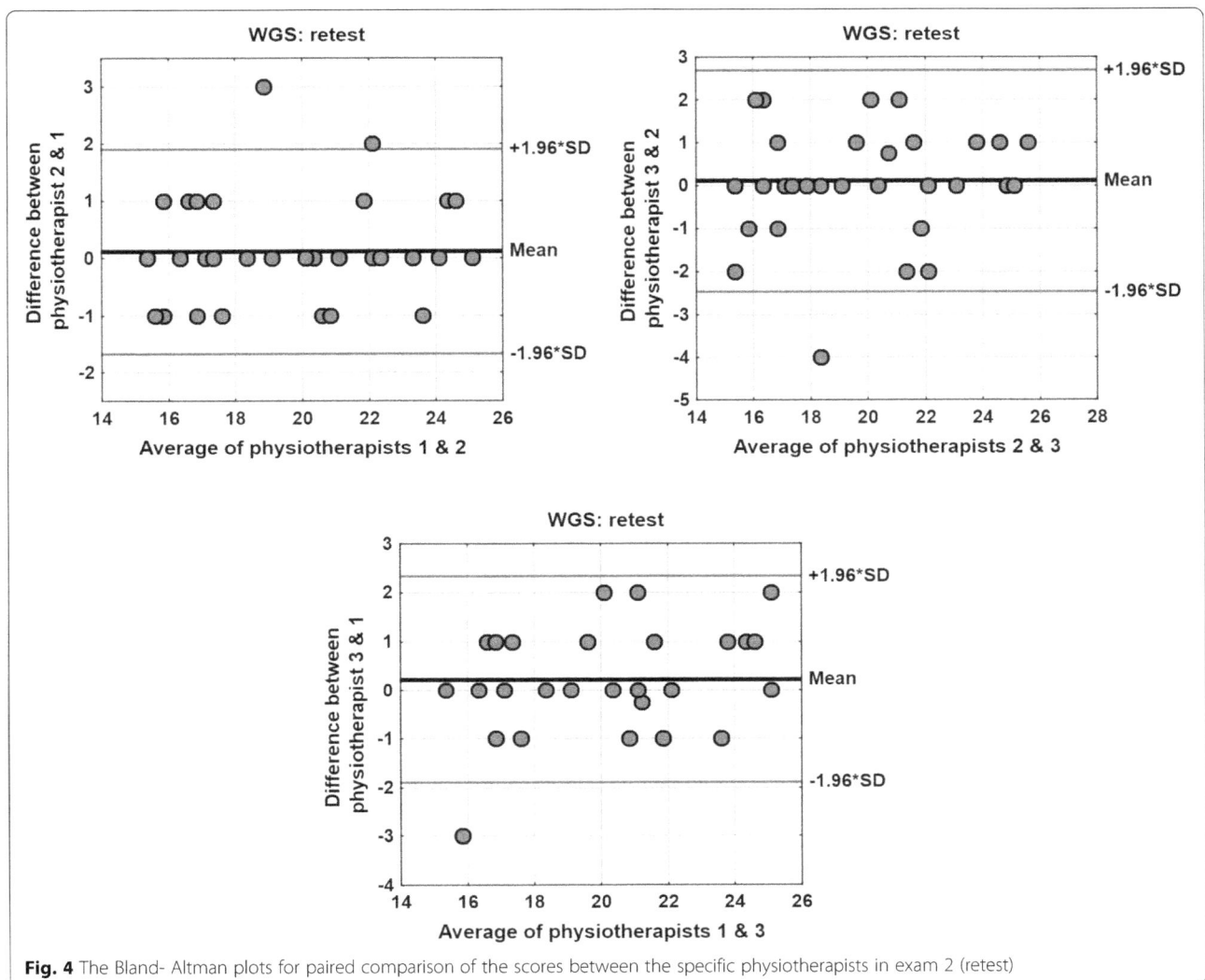

Fig. 4 The Bland- Altman plots for paired comparison of the scores between the specific physiotherapists in exam 2 (retest)

established that the OGS presented very good intra-rater reliability for the hip ($r = 0.73$), knee ($r = 0.77$) and ankle/foot complex ($r = 0.79$), and good reliability for the pelvis ($r = 0.59$). Very good inter-rater reliability was identified for the knee ($r = 0.65$), and ankle/foot complex ($r = 0.68$), while good reliability was shown for the hip ($r = 0.48$). All of the above relationships were statistically significant [29]. Similar issues were investigated by Dickens and Smith who evaluated reliability of a visual assessment of gait based on the Physician Rating Scale in children with hemiplegic cerebral palsy. Evaluation of the Visual Gait Assessment Scale (VGAS), in this case performed by two expert raters, was based on video material showing 31 hemiplegic children, ranging in age from 5 to 17 years. The version used in the study was developed with the aim to evaluate the position of hip, knee, ankle and foot in the sagittal plane. The highest intra-rater reliability was demonstrated in the case of initial contact and foot contact during the stance phase. On the other hand, better inter-rater

reliability was reported for foot contact during stance and heel-off during the terminal stance. Conversely, poor reliability was found for hip parameters, particularly in the swing phase [11]. Likewise, Brown and colleagues evaluated reliability of the VGAS for children with hemiplegic cerebral palsy when used by experienced and inexperienced observers. Four experienced and six inexperienced observers viewed videotaped footage of four children with hemiplegic cerebral palsy on two separate occasions. The experienced observers generally had higher inter-observer and intra-observer reliability than the inexperienced observers. Both groups showed higher agreement for assessments made at the ankle and foot than at the knee and hip. The authors argue that VGAS can be used by inexperienced observers but is limited to observations in the sagittal plane and by poor reliability at the knee and hip for experienced and inexperienced observers [30].

The present findings suggest that WGS, originally designed for gait assessment in adults after stroke, can in fact be successfully used in children with spastic hemiplegic cerebral palsy. This provides encouragement for the authors to carry out further research focused on detailed analysis of psychometric properties of the new, paediatric version of WGS applied in this group of patients.

Conclusion

The findings show very good intra- and inter-observer reliability of the modified WGS. The new, ordinal, paediatric version of WGS, proposed by the authors, seems to be useful as an additional tool that can be used in qualitative observational gait assessment of children with spastic hemiplegic cerebral palsy. Practical dimension of the study lies in the fact that it proposes a simple, easy-to-use tool for a global gait assessment in children with spastic hemiplegic cerebral palsy. However, further research is needed to validate the modified WGS by comparing it to other observational scales and objective 3-dimensional spatio-temporal and kinematic gait parameters.

Abbreviations

CV: Intra-subject coefficient of variation; ICC: Intra-class correlation coefficient; WGS: Wisconsin Gait Scale

Funding

This research did not receive any specific grant from funding agencies in the public, commercial, or not-for-profit sectors.

Authors' contributions

AG: conceptualized and designed the study, ran the data collection, performed the analysis, drafted the initial manuscript, and approved the final manuscript as submitted. MD: carried out the analyses, drafted the initial manuscript, and approved the final version as submitted. AK: supervised the project and reviewed and revised the manuscript making important intellectual contributions. GP: coordinated and supervised data collection, critically reviewed the manuscript, and approved the final manuscript as submitted. KBM and MS: ran the data collection, performed the analysis and approved the final manuscript. AWN and MS: supervised data analyses and reviewed and revised the manuscript. All authors read and approved the final manuscript.

Competing interests

The authors declare that they have no competing interests.

Author details

[1]Institute of Physiotherapy, University of Rzeszów, Warszawska 26 a, 35-205 Rzeszów, Poland. [2]Rzeszów University of Technology, Rzeszów, Poland.

References

1. Tan SS, Wiegerink DJ, Vos RC, Smits DW, Voorman JM, Twisk JW, et al. Developmental trajectories of social participation in individuals with cerebral palsy: a multicentre longitudinal study. Dev Med Chilc Neurol. 2014;56(4):370–7.
2. Vos RC, Becher JG, Ketelaar M, Smits DW, Voorman JM, Tan SS, et al. Developmental trajectories of daily activities in children and adolescents with cerebral palsy. Pediatrics. 2013;132(4):e915–e23.
3. Maltais DB, Wiart L, Fowler E, Verschuren O, Damiano DL. Health-related physical fitness for children with cerebral palsy. J Child Neurol. 2014;29: 1091–100.
4. Badia M, Riquelme I, Orgaz B, Acevedo R, Longo E, Montoya P. Pain, motor function and health-related quality of life in children with cerebral palsy as reported by their physiotherapists. BMC Pediatr. 2014;27:192.
5. Zhou J, Butler EE, Rose J. Neurologic correlates of gait abnormalities in cerebral palsy: implications for treatment. Front Hum Neurosci. 2017;17:103.
6. Rathinam C, Bateman A, Peirson J, Skinner J. Observational gait assessment tools in paediatrics- a systematic review. Gait Posture. 2014;40:279–85.
7. Bella GP, Rodrigues NB, Valenciano PJ, Silva LM, Souza RC. Correlation among the visual gait assessment scale, Edinburgh visual gait scale and observational gait scale in children with spastic diplegic cerebral palsy. Rev Bras Fisioter. 2012;16:134–40.
8. Borel S, Schneider P, Newman CJ. Video analysis software increases the interrater reliability of video gait assessments in children with cerebral palsy. Gait Posture. 2011;33:727–9.
9. Harvey A, Gorter JW. Video gait analysis for ambulatory children with cerebral palsy: why, when, where and how! Gait Posture. 2011;33:501–3.
10. Boyd R, Graham K. Objective measurement of clinical findings in the use of botulinum toxin type a for the management of children with cerebral palsy. Eur J Neurol. 1999;6:23–35.
11. Dickens WE, Smith MF. Validation of a visual gait assessment scale for children with hemiplegic cerebral palsy. Gait Posture. 2006;23:78–82.
12. Toro B, Nester CJ, Farren PC. The development and validity of the Salford gait tool: an observation-based clinical gait assessment tool. Arch Phys Med Rehabil. 2007;88:321–7.
13. Viehweger E, Zürcher Pfund L, Hélix M, Rohon MA, Jacquemier M, Scavarda D, Jouve JL, Bollini G, Loundou A, Simeoni MC. Influence of clinical and gait analysis experience on reliability of observational gait analysis (Edinburgh gait score reliability). Ann Phys Rehabil Med. 2010;53(9):535–46.
14. Rodriquez AA, Black PO, Kile KA, Sherman J, Stellberg B, McCormnick J, Roszkowski J, Swiggum E. Gait training efficacy using a home-based practice model in chronic hemiplegia. Arch Phys Med Rehabil. 1996;77: 801–5.
15. Guzik A, Drużbicki M, Przysada G, Kwolek A, Brzozowska-Magoń A, Wolan-Nieroda A. Analysis of consistency between temporospatial gait parameters and gait assessment with the use of Wisconsin gait scale in post-stroke patients. Neurol Neurochir Pol. 2017;51:60–5.
16. Yaliman A, Kesiktas N, Ozkaya M, Eskiyurt N, Erkan O, Yilmaz E. Evaluation of intrarater and interrater reliability of the Wisconsin gait scale with using the video taped stroke patients in a Turkish sample. NeuroRehabilitation. 2014; 34:253–8.
17. Wellmon R, Degano A, Rubertone JA, Campbell S, Russo KA. Interrater and intrarater reliability and minimal detectable change of the Wisconsin gait scale when used to examine videotaped gait in individuals post-stroke. Arch Physiother. 2015;5:11.
18. Lu X, Hu N, Deng S, Li J, Qi S, Bi S. The reliability, validity and correlation of two observational gait scales assessed by video tape for Chinese subjects with hemiplegia. J Phys Ther Sci. 2015;27:3717–21.
19. Wang X, Wang Y. Gait analysis of children with spastic hemiplegic cerebral palsy. Neural Regen Res. 2012;7:1578–84.
20. Dobson F, Morris ME, Baker R, Graham HK. Gait classification in children with cerebral palsy: a systematic review. Gait Posture. 2007;25:140–52.
21. Gor-García-Fogeda MD, Cano de la Cuerda R, Carratalá Tejada M, Alguacil-Diego IM. Molina-Rueda F Observational Gait Assessments in People With Neurological Disorders: A Systematic Review. Arch Phys Med Rehabil. 2016; 97:131–40.
22. Strączyńska A, Radzimińska A, Weber-Rajek M, Strojek K, Goch A. Functional assessment of children with cerebral palsy – current report. Adv in Rehab. 2015;3:43–9.
23. Liptak GS, Accardo PJ. Health and social outcomes of children with cerebral palsy. J Pediatr. 2004;145:36–41.
24. Dickinsen HO, Parkinson KN, Ravens-Sieberer U, et al. Self-reported quality of life of 8–12-year-old children with cerebral palsy: a cross-sectional European study. Lancet. 2007;369:2172–8.
25. Berg M, Jahnsen R, Frey Frøslie K, Hussain A. Reliability of the pediatric evaluation of disability inventory (PEDI). Phys Occup Ther Pediatr. 2004;24:61–77.
26. Rosa-Rizzotto M. Visonà Dalla Pozza L, Corlatti a, et al. a new scale for the assessment of performance and capacity of hand function in children with hemiplegic cerebral palsy: reliability and validity studies. Eur J Phys Rehabil Med. 2014;50:543–56.
27. Wallen M, Bundy A, Pont K, Ziviani J. Psychometric properties of the pediatric motor activity log used for children with cerebral palsy. Dev Med Child Neurol. 2009;51:200–8.
28. Guzik A, Drużbicki M, Przysada G, Kwolek A, Brzozowska-Magoń A, Wyszyńska J, Podgórska-Bednarz J. Assessment of test-retest reliability and internal consistency of the Wisconsin gait scale in hemiparetic post-stroke patients. Adv in Rehab. 2016;3:41–53.

13

Total and regional bone mineral and tissue composition in female adolescent athletes: comparison between volleyball players and swimmers

João Valente-dos-Santos[1,2,3,4] iD, Óscar M. Tavares[5], João P. Duarte[1,6,7], Paulo M. Sousa-e-Silva[1,6], Luís M. Rama[1,6], José M. Casanova[8], Carlos A. Fontes-Ribeiro[9,10], Elisa A. Marques[11], Daniel Courteix[12,13], Enio R. V. Ronque[14], Edilson S. Cyrino[14], Jorge Conde[15] and Manuel J. Coelho-e-Silva[1,6*]

Abstract

Background: Exploring the osteogenic effect of different bone-loading sports is particular relevant to understand the interaction between skeletal muscle and bone health during growth. This study aimed to compare total and regional bone and soft-tissue composition between female adolescent swimmers ($n=20$, 15.71 ± 0.93 years) and volleyball players ($n=26$, 16.20 ± 0.77 years).

Methods: Dietary intake was obtained using food frequency questionnaires. Body size was given by stature, sitting height, and body mass. Six skinfolds were measured. Bone mineral content (BMC) and density (BMD), lean soft tissue, and fat tissue were assessed using dual-energy X-ray absorptiometry. Pearson's product moment correlation coefficients were calculated to examine the relationships among variables, by type of sport. Comparisons between swimmers and volleyball players were performed using student t-tests for independent samples and multivariate analysis of covariance (controlling for age, training history and body size).

Results: Swimmers (BMC: 2328 ± 338 g) and volleyball players (BMC: 2656 ± 470 g) exceeded respectively by 2.1 and 2.8 standard deviation scores the average of international standards for whole body BMC of healthy adolescents. Years of training in swimmers were positively related to the upper limbs BMC ($r=+0.49$, $p<0.05$). In volleyball players, years of training correlated significantly with lower limbs BMD ($r=+0.43$, $p<0.05$). After adjustments for potential confounders, moderate differences (ES-$r=0.32$) between swimmers and volleyball players were noted in BMD at the lower limbs (volleyball players: $+0.098$ g·cm^{-2}, $+7.8\%$).

Conclusions: Youth female athletes who participate in high-intensity weight-loading activities such as volleyball exhibit moderately higher levels of BMD at the lower limbs compared to non-loading sports such as swimming.

Keywords: DXA, Impact and non-impact loading sports, Exercise, Bone health, Body composition

* Correspondence: mjcesilva@hotmail.com
[1]CIDAF (UID/DTP/04213/2016), University of Coimbra, Coimbra, Portugal
[6]Faculty of Sports Sciences and Physical Education, University of Coimbra, Coimbra, Portugal
Full list of author information is available at the end of the article

Background

As life expectancy continues to rise, osteoporosis becomes an increasingly important healthcare concern due its economic impact and harmful effects on human health, especially among women [1]. Adult bone structure is largely determined during the two first decades of life; thus factors that stimulate bone formation during childhood and adolescence have a major role in the prevention of osteoporosis later in life [2]. Particularly, sex, ethnicity, hormones, alcohol consumption, tobacco, nutrition, and exercise are among the most significant contributing factors that can influence bone acquisition during early life [3].

During the period of growth, physical activity (mostly weight-bearing activities) is a particularly relevant factor for achieving an optimum peak bone mass level, due to the positive osteogenic response [4, 5]. In a cross-sectional study, Ginty et al. [6] demonstrated that high-impact loading activities (such as jogging, playing tennis, football, rugby, basketball, and exercising with weights) for 1 h or more a day was associated with greater size-adjusted whole body (+3.4%) and total hip (+8.5%) bone mineral content (BMC) among male adolescents, compared to those with a median of 7 min·day of participation in high-impact loading activities. Although weight-bearing physical activity during childhood and adolescence has been widely recognized to be beneficial for bone health [7], previous studies have focused predominantly on assessing the combined effect of different high-impact loading sports (mixing participants from different sports into the same bone-loading category) [8, 9]. Thus, the osteogenic effect of specific sports is less well understood.

Muscle and bone are inextricably linked not only mechanically but also genetically and molecularly. Recent studies demonstrated a molecular "cross talk" between muscle and bone, as both tissues release endocrine, paracrine, and autocrine factors that may mediate intercellular communication [10]. Although non-impact loading sports, such as swimming, are widely recognized to have no substantial positive effect on bone health [11, 12], they stimulate muscle contraction in a variety of muscles that can induce hypertrophy and also may potentially stimulate the molecular "cross talk" between muscle and bone [13]. Thus, exploring the effect of sports with clearly different bone-loading mechanisms, such as volleyball and swimming, may help to better understand the interaction between skeletal muscle and bone during growth.

Sex differences in bone quality and strength are well described [14]. By late puberty, boys have higher bone strength than girls, which is due mainly to the larger bone size in boys than in girls [15]. During aging, men have a greater periosteal apposition that increases bone size and offsets bone loss more than in women, yielding fewer males than females at risk for fracture in old age [16]. Thus, the relationship between physical activity and bone health is particularly relevant among females compared to males because they are at increased risk for osteoporosis and fracture later in life. At present the most effective sport modality for bone health promotion in girls is unknown, largely because of the confounding effects of biological maturation on bone development during adolescence [17, 18].

The aim of the current study was to compare total and regional bone (mineral content and density) and soft-tissue composition (fat and lean mass) between female adolescent swimmers and volleyball players. As the positive impact of sports participation on bone mass can be tempered by nutritional factors (such as calcium, protein and total caloric intake), differences in dietary intake were controlled for. It was hypothesized that volleyball players would have higher whole-body and regional BMC and bone mineral density (BMD) than swimmers; no differences in fat mass and lean mass were expected between sports.

Methods

Participants and procedures

The sample was composed of 46 female athletes (swimmers: $n=20$; volleyball players: $n=26$; Additional file 1) aged 14.5-17.4 years who were recruited voluntarily from seven competitive clubs in the Portuguese Midlands. The following inclusion criteria were considered: (i) chronological age less than 17.5 years; (ii) reaching menarche >1 year before testing; (iii) a minimum of 2 years of competitive participation at the national level in the sport; (iv) absence of medication usage that could affect bone metabolism; (v) absence of bone fractures.

All procedures were approved by the Ethics Committee of the Faculty of Sport Sciences and Physical Education of the University of Coimbra (CE/FCDEF-UC/00102014). The study was conducted in accordance with the Declaration of Helsinki for human studies of the World Medical Association. Participants were informed of the objectives and methodology and also that participation was voluntary and that they could withdraw from the experiment at any time. Parents or legal guardians and each participant signed an informed consent document. All measurements were completed in the same laboratory. The primary outcomes were whole-body and regional BMC, BMD, fat mass, and lean mass, measured by dual-energy X-ray absorptiometry (DXA) scans. Secondary outcomes included: (i) chronological age, calculated to the nearest 0.1 year by subtracting birth date from date of assessment; (ii) age at menarche, retrospectively self-reported; (iii) athlete's training experience, obtained from coaches; (iv) dietary intake, obtained using food frequency questionnaires; (v) and, a brief anthropometric battery. For descriptive purposes, characteristics of the total sample are presented in Additional file 2 and Additional file 3.

Training history
Information about formal years of participation and annual training sessions were obtained from coaches who maintained individual registration records. Swimmers participated in 4-6 training sessions per week (60-120 min·session^{-1}) and 1-2 competitions per month. Volleyball players participated in 3-4 training sessions per week, usually 90 min·session^{-1} and 1 game·week, usually Saturdays or Sundays. Competition calendars were usually October-May for swimming and September-July for volleyball.

Dietary intake
Dietary intake was obtained using a structured semi-quantitative food frequency questionnaire [19] over the previous 12 months, comprised of 86 food items or beverage categories. This is a validated dietary instrument used frequently in Portugal and is based on the frequency of consumption of the main sources of proteins (%Kcal), carbohydrates (%Kcal), total fat (%Kcal), saturated fat (%Kcal), monounsaturated fat (%Kcal), polyunsaturated fatty (%Kcal), cholesterol (mg), fiber (g), ethanol (g), and calcium (mg). Variables taken into consideration in the study (i.e., protein, cholesterol and calcium) are in accordance with previous literature [17, 20, 21].

Body size and skinfolds
The same experienced technician performed anthropometry according to recommended and standardized procedures [22]. Stature (Harpenden stadiometer, model 98.603, Holtain, Crosswell, UK) and sitting height (Harpenden sitting height table, model 98.607, Holtain, Crosswell, UK) were measured to the nearest 0.1 cm (leg length was calculated as the difference between the two). Body mass was measured to the nearest 0.1 kg using a SECA balance (model 770, Hanover, MD, USA). Stature and body mass were expressed as sex-age-specific z-scores for a reference population [23]. Individual z-scores were calculated based on the LMS parameters (Lambda for the skew, Mu for the median, and Sigma for the generalized coefficient of variation) constructed for the Centers for Disease Control and Prevention 2000 growth charts [24]. Corresponding percentiles were obtained from standard normal distribution tables. Seven skinfolds (tricipital, bicipital, subscapular, suprailiac, abdominal, anterior thigh and medial calf) were measured to the nearest 1 mm using a Lange caliper (Beta Technology,

Ann Arbor, MI, USA). Technical errors of measurement for stature (0.29 cm), sitting height (0.30 cm), weight (0.19 kg), and skinfolds (0.74-1.04 mm) were well within the range of several health surveys in the United States and a variety of field surveys [25].

Dual-energy x-ray absorptiometry
Absorptiometry (fan-beam Lunar DPX-PRO) was used to measure total body BMC (g), BMD (g·cm^{-2}), fat mass, and lean mass using standard or thick mode depending on body stature. Participants were placed in the supine position on the scanning table with the body aligned along the central horizontal axis. Arms were positioned parallel to, but not touching the body. Forearms were pronated with hands flat on the bed. Legs were fully extended, and feet were secured with a canvas and Velcro support to avoid foot movement during the scan acquisition. One skilled technician performed and analyzed all scans following the manufacturer's guidelines (V 13.6 software) for patient positioning. Identical scanning parameters were used for each scan, and the output report considered bone area, BMC, BMD, lean soft tissue, and fat tissue. The regions of interest were manually positioned according to International Society for Clinical Densitometry guidelines and were apportioned as subhead (clavicle as reference), trunk, upper limbs and lower limbs. Scan analysis was performed using the Lunar Encore software (Version 13.6). The machine's calibration was checked and passed on a daily basis using the Lunar calibration epoxy resin phantom.

Data analysis
Descriptive statistics (mean, standard deviation, and range) were calculated for the total sample. Kolmogorov-Smirnov test was used to check variable distributions. When the assumptions of normality were violated, log-transformations were performed to reduce nonuniformity of error. Student t-tests for independent samples were used to compare athlete's physical characteristics by sport. Cohen's d effect sizes and thresholds (0.2, 0.6, 1.2, 2.0, 4.0 for trivial, small, moderate, large, very large and extremely large) were used to evaluate the magnitude of differences [26]. Pearson's product moment correlation coefficients ($r_{y,x}$) were calculated to examine the magnitude and direction of relationships among variables extracted from DXA (Y_i) with age, training experience, and body size descriptors (X_i), by type of sport. The magnitude of correlations was interpreted as follows [26]: trivial ($r<0.1$), small ($0.1<r<0.3$), moderate ($0.3<r<0.5$), large ($0.5<r<0.7$), very large ($0.7<r<0.9$), and nearly perfect ($r>0.9$). Multivariate analysis of covariance (MANCOVA) was used to determine significant

differences between groups in total and regional bone and soft-tissue composition (fat and lean mass), after adjustments for age, training experience, and body size. The effect sizes for correlations (ES-r) were estimated using the square root of the ratio of the F-ratio squared and the difference between the F-value squared and degrees of freedom [27]. Coefficients were interpreted as follows: trivial ($r<0.1$), small ($0.1<r<0.3$), moderate ($0.3<r<0.5$), large ($0.5<r<0.7$), very large ($0.7<r<0.9$), and nearly perfect ($r>0.9$) [26]. Statistical significance was set to a p-value < 0.05. Statistical analyses were performed using the software IBM SPSS v.23 for Mac OS (SPSS Inc., IBM Company, NY, USA) and *GraphPad* Prism software (GraphPad Software, Inc., La Jolla, CA, USA).

Results

Current age, age at menarche, training history, anthropometry, and dietary intake of swimmers and volleyball players are presented in Table 1. Swimmers and volleyball players did not differ significantly in chronological age but differed moderately in age at menarche [d=0.65 (t=2.121, $p<0.05$)]; volleyball players experienced the first menstruation 0.72 years earlier than swimmers. Swimmers had significantly more years of training [d=1.69 (t=-3.836, $p<0.01$)] and annual number of training

sessions (i.e., training volume) [d=6.30 (t=20.814, $p<0.01$)] compared to volleyball players. Athletes had mean statures and mean body masses that approximate, respectively, the 53th and 68th age-specific percentiles for U.S. girls [23]. Mean BMI-for-age exceeded the ≥50th percentile in both groups (swimmers: 60th percentile; volleyball players: 73rd percentiles) [23]. Volleyball players were heavier (body mass: d=-0.79 (t=-2.596, $p<0.01$), with more subcutaneous adipose tissue than swimmers (suprailiac, abdominal and anterior thigh skinfolds: d=-0.67 to -1.06 (t=-2.233 to -3.556, p=0.031 to $p<0.01$). Volleyball players also had higher levels of cholesterol intake [d=0.87 (t=-2.485, $p<0.018$)] than swimmers.

Table 2 and Fig. 1 comprises the descriptive statistics for DXA whole body and regional body composition of swimmers and volleyball players. Overall, swimmers (BMC: 2328±338 g) and volleyball players (BMC: 2656 ±470 g) exceeded in 2.1 and 2.8 standard deviation scores, respectively, the average of international standards for whole body BMC of healthy adolescents of the same race, gender, stature and body mass [28]. Volleyball players had significantly greater BMC and BMD in the whole body [+12.4%: d=-0.80 (t=-2.637, $p<0.05$) and +5.5%: d=-0.80 (t=-2.574, $p<0.05$), respectively], subhead [+13.8%: d=-0.83 (t=-2.724, $p<0.01$) and +6.5%: d=-0.89

Table 1 Means and standard deviations by type of sport (swimmers vs. volleyball players) on age, training experience, dietary intake, body size and skinfolds

Dependent variables Y_i	X: Sport		Comparisons[b]				
	Swimming (n=20)	Volleyball (n=26)	mean difference (95%CI)	t-student		Magnitude effects	
				t-value	p	d	(description)
Y_1: Chronological age (years)	15.71±0.93	16.20±0.77	-0.49 (-1.00; 0.02)	-1.957	0.057	-0.59	(small)
Y_2: Age at menarche (years)	13.31±1.33	12.59±0.95	0.72 (0.04; 1.39)	2.121	0.040	0.65	(moderate)
Y_3: Years of training (years)	8.9±3.9	4.1±1.8	4.8 (2.9; 6.7)	-3.836	<0.01	1.69	(large)
Y_4: Annual number of training sessions (#)	298±34	115±26	182 (164; 200)	20.814	<0.01	6.30	(extremely large)
Y_5: Energy intake [a] (Kcal/day)	2557±1188	3036±1188	-480 (-1305; 346)	-1.183	0.245	-0.42	(small)
Y_6: Proteins [a] (%Kcal)	18.1±2.8	20.5±5.2	-2.4 (-5.5; 0.7)	-1.590	0.128	-0.62	(moderate)
Y_7: Cholesterol [a] (mg)	353±174	527±241	-174 (-317; -32)	-2.485	0.018	-0.87	(moderate)
Y_8: Calcium [a] (mg)	1141±556	1334±455	-192 (-550; 166)	-1.091	0.283	-0.39	(small)
Y_9: Stature (cm)	161.3±4.4	164.2±6.0	-2.9 (-6.1; 0.3)	-1.821	0.075	-0.55	(small)
Y_{10}: Body mass (kg)	55.0±5.6	61.0±9.0	-6.0 (-10.6; -1.3)	-2.596	0.013	-0.79	(moderate)
Y_{11}: Skinfold triceps (mm)	17.9±6.0	20.4±3.9	-2.5 (-5.7; 0.6)	-1.642	0.111	-0.52	(small)
Y_{12}: Skinfold subscapular (mm)	12.4±4.2	13.3±3.5	-1.0 (-3.3; 1.3)	-0.868	0.390	-0.24	(small)
Y_{13}: Skinfold suprailiac (mm)	17.8±5.5	22.7±6.9	-4.9 (-8.7; -1.1)	-2.581	0.013	-0.79	(moderate)
Y_{14}: Skinfold abdominal (mm)	17.6±6.1	22.0±7.1	-4.5 (-8.5; -0.4)	-2.233	0.031	-0.67	(moderate)
Y_{15}: Skinfold thigh anterior (mm)	18.7±6.8	25.1±5.6	-6.5 (-10.1; -2.8)	-3.556	0.001	-1.06	(moderate)
Y_{16}: Skinfold calf medial (mm)	17.9±5.3	17.7±4.8	0.20 (-2.8; 3.2)	0.113	0.910	0.04	(trivial)

95%CI 95% confidence intervals
[a]20 swimmers and 15 volleyball players completed the food questionnaire
[b]Results of comparisons between groups on chronological age, age at menarche, training experience, outputs obtained from the food questionnaire and anthropometry, mean differences, results of t-student test for independent samples and magnitude effect size (Cohen's *d*)

Table 2 Means and standard deviations by type of sport (swimmers vs. volleyball players) on variables extracted from dual-energy x-ray absorptiometry

Dependent variables Y_i	X: Sport		Comparisons [a]				
	Swimming (n=20)	Volleyball (n=26)	mean difference (95%CI)	t-student		Magnitude effects	
				t-value	p	d	(description)
Bone mineral content (g)							
Y_1: Whole body	2328±338	2656±470	-328 (-578; -77)	-2.637	0.012	-0.80	(moderate)
Y_2: Subhead	1856±284	2154±420	-298 (-518; -77)	-2.724	0.009	-0.83	(moderate)
Y_3: Trunk	786±153	926±213	-140 (-254; -27)	-2.491	0.017	-0.76	(moderate)
Y_4: Upper limbs	290±36	300±64	-10 (-42; 22)	-0.626	0.534	-0.19	(trivial)
Y_5: Lower limbs	781±106	928±164	-147 (-232; -62)	-3.476	0.001	-1.06	(moderate)
Bone mineral density (g·cm^{-2})							
Y_6: Whole body	1.118±0.079	1.184±0.089	-0.065 (-0.116; -0.014)	-2.574	0.013	-0.80	(moderate)
Y_7: Subhead	0.995±0.070	1.064±0.086	-0.069 (-0.116; -0.021)	-2.893	0.006	-0.89	(moderate)
Y_8: Trunk	0.950±0.067	1.028±0.091	-0.078 (-0.127; -0.030)	-3.233	0.002	-0.98	(moderate)
Y_9: Upper limbs	0.801±0.049	0.812±0.066	-0.011 (-0.046; 0.024)	-0.616	0.541	-0.19	(trivial)
Y_{10}: Lower limbs	1.155±0.103	1.235±0.123	-0.080 (-0.149; -0.011)	-2.344	0.024	-0.71	(moderate)
Lean soft tissue (kg)							
Y_{11}: Whole body	38.6±3.0	38.7±3.4	-0.1 (-2.0; 1.8)	-0.109	0.914	-0.03	(trivial)
Y_{12}: Trunk	18.7±1.7	17.9±1.6	0.8 (-0.2; 1.8)	1.596	0.118	0.59	(small)
Y_{13}: Upper limbs	4.4±0.4	4.1±0.7	0.3 (0.1; 0.6)	2.096	0.043	0.52	(small)
Y_{14}: Lower limbs	12.7±1.1	13.6±1.4	-0.8 (-1.6; -0.1)	-2.217	0.032	-0.72	(moderate)
Fat tissue (kg)							
Y_{15}: Whole body	12.5±4.4	17.7±7.1	-5.2 (-8.8; -1.5)	-2.853	0.007	-0.87	(moderate)
Y_{16}: Trunk	6.2±2.3	8.5±3.8	-2.4 (-4.3; -0.4)	-2.456	0.018	-0.73	(moderate)
Y_{17}: Upper limbs	1.1±0.9	1.5±0.8	-0.4 (-0.9; 0.1)	-1.602	0.116	-0.48	(small)
Y_{18}: Lower limbs	8.0±4.4	7.0±2.6	0.9 (-1.3; 3.2)	0.865	0.394	0.29	(small)

95%CI 95% confidence intervals
[a]Results of comparisons between groups on variables extracted from the dual energy x-ray absorptiometry, mean differences, results of t-student test for independent samples and magnitude effect size (Cohen's *d*)

(t=-2.893, *p*<0.01), respectively], trunk [+15.1%: d=-0.76 (t=-2.491, *p*<0.05) and +7.6%: d=-0.98 (t=-3.233, *p*<0.01, respectively] and lower limbs [15.8%: d=-1.06 (t=-3.476, *p*<0.01) and +6.4%: d=-0.71 (t=-2.344, *p*<0.05), respectively] than swimmers. In addition, volleyball players had significantly greater lean soft tissue in the lower limbs [+5.9%: d=-0.72 (t=-2.217, *p*<0.05)], whole body [+29.4%: d=-0.87 (t=-2.853, *p*<0.01)], and trunk fat tissue [+28.2%: d=-0.73 (t=-2.456, *p*<0.05)].

Table 3 summarizes the interrelationship between age, training experience, and body size descriptors with variables extracted from DXA, by type of sport. In swimmers, BMC, BMD (whole body, subhead, trunk, and upper limbs) and fat tissue (whole body, trunk, and lower limbs) are moderately to largely correlated with CA (*r*=+0.46 to +0.59, *p*<0.05). No significant associations were noted within the same variables for volleyball players. With one exception – lower limbs lean soft tissue in volleyball players (*r*=+0.40, *p*<0.05) – no correlations were found between age at menarche and total and

regional bone mineral and tissue composition. Training experience in swimmers is positively related to the upper limbs BMC (*r*=+0.49, p<0.05) and fat tissue (*r*=+0.49, *p*<0.05), and lower limbs fat tissue (*r*=+0.52, *p*<0.05). In volleyball players, years of training only correlated significantly with lower limbs BMD (*r*=+0.43, *p*<0.05). Correlations between stature and BMC in swimmers are large to very large (*r*=+0.64 to +0.82, *p*<0.01) and are generally higher than those for BMD (*r*=+0.57 to +0.66, *p*<0.01) and lean soft tissue (whole body: *r*=+0.52, *p*<0.05; lower limbs: *r*=+0.70, *p*<0.01). The BMC [with one exception: lower limbs (*r*=+0.46, *p*<0.05)] and BMD of volleyball players are not significantly related to stature. In contrast to bone mineral parameters, stature is largely related to lean soft tissue (whole body: *r*=+0.63, *p*<0.01; trunk: *r*=+0.64, *p*<0.01; lower limbs: *r*=+0.61, *p*<0.01). Although the correlation data between body mass and variables extracted from DXA for swimmers and volleyball players are somewhat different, they reflect moderate to very large [BMC, BMD, lean soft tissue

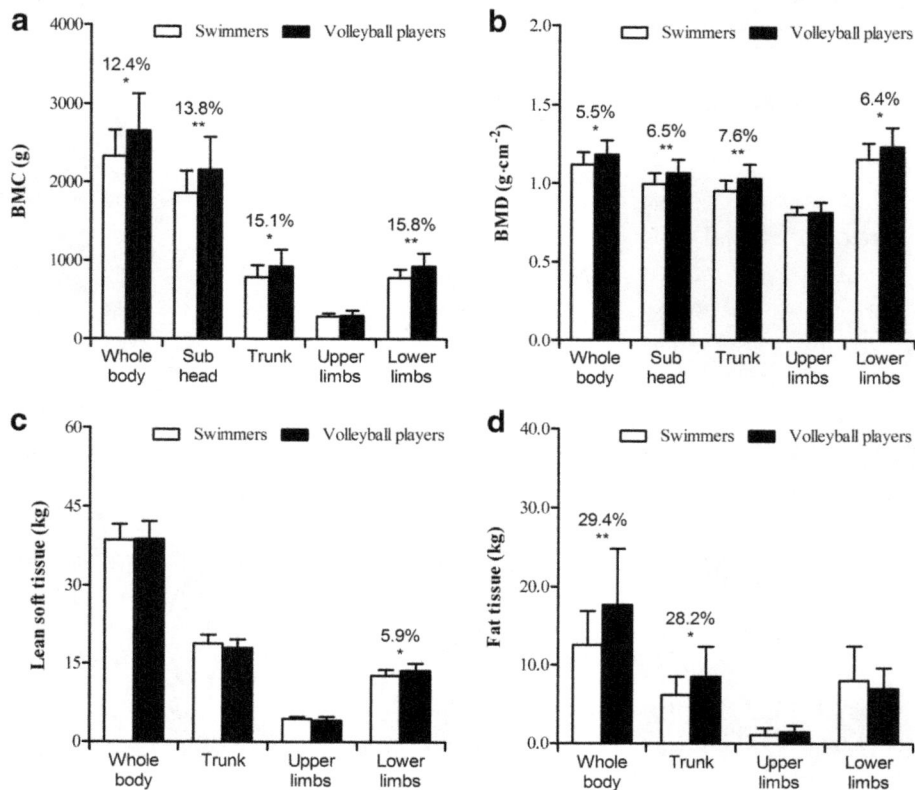

Fig. 1 Bone mineral content (BMC, panel **a**), bone mineral density (BMD, panel **b**), lean soft tissue (panel **c**) and fat tissue (panel **d**) in female swimmers (white bars) and volleyball players (black bars). * indicates difference between the groups ($p<0.05$), ** $p<0.01$

(whole body, upper and lower limbs) and fat tissue (whole body and trunk)] and moderate to nearly perfect [BMC, BMD (whole body, subhead and trunk), lean soft tissue (whole body, upper and lower limbs), and fat tissue] positive associations ($p<0.05$), respectively.

Sport-related variation for total and regional bone and soft-tissue composition, when chronological age, age at menarche, training experience, stature and body mass were statistically controlled by MANCOVA is presented in Table 4. Moderate differences (ES-r=0.32) between swimmers and volleyball players persisted for BMD at the lower limbs (0.098 g·cm^{-2}, 7.8%).

Discussion

This study showed that volleyball players presented greater BMC and BMD, in the whole body, and greater lean soft tissue in the lower limbs with respect to swimmers. Although swimming stimulates muscle hypertrophy [29], our results showed that swimmers had moderately less skinfold thickness (a measure of subcutaneous fat), whole body and trunk fat tissue. Differences between groups in lean mass were mostly small. Thus, the mechanical and non-mechanical stimuli associated with swimming may not be sufficient to trigger

the responsiveness of bone cells. After adjustments for potential confounders (i.e., chronological age, age at menarche, years of training, stature, and body mass) the bone content, lean soft tissue and fat tissue were similar between groups. Differences persisted for the lower limbs, with volleyball players presenting higher BMD compared to swimmers.

A secular decline in the age at menarche occurred in the Portuguese population [30]. Findings suggest that the decline is associated, to a large extent, with a reduction in the number of girls who mature late [25]. Allowing for normal variability, training is not related to age at menarche in athletes [31] and variation in mean ages at menarche within a sport is especially evident in swimmers and volleyball players [25]. Mean ages at menarche were 13.31±1.33 years and 12.59±0.95 years for swimmers and volleyball players, respectively. Volleyball players approximates the mean age of menarche for Portuguese school girls calculated using recall methods (i.e., 12.53±1.27 years) [30]. Although there is a difference of 0.72 years between groups' means, about two-thirds of the present sample attains menarche between 12.0 and 14.0 years. The limited variability may explain the reduced interrelationships between age at menarche with

Table 3 Correlations between age, training experience, and body size descriptors (Xi) with variables extracted from dual-energy x-ray absorptiometry (Yi) by type of sport (swimmers and volleyball players)

	Correlation (Xi, Yi)									
	X1: Chronological age		X2: Age at menarche		X3: Years of training		X4: Stature		X5: Body mass	
	Swimming (n=20)	Volleyball (n=26)	Swimming (n=20)	Volleyball (n=26)	Swimming (n=20)	Volleyball (n=26)	Swimming (n=20)	Volleyball (n=26)	Swimming (n=20)	Volleyball (n=26)
	r (95%CI)	r (95%CI)	r (95%CI)	r (95%CI)	r (95%CI)	r (95%CI)	r (95%CI)	r (95%CI)	r (95%CI)	r (95%CI)
Bone mineral content (g)										
Y_1: Whole body	0.51* (0.11; 0.76)	0.20 (-0.14; 0.55)	0.11 (-0.31; 0.46)	0.18 (-0.25; 0.49)	0.31 (-0.05; 0.64)	0.19 (-0.23; 0.65)	0.81** (0.53; 0.92)	0.32 (-0.21; 0.63)	0.85** (0.69; 0.94)	0.71** (0.32; 0.87)
Y_2: Subhead	0.53* (0.14; 0.78)	0.16 (-0.14; 0.52)	0.14 (-0.30; 0.49)	0.19 (-0.23; 0.50)	0.31 (-0.05; 0.65)	0.18 (-0.24; 0.65)	0.82** (0.57; 0.93)	0.35 (-0.17; 0.64)	0.87** (0.71; 0.95)	0.73** (0.33; 0.89)
Y_3: Trunk	0.48* (0.06; 0.75)	0.11 (-0.24; 0.49)	0.14 (-0.33; 0.48)	0.12 (-0.24; 0.49)	0.26 (-0.10; 0.61)	0.14 (-0.26; 0.60)	0.82** (0.56; 0.92)	0.26 (-0.35; 0.61)	0.86** (0.71; 0.93)	0.76** (0.34; 0.88)
Y_4: Upper limbs	0.59** (0.25; 0.82)	0.14 (-0.13; 0.46)	0.15 (-0.36; 0.56)	0.11 (-0.39; 0.52)	0.49* (0.08; 0.74)	0.28 (-0.12; 0.67)	0.64** (0.38; 0.81)	0.25 (-0.25; 0.58)	0.76** (0.57; 0.90)	0.48* (0.01; 0.75)
Y_5: Lower limbs	0.52* (0.15; 0.78)	0.22 (-0.05; 0.53)	0.11 (-0.28; 0.49)	0.27 (-0.14; 0.57)	0.29 (-0.09; 0.62)	0.17 (-0.25; 0.65)	0.80** (0.52; 0.92)	0.46* (0.07; 0.70)	0.82** (0.64; 0.93)	0.68** (0.29; 0.86)
Bone mineral density (g·cm⁻²)										
Y_6: Whole body	0.46* (0.06; 0.75)	0.21 (-0.24; 0.62)	-0.03 (-0.35; 0.31)	0.19 (-0.29; 0.53)	0.33 (-0.11; 0.69)	0.36 (-0.05; 0.72)	0.63** (0.22; 0.83)	0.01 (-0.47; 0.41)	0.67** (0.36; 0.86)	0.41* (0.01; 0.69)
Y_7: Subhead	0.50* (0.11; 0.80)	0.13 (-0.28; 0.56)	0.04 (-0.29; 0.39)	0.21 (-0.26; 0.56)	0.31 (-0.17; 0.69)	0.37 (-0.04; 0.75)	0.66** (0.30; 0.86)	0.10 (-0.41; 0.47)	0.70** (0.43; 0.87)	0.49* (0.06; 0.75)
Y_8: Trunk	0.52* (0.09; 0.80)	0.08 (-0.30; 0.50)	0.08 (-0.30; 0.39)	0.09 (-0.40; 0.46)	0.28 (-0.20; 0.68)	0.36 (-0.06; 0.74)	0.65** (0.26; 0.85)	0.04 (-0.50; 0.46)	0.69** (0.42; 0.85)	0.57** (0.10; 0.77)
Y_9: Upper limbs	0.51* (0.17; 0.73)	0.08 (-0.42; 0.54)	-0.07 (-0.44; 0.30)	0.33 (-0.28; 0.71)	0.45* (0.05; 0.71)	0.21 (-0.11; 0.56)	0.57** (0.26; 0.79)	-0.23 (-0.63; 0.13)	0.67** (0.39; 0.91)	0.24 (-0.16; 0.58)
Y_{10}: Lower limbs	0.40 (0.01; 0.81)	0.13 (-0.27; 0.53)	0.01 (-0.35; 0.44)	0.20 (-0.21; 0.54)	0.27 (-0.21; 0.68)	0.43* (-0.03; 0.77)	0.59** (0.28; 0.81)	0.19 (-0.34; 0.55)	0.63** (0.34; 0.83)	0.37 (-0.13; 0.72)
Lean soft tissue (kg)										
Y_{11}: Whole body	0.18 (-0.32; 0.54)	0.30 (-0.02; 0.61)	0.08 (-0.58; 0.56)	0.38 (0.07; 0.65)	0.02 (-0.38; 0.38)	0.38 (0.02; 0.66)	0.52* (0.05; 0.79)	0.63** (0.40; 0.88)	0.46* (0.07; 0.72)	0.42* (0.01; 0.67)
Y_{12}: Trunk	-0.05 (-0.57; 0.41)	0.29 (-0.13; 0.62)	0.08 (-0.53; 0.54)	0.34 (0.04; 0.69)	-0.08 (-0.45; 0.36)	0.37 (0.09; 0.62)	0.21 (-0.46; 0.71)	0.64** (0.44; 0.80)	0.20 (-0.41; 0.63)	0.32 (-0.11; 0.60)
Y_{13}: Upper limbs	0.41 (-0.04; 0.69)	0.14 (-0.15; 0.45)	0.12 (-0.48; 0.54)	0.13 (-0.27; 0.50)	0.33 (-0.08; 0.65)	0.30 (-0.06; 0.62)	0.31 (0.01; 0.62)	0.17 (-0.23; 0.57)	0.51* (0.17; 0.74)	0.41* (-0.06; 0.70)
Y_{14}: Lower limbs	0.19 (-0.34; 0.61)	0.30 (0.02; 0.57)	0.26 (-0.20; 0.67)	0.40* (-0.02; 0.70)	-0.08 (0.47; 0.29)	0.24 (-0.16; 0.58)	0.70** (0.36; 0.88)	0.61** (0.35; 0.79)	0.56** (0.22; 0.77)	0.41* (0.03; 0.67)
Fat tissue (kg)										
Y_{15}: Whole body	0.48* (0.01; 0.75)	0.04 (-0.24; 0.37)	0.06 (-0.45; 0.53)	-0.02 (-0.27; 0.22)	0.41 (0.09; 0.70)	-0.06 (-0.57; 0.38)	0.41 (-0.15; 0.78)	0.14 (-0.38; 0.51)	0.84** (0.61; 0.95)	0.94** (0.77; 0.97)
Y_{16}: Trunk	0.48* (0.03; 0.74)	0.08 (-0.21; 0.39)	0.04 (-0.47; 0.51)	-0.02 (-0.24; 0.21)	0.44 (0.15; 0.72)	-0.07 (-0.55; 0.35)	0.43 (-0.12; 0.78)	0.15 (-0.39; 0.52)	0.85** (0.63; 0.95)	0.93** (0.74; 0.97)
Y_{17}: Upper limbs	0.38 (0.01; 0.81)	-0.05 (-0.36; 0.27)	0.20 (-0.24; 0.53)	-0.04 (-0.35; 0.20)	0.49* (0.35; 0.72)	-0.01 (-0.59; 0.42)	-0.27 (-0.66; 0.63)	0.17 (-0.30; 0.50)	0.05 (-0.46; 0.84)	0.86** (0.60; 0.94)
Y_{18}: Lower limbs	0.46* (0.05; 0.74)	0.02 (-0.26; 0.34)	0.16 (-0.33; 0.63)	-0.01 (-0.32; 0.27)	0.52* (0.15; 0.83)	-0.03 (-0.55; 0.38)	0.23 (-0.26; 0.64)	0.11 (-0.36; 0.47)	0.53 (0.03; 0.82)	0.88** (0.67; 0.95)

r correlation coefficients, 95%CI 95% confidence intervals
*p < 0.05, **p < 0.01

variables extracted from DXA (see Table 3), suggesting that they are somewhat independent.

The current sample has a mean stature and mean body mass which approximate, respectively, the 53th and 68th age-specific percentiles for U.S. girls [23]. The trend for elevated mass-for-stature likely reflects the advanced maturity status of the athletes [31]. Mean BMI-for-age exceeded the ≥50th percentile in both groups (swimmers: 60th percentile; volleyball players: 73rd percentiles) [23]. This was consistent with observations for other samples of youth swimmers and volleyball players [25, 32]. In the current study, dietary data suggested differences only for cholesterol intake with higher amounts being consumed by volleyball players

Table 4 Estimated marginal means controlling for age, training experience, and body size descriptors to examine variation associated to type of sport in variables extracted from dual-energy x-ray absorptiometry

Dependent variables Yi	X: Sport		MANCOVA[b]		Magnitude effect	
	Swimming[a] (n=20)	Volleyball[a] (n=26)	F	p	ES-r	(descriptive)
Bone mineral content (g)						
Y_1: Whole body	2476±84	2615±69	1.113	0.298	0.167	(small)
Y_2: Subhead	1982±71	2118±58	1.496	0.229	0.192	(small)
Y_3: Trunk	858±37	897±30	0.461	0.501	0.110	(small)
Y_4: Upper limbs	296±14	304±11	0.153	0.698	0.063	(small)
Y_5: Lower limbs	830±28	916±23	3.822	0.058	0.298	(small)
Bone mineral density (g·cm^{-2})						
Y_6: Whole body	1.132±0.024	1.190±0.019	2.414	0.128	0.241	(small)
Y_7: Subhead	1.005±0.021	1.069±0.018	3.648	0.063	0.293	(small)
Y_8: Trunk	0.965±0.021	1.020±0.018	2.617	0.114	0.251	(small)
Y_9: Upper limbs	0.800±0.017	0.821±0.014	0.656	0.423	0.130	(small)
Y_{10}: Lower limbs	1.160±0.030	1.258±0.025	4.306	0.045	0.315	(moderate)
Lean soft tissue (kg)						
Y_{11}: Whole body	39.0±0.8	39.1±0.6	0.006	0.937	0.032	(trivial)
Y_{12}: Trunk	18.7±0.5	18.2±0.4	0.518	0.476	0.114	(small)
Y_{13}: Upper limbs	4.4±0.2	4.1±0.1	1.537	0.223	0.195	(small)
Y_{14}: Lower limbs	13.0±0.3	13.7±0.2	2.769	0.104	0.257	(small)
Fat tissue (kg)						
Y_{15}: Whole body	15.9±0.7	15.7±0.6	0.017	0.896	0.032	(trivial)
Y_{16}: Trunk	8.1±0.4	7.6±0.3	0.616	0.437	0.126	(small)
Y_{17}: Upper limbs	1.1±0.2	1.5±0.2	1.620	0.211	0.200	(small)
Y_{18}: Lower limbs	8.4±0.9	6.9±0.7	1.334	0.255	0.182	(small)

ES-r effect size correlation
[a]Data presented as estimated marginal means ± standard error
[b]MANCOVA models adjusted by chronological age, age at menarche, years of training, stature, and body mass

compared to swimmers. Volleyball players were significantly heavier (+6 kg) but not taller than swimmers. Differences between groups in the components assessed by whole-body DXA were moderate for mineral content (328 g) and fat tissue (5200 g) and trivial for lean soft tissue (100 g). Allowing for the limitation of the comparison, swimmers and volleyball players exceeded in 2.1 and 2.8 standard deviation scores, respectively, the average of international standards for whole body BMC of healthy adolescents [28]. This suggests greater BMC of female adolescent swimmers and volleyball players compared to healthy female adolescents, likely with positive effects on bone health later in life.

Reduced lean mass constitutes one of the most relevant determinants of risk for low BMD in female adolescent runners [33], while lean mass is related to BMD gains and bone geometry changes in female soccer players [18]. As previously described, part of the osteogenic effect attributed to sport participation may be related to the increase in muscle mass, and subsequent

effect on bone cells [12, 34]. Correlations between primary and secondary outcomes in swimmers and volleyball players are summarized in Table 3. Results indicate the complexities involved in attempting to partition out the contribution of age, training and body size, which are often overlooked in comparisons of bone and soft tissue between athletes of different sports.

Bone is a component of body composition that is a focus of attention specifically in the context of preventing osteoporosis later in life [1, 2]. In general, the more mineral accumulated in the skeleton during growth and maturation, the better off the individual will be several decades later when mineral content of the skeleton begins to decline [2, 21]. Evidence from cross-sectional studies suggested that the peak of bone mass acquisition is reached during adolescent years and significantly affects the BMC observed in adulthood [2, 12, 34]. It has been noted that active adolescent males had 8-10% more adjusted BMC at the total body, total hip and femoral neck ($p < 0.05$) in young adulthood and active adolescent females had 9-10% more adjusted BMC at the total hip and femoral neck [21]. In the present study, years of training were positively related to the upper limbs BMC ($r=+0.49$, $p<0.05$) in swimmers and with lower limbs BMD ($r=+0.43$, $p<0.05$) in volleyball players. All together, this would suggest that the adoption of routines of physical activity including exercise and sport participation during adolescence may itself mediate enhanced skeleton formation, and these benefits are maintained into young adulthood, which may help prevent musculoskeletal diseases, such as osteoporosis, during old age.

The lower values of BMD in swimmers when compared to other sports have been investigated over the last years [29]. Although the mechanisms are not entirely clear, recent evidence point to several possible explanations. It has been theorized that muscle forces produced during sports such as swimming and cycling may not exceed the minimum effective strain stimulus threshold to induce an osteogenic effect [35, 36]. The most relevant aspect of the non-significant effect of swimming on bone gains is due its movement in a "hypogravity" environment [12, 33] for large amount of time per week [18]. The extensive time spent in the water by swimmers may also limit the time they have available to perform other sports, including weight-bearing activities during the day.

The apparent benefits of high-impact loading sport (i.e., volleyball) on BMC and BMD in the present study seemed to be specific to the trunk and lower limbs while differences between volleyball players and swimmers for bone mineral parameters in the upper limbs were trivial. Mechanical loading leads to bone remodelling, adapting the bone structure in response to the mechanical demands [12]. The stress generated by physical exercise on bone stimulates the collagen alignment in the sites directly affected by the activity, leading to higher bone strength [34]. The high quantity of jumps required during a volleyball practice may explain, at least in part, the differences observed for BMD at the lower limbs compared to swimmers. Ferry et al. [18] noted the same effect on lower limbs among girls engaged in soccer practice, in which jumps, kicks, and sprints are commonly performed. In addition, bone cells become desensitized to prolonged mechanical stimulation [37], thus incorporating periods of rest between short vigorous skeletal loading sessions may be a valid strategy to promote osteogenesis. Volleyball practice is characterized by intermittent movement (acceleration and jumps), which may also explain the higher bone mass observed in the female volleyball players compared to swimmers.

A major strength of this study was the inclusion of under-researched late-adolescent female athletes (i.e.,

volleyball players and swimmers). A further strength of the study was the use of DXA which is considered the safest and most appropriate imaging modality to access body composition and bone status. However, the current investigation is also not without limitations. First, the cross-sectional design prevents comment on causation. The sample size is fairly small, and we were unable to control for participation in other sports, or factors known to affect bone mineral density. Second, no regional site scans at the lumbar spine and proximal femur were performed, and no accurate geometrical properties were captured by DXA. Further research might attempt to control for the influences of biological maturity when seeking to determine the effects of specific physical activities on bone health among young female athletes. This will help inform programs and strategies to enhance bone health during the adolescent period of growth and development, leading to prevention of osteoporosis in later years.

Conclusions

In conclusion, volleyball players had greater BMD at the lower limbs when compared to swimmers. The results support the fact that 3 to 4 times per week of high impact loading activities are associated with higher bone mineral density at regions of interest. The observed skeletal benefits may also translate in positive changes in bone geometry and quality, this providing a substantial increase in bone strength. This observational study provides practical implications for inactive young individuals, young athletes of non-impact loading sports (including swimming) and coaches who can benefit from complementing training routines with osteogenic weight-bearing activities [29], such as resistance, strength and plyometric training.

Abbreviations

MANCOVA: multivariate analysis of covariance; BMC: bone mineral content; BMD: bone mineral density; CI: confidence intervals; DXA: Dual-energy X-ray absorptiometry; ES-r: effect size correlations; K-S: Kolmogorov-Smirnov; SEM: standard error of the mean

Acknowledgments

The early contribution of Filipe Simões (†2013) in the current project is remembered. Our thanks also go to Alexandra Silva, Nuno Amado and Shirley Souza for their participation in the data collection. The authors gratefully acknowledge the effort of the participants, their parents and coaches.

Funding

CIDAF is supported by the Portuguese Foundation for Science and Technology (uid/dtp/04213/2016). JVdS (SFRH/BPD/100470/2014) and JPD (SFRH/BD/101083/2014) were partially supported by the Portuguese Foundation for Science and Technology. No other current funding sources for this study. The Portuguese Foundation for Science and Technology played no role in the design, collection, analysis or interpretation of the data, nor in the preparation of the manuscript or decision to submit the manuscript for publication.

Authors' contributions

Conceived and designed the experiments: JVS OMT LMR CAFR DC JC MJCS. Performed the experiments: OMT JPD PMSS MJCS. Analyzed the data: JVdS LMR JMC DC ERVR ESC MJCS. Data interpretation: JVdS JPD PMSS JMC CAFR EAM ERVR ESC JC. Wrote the paper: JVdS OMT JPD EAM DC MJCS. Revised manuscript content: OMT JPD PMSS LMR JMC CAFR EAM DC ERVR ESC JC. All authors read and approved the final manuscript.

Competing interests

The authors declare that they have no competing interest.

Author details

[1]CIDAF (UID/DTP/04213/2016), University of Coimbra, Coimbra, Portugal. [2]Portuguese Foundation for Science and Technology (SFRH/BPD/100470/2014), Lisbon, Portugal. [3]Institute for Biomedical Imaging and Life Sciences (IBILI), Faculty of Medicine, University of Coimbra, Coimbra, Portugal. [4]Faculty of Physical Education and Sport, Lusófona University of Humanities and Technologies, Lisbon, Portugal. [5]Department of Medical Imaging and Radiation Therapy, School of Health and Technology, Polytechnical Institute of Coimbra, Coimbra, Portugal. [6]Faculty of Sports Sciences and Physical Education, University of Coimbra, Coimbra, Portugal. [7]Portuguese Foundation for Science and Technology (SFRH/BD/101083/2014), Lisbon, Portugal. [8]Faculty of Medicine, University of Coimbra, Coimbra, Portugal. [9]Laboratory of Pharmacology and Experimental Therapeutics, Institute for Biomedical Imaging and Life Sciences (IBILI), Faculty of Medicine, University of Coimbra, Coimbra, Portugal. [10]Center for Neuroscience and Cell Biology (CNC), Institute for Biomedical Imaging and Life Sciences (IBILI), Faculty of Medicine, University of Coimbra, Coimbra, Portugal. [11]Research Center in Sports Sciences, Health Sciences and Human Development (CIDESD), University Institute of Maia (ISMAI), Maia, Portugal. [12]Laboratory of Metabolic Adaptations to Exercise in Physiological and Pathological conditions (AME2P), Université Clermont Auvergne, Clermont-Ferrand, France. [13]School of Exercise Science, Faculty of Health, Australian Catholic University, East Melbourne, Victoria, Australia. [14]Metabolism, Nutrition, and Exercise Laboratory (GEPEMENE), State University of Londrina (UEL), Londrina, Brazil. [15]School of Health and Technology, Polytechnical Institute of Coimbra, Coimbra, Portugal.

References

1. Johnell O, Kanis JA. An estimate of the worldwide prevalence and disability associated with osteoporotic fractures. Osteoporos Int. 2006;17(12):1726–33.
2. Rizzoli R, Bianchi ML, Garabedian M, McKay HA, Moreno LA. Maximizing bone mineral mass gain during growth for the prevention of fractures in the adolescents and the elderly. Bone. 2010;46(2):294–305.
3. Bonjour JP, Chevalley T, Rizzoli R, Ferrari S. Gene-environment interactions in the skeletal response to nutrition and exercise during growth. Med Sport Sci. 2007;51:64–80.
4. Behringer M, Gruetzner S, McCourt M, Mester J. Effects of weight-bearing activities on bone mineral content and density in children and adolescents: a meta-analysis. J Bone Miner Res. 2014;29(2):467–78.
5. Wallace IJ, Kwaczala AT, Judex S, Demes B, Carlson KJ. Physical activity engendering loads from diverse directions augments the growing skeleton. J Musculoskelet Neuronal Interact. 2013;13(3):283–8.
6. Ginty F, Rennie KL, Mills L, Stear S, Jones S, Prentice A. Positive, site-specific associations between bone mineral status, fitness, and time spent at high-impact activities in 16- to 18-year-old boys. Bone. 2005;36(1):101–10.
7. Boreham CA, McKay HA. Physical activity in childhood and bone health. Br J Sports Med. 2011;45(11):877–9.
8. Gruodyte R, Jurimae J, Cicchella A, Stefanelli C, Passariello C, Jurimae T. Adipocytokines and bone mineral density in adolescent female athletes. Acta Paediatr. 2010;99(12):1879–84.
9. Nichols JF, Rauh MJ, Barrack MT, Barkai HS. Bone mineral density in female high school athletes: interactions of menstrual function and type of mechanical loading. Bone. 2007;41(3):371–7.
10. Pedersen BK, Febbraio MA. Muscles, exercise and obesity: skeletal muscle as a secretory organ. Nat Rev Endocrinol. 2012;8(8):457–65.
11. Scofield KL, Hecht S. Bone health in endurance athletes: runners, cyclists, and swimmers. Current Sports Med Rep. 2012;11(6):328–34.
12. Tenforde AS, Fredericson M. Influence of sports participation on bone health in the young athlete: a review of the literature. PMR. 2011;3(9):861–7.
13. Sartori R, Sandri M. BMPs and the muscle-bone connection. Bone. 2015;80:37–42.
14. Seeman E. Clinical review 137: Sexual dimorphism in skeletal size, density, and strength. J Clin Endocrinol Metab. 2001;86(10):4576–84.
15. Kirmani S, Christen D, van Lenthe GH, Fischer PR, Bouxsein ML, McCready LK, et al. Bone structure at the distal radius during adolescent growth. J Bone Miner Res. 2009;24(6):1033–42.
16. Duan Y, Turner CH, Kim BT, Seeman E. Sexual dimorphism in vertebral fragility is more the result of gender differences in age-related bone gain than bone loss. J Bone Miner Res. 2001;16(12):2267–75.
17. Burt LA, Naughton GA, Greene DA, Courteix D, Ducher G. Non-elite gymnastics participation is associated with greater bone strength, muscle size, and function in pre- and early pubertal girls. Osteoporos Int. 2012;23(4):1277–86.
18. Ferry B, Lespessailles E, Rochcongar P, Duclos M, Courteix D. Bone health during late adolescence: effects of an 8-month training program on bone geometry in female athletes. Joint Bone Spine. 2013;80(1):57–63.
19. Lopes C, Aro A, Azevedo A, Ramos E, Barros H. Intake and adipose tissue composition of fatty acids and risk of myocardial infarction in a male Portuguese community sample. J Am Diet Assoc. 2007;107(2):276–86.
20. Agostinete RR, Duarte JP, Valente-dos-Santos J, Coelho-e-Silva MJ, Tavares OM, Conde JM, et al. Bone tissue, blood lipids and inflammatory profiles in adolescent male athletes from sports contrasting in mechanical load. PLoS One. 2017;12(6):e0180357.
21. Baxter-Jones AD, Kontulainen SA, Faulkner RA, Bailey DA. A longitudinal study of the relationship of physical activity to bone mineral accrual from adolescence to young adulthood. Bone. 2008;43(6):1101–7.
22. Lohman T, Roche AF, Martorell R. Anthropometric standardization reference manual. Human Kinetics: Champaign; 1988.
23. Kuczmarski RJ, Ogden CL, Guo SS, Grummer-Strawn LM, Flegal KM, Mei Z, et al. 2000 CDC growth charts for the United States: methods and development. Vital Health Stat. 2002;11:1–186.
24. Flegal KM, Cole TJ. Construction of LMS parameters for the Centers for Disease Control and Prevention 2000 growth charts. Natl Health Stat Rep. 2013;63:1–3.
25. Malina RM, Bouchard C, Bar-Or O. Growth, maturation, and physical activity. Human Kinetics: Champaign; 2004.
26. Hopkins WG, Marshall SW, Batterham AM, Hanin J. Progressive statistics for studies in sports medicine and exercise science. Med Sci Sports Exerc. 2009; 41(1):3–13.
27. Rosnow RL, Rassithal R. Computing contrast, effect sizes and conternulls on other people is published data: General procedures for research consumer. Psychol Methods. 1996;1:331–40.
28. Baxter-Jones AD, Burrows M, Bachrach LK, Lloyd T, Petit M, Macdonald H, et al. International longitudinal pediatric reference standards for bone mineral content. Bone. 2010;46(1):208–16.
29. Gomez-Bruton A, Gonzalez-Aguero A, Gomez-Cabello A, Matute-Llorente A, Casajus JA, Vicente-Rodriguez G. The effects of swimming training on bone tissue in adolescence. Scand J Med Sci Sports. 2015;25(6):589–602.
30. Padez C, Rocha MA. Age at menarche in Coimbra (Portugal) school girls: a note on the secular changes. Ann Hum Biol. 2003;30(5):622–32.
31. Malina RM, Rogol AD, Cumming SP, Coelho e Silva MJ, Figueiredo AJ. Biological maturation of youth athletes: assessment and implications. Br J Sports Med. 2015;49(13):852–9.
32. Santos DA, Dawson JA, Matias CN, Rocha PM, Minderico CS, Allison DB, et al. Reference values for body composition and anthropometric measurements in athletes. PLoS One. 2014;9(5):e97846.
33. Tenforde AS, Fredericson M, Sayres LC, Cutti P, Sainani KL. Identifying sex-specific risk factors for low bone mineral density in adolescent runners. Am J Sports Med. 2015;43(5):1494–504.
34. Kini U, Nandeesh BN. Physiology of Bone Formation, Remodeling, and Metabolism. In: Fogelman I, Gnanasegaran G, van der Wall H, editors. Radionuclide and Hybrid Bone Imaging. Berlin: Springer; 2012. p. 29–57.
35. Fehling PC, Alekel L, Clasey J, Rector A, Stillman RJ. A comparison of bone mineral densities among female athletes in impact loading and active loading sports. Bone. 1995;17(3):205–10.
36. Heinonen A, Oja P, Kannus P, Sievanen H, Manttari A, Vuori I. Bone mineral density of female athletes in different sports. Bone Miner. 1993;23(1):1–14.
37. Umemura Y, Ishiko T, Yamauchi T, Kurono M, Mashiko S. Five jumps per day increase bone mass and breaking force in rats. J Bone Miner Res. 1997;12(9): 1480–5.

14

Residents' breastfeeding knowledge, comfort, practices, and perceptions

Elizabeth Esselmont[1,2], Katherine Moreau[1], Mary Aglipay[3] and Catherine M. Pound[1,2]*

Abstract

Background: Physicians have a significant impact on new mothers' breastfeeding practices. However, physicians' breastfeeding knowledge is suboptimal. This knowledge deficit could be the result of limited breastfeeding education in residency. This study aimed to explore pediatric residents' breastfeeding knowledge, comfort level, clinical practices, and perceptions. It also investigated the level and type of education residents receive on breastfeeding and their preferences for improving it.

Methods: Descriptive, cross-sectional, self-reported online questionnaires were sent to all residents enrolled in a Canadian general pediatric residency program, as well as to their program directors. Resident questionnaires explored breastfeeding knowledge, comfort level, clinical practices, perceptions, educational experiences and educational preferences. Program director questionnaires collected data on current breastfeeding education in Canadian centers. For the resident survey, breastfeeding knowledge was calculated as the percent of correct responses. Demographic factors independently associated with overall knowledge score were identified by multiple linear regression. Descriptive statistics were used for the program director survey.

Results: Overall, 201 pediatric residents, and 14 program directors completed our surveys. Residents' mean overall breastfeeding knowledge score was 71% (95% CI: 69-79%). Only 4% (95% CI: 2-8%) of residents were very comfortable evaluating latch, teaching parents breastfeeding positioning, and addressing parents' questions regarding breastfeeding difficulties. Over a quarter had not observed a patient breastfeed. Nearly all agreed or strongly agreed that breastfeeding promotion is part of their role. Less than half reported receiving breastfeeding education during residency and almost all wanted more interactive breastfeeding education. According to pediatric program directors, most of the breastfeeding education residents receive is didactic. Less than a quarter of program directors felt that the amount of breastfeeding education provided was adequate.

Conclusion: Pediatric residents in Canada recognize that they play an important role in supporting breastfeeding. Most residents lack the knowledge and training to manage breastfeeding difficulties but are motivated to learn more about breastfeeding. Pediatric program directors recognize the lack of breastfeeding education.

Keywords: Assessment, Postgraduate medical education, Residency, Breastfeeding

* Correspondence: cpound@cheo.on.ca
[1]University of Ottawa, 451 Smyth Road, Ottawa, ON K1H 8M5, Canada
[2]Children's Hospital of Eastern Ontario, 401 Smyth Road, Ottawa, ON K1H 8L1, Canada
Full list of author information is available at the end of the article

Background

Infants, mothers, families, and society benefit from breastfeeding [1]. Breastfeeding decreases the incidence of infectious diseases [2, 3], enhances performance on neurocognitive testing [4, 5], decreases the risk of breast [6, 7] and ovarian cancers [6] in mothers, and strengthens the mother-infant bond [8]. Both the American Academy of Pediatrics and the Canadian Pediatric Society advocate for physicians to be knowledgeable about breastfeeding in order to successfully address and manage breastfeeding issues [1, 9]. Yet, multiple studies have shown that physicians' knowledge of breastfeeding continues to be inadequate and thus, they are unable to counsel mothers appropriately [10–19].

A lack of physician support negatively affects breastfeeding duration [20–23]. As such, there is a need to provide breastfeeding education to residents. A recent study showed that Canadian physicians' breastfeeding knowledge is suboptimal, and that breastfeeding education in residency is limited [18]. Although this study provided useful information about specific knowledge gaps among Canadian physicians, it included only a small number of pediatric residents. Therefore, we undertook the present Canadian study to explore: (a) residents' breastfeeding knowledge, comfort level, clinical practices, and perceptions; (b) the level and type of education residents receive on breastfeeding and their preferences for improving it; and (c) whether demographic variables are associated with residents' breastfeeding knowledge, comfort level, clinical practices, and perceptions. We also surveyed pediatric program directors in Canada to gather additional information on the level of breastfeeding education in their programs.

Methods

Study design and participant criteria

We conducted a descriptive, cross-sectional, self-reported, online survey of all general pediatric residents enrolled in years 1 to 4 of a Canadian residency training program in March 2014. There were 638 general pediatric residents enrolled in Canadian programs for the 2013-2014 academic year. Residents were excluded if they had already entered a pediatric subspecialty training program or if they had previously been enrolled in a residency training program outside of Canada. We also conducted a descriptive, cross-sectional, self-reported, online survey of the 17 pediatric residency program directors across Canada.

Sample size

We based our sample size calculation on the response rate (30%) of a previous national breastfeeding study as well as other studies involving physicians [18, 24]. Given that 637 residents were eligible for the study, a response rate of 30% would equate to 191 participants. This would allow us to estimate a proportion (assuming a true value of 50%) to within plus or minus 7.1% with 95% confidence. We expected all 17 Canadian program directors to participate.

Survey instruments

Resident survey

The resident survey included the following six domains: breastfeeding knowledge, comfort level, clinical practices, perceptions, educational experiences, and educational preferences. To develop questions for the knowledge domain, we drew on items from the American Academy of Pediatrics' online breastfeeding curriculum pre- and post- knowledge tests [25, 26] as well those from a previous physician survey on breastfeeding [18]. We obtained permission from both these sources prior to using their items. We also ensured that all survey questions reflected the National Board of Medical Examiners guidelines for valid one-best answer knowledge questions [27]. Five International Board-Certified Lactation consultants and 12 subspecialty pediatric residents reviewed the survey for clarity and feasibility. We then modified the survey based on the feedback received from these individuals.

The final survey consisted of 35 closed-ended questions. These questions included ten multiple-choice items for the knowledge domain. We defined a priori an overall knowledge score of 70% (7/10 questions correct) as acceptable because this cut-off score was used in the previous national physician breastfeeding survey [18]. The survey also included three questions for each of the comfort level, clinical practices, perceptions, educational experiences, and educational preferences domains. The remaining questions addressed participant eligibility and demographics.

Program director survey

A three-question program director survey was also developed by the study team to gather data on current breastfeeding education in Canadian pediatric residency programs. The following questions were included: (1) In total, how much time does your program devote to educating residents about the assessment and management of breastfeeding difficulties? (2) What modalities are used to educate residents in your program about breastfeeding? (3) To what extent do you agree that the amount of breastfeeding education currently provided to residents in your program is adequate? Given the exploratory nature of these questions and the brevity of the survey, validity evidence was not established for this survey.

Data collection

The Children's Hospital of Eastern Ontario Research Ethics Board approved this study. All pediatric program directors consented for residents in their programs to participate. Each program director provided the study

131

team with the contact information of one resident representative, who distributed the online resident survey. This survey was available in Canada's two official languages (French and English). The online program director survey was sent directly to all program directors via e-mail.

Statistical analysis

For the resident survey, descriptive statistics were used to summarize the respondents' demographic characteristics, educational experiences, comfort level, clinical practice, perceptions, and educational preferences. Breastfeeding knowledge was calculated as the percent of correct responses. Multiple linear regression was used to identify demographic factors that were independently associated with the overall knowledge score. All demographic variables were included in the multivariate model. Missing data were handled via list-wise deletion. The identification of demographic factors associated with knowledge was the primary goal of the modeling so only main effects (no interactions) were assessed. Associations between residents' comfort level and these demographic factors were tested using chi-squared tests and Fisher's exact test where appropriate. A p-value of < 0.05 was considered statistically significant. The analyses were performed using SPSS (IBM Corp. Version 21.0.). Descriptive statistics were also used to summarize time spent on breastfeeding education in Canadian pediatric residency programs, levels of education provided and program directors perceptions regarding the adequacy of breastfeeding teaching provided to their residents.

For the program director survey, descriptive statistics were used to summarize time spent on breastfeeding education in Canadian pediatric residency programs, levels of education provided, and program directors' perceptions regarding the adequacy of the breastfeeding education.

Results

Resident survey

Respondent characteristics

The majority of respondents were female (88%) and under the age of 30 (70%). Of the respondents, 18% of had children. Table 1 provides additional characteristics of the respondents.

Knowledge

The average overall knowledge score of pediatric residents was 71% (95%CI: 69-73%). Table 2 summarizes residents' results on each question in the knowledge domain of the questionnaire. Multiple linear regression results are shown in Table 3. Residents who had one or more children and residents who reported receiving breastfeeding education scored an average of 11.6 points higher (95% CI: 3.1-22.7; $p = 0.01$) and an average of 4.8 points higher (95% CI: -0.07-9.7; $p = 0.05$) (on a 100-point scale), respectively, on the knowledge domain of the questionnaire.

Table 1 Participant Demographics

Characteristic	Total n (%)
Age (years) [a]	
< 30	140 (70)
30-50	60 (30)
Current Year of Residency Training	
First	57 (28)
Second	53 (26)
Third	57 (28)
Fourth	34 (17)
Province / Territory of Residency Program[b]	
Western Provinces (BC, AB, SK, MB)[c]	49 (25)
Ontario	75 (38)
Quebec	57 (29)
Atlantic Provinces (NS, NFLD)[d]	19 (10)
Breastfeeding learning (check all that apply)	
Personal experience	54 (27)
Medical school	78 (39)
Residency	134 (67)
Course	9 (5)
Self-directed learning	70 (35)
Other	17 (9)
Breastfeeding education during residency	97 (48)
Certification in breastfeeding support	1 (0.5)
Has one or more children	36 (18)

[a]Missing 1 response
[b]Missing 1 response
[c]BC: British Columbia, AB: Alberta, SK: Saskatchewan, MB: Manitoba
[d]NS: Nova Scotia, NFLD: Newfoundland

Comfort level

Seven percent of residents were very comfortable evaluating an infant's latch at the breast while 10% were very comfortable teaching a parent to position an infant at the breast. Nine percent were very comfortable addressing parents' questions about breastfeeding difficulties and 4 % of residents were very comfortable at all three of these skills. Older age (30-50 years old versus less than 30), higher year of residency training, personal experience with breastfeeding, having one or more children, and possessing certification in breastfeeding were all associated with higher levels of comfort with these skills ($p < 0.05$).

Clinical practices supporting breastfeeding

A total of 28% of residents had not observed a patient breastfeed in the hospital or office setting; 74% had observed a patient breastfeed 4 times or less in the same setting. In addition, 75 and 96% of residents reported having never taught a new mother breastfeeding techniques (e.g., latch, positioning at the breast), and how to use a breast pump, respectively.

Table 2 Frequency Distribution of Correct Response on Residents' Survey (*N* = 201)

Question	Correct Answer	Respondents with Correct Answer (*n* %)
A mother complains that her otherwise healthy and thriving 6 week old infant has been breastfeeding almost every 1-2 h for a day or two. What do you explain to her?	The baby requires more milk because he/she is growing and frequent breastfeeding is his/her way to increase milk supply.	145 (72.9)[a]
A mother with a 3-day-old baby presents with sore nipples. The problem began with the first feeding and has persisted with every feeding. What is the most likely source of the problem? (AAP)[b]	Poor attachment to the breast	175 (87.1)
Which of the following is a correct statement about the latch during breastfeeding? (AAP)	The baby needs to be latched so that he compresses the milk sinuses when suckling at the breast[e]	52 (25.9)
The mother of a breastfed 3-month-old will be away from her baby overnight for a business trip. She has an electric pump, but will not have a refrigerator available to her during the trip. Of the following, which is the BEST advice to give her regarding pumping and storing of her breast milk during the time of separation? (AAP)	She should pump the milk and store it with ice in a cooler at approximately refrigerator temperature (< 4 °C)	102 (50.7)
What increases milk production? (AAP)	More frequent milk removal	175 (87.5)[c]
During the postpartum stay, a breastfeeding mother reports that she is having difficulty getting her infant to breastfeed. What is the best way to manage this situation? (AAP)	Request assistance for the mother at the infant's next feeding to evaluate the breastfeeding technique	192 (96.0)[d]
What is severe engorgement most often due to? (AAP)	Infrequent feedings	140 (69.7)
An otherwise healthy, well-hydrated 5-day old breastfeeding infant is admitted to the hospital with jaundice. In addition to treating the child with phototherapy, which of the following would you first recommend?	Feed the infant more frequently and ensure the mother knows how and when to use a breast pump	153 (76.1)
In a baby who is breastfeeding effectively, what is the position of the baby's tongue?	The tongue is easily visible	102 (50.7)
What is the first thing you would do if a breastfeeding mother complains that her nipples are cracked and sore?	Assess baby's position and latch	192 (95.5)

[a]Missing 2 responses
[b]AAP: American Academy of Pediatrics
[c]Missing 1 response
[d]Missing 1 response
[e]This answer, taken verbatim from the American Academy of Pediatrics, is only partially correct as milk sinuses have been demonstrated to be absent from the breast as per Ramsay et al. study [29]

Perceptions

Ninety-four percent of respondents agreed or strongly agreed that breastfeeding promotion is part of their role as a pediatric resident; 54% agreed or strongly agreed that is the responsibility of the child's primary physician to perform an evaluation of breastfeeding in the first 3 to 5 days after birth, and 92% of residents agreed or strongly agreed that physicians can influence how long a mother decides to breastfeed.

Quality of education

Less than half (48%) of pediatric residents reported receiving breastfeeding education during their residency. The teaching provided was most often didactic. Only 16% of pediatric residents had the opportunity to follow a lactation consultant during their residency. Only 5% of pediatric residents reported receiving teaching in the form of interactive workshops with breastfeeding mothers.

Educational preferences

Almost all residents (93%) agreed or strongly agreed that more breastfeeding education should be incorporated into

pediatric residency training. Most residents felt that 4-8 h of breastfeeding teaching throughout residency would be the optimal amount. The two teaching methods that residents believed would be most effective for helping them learn about breastfeeding were following a lactation consultant (81%) and interactive workshops with breastfeeding mothers (71%).

Program directors' survey

Information on 14 residency programs was obtained from the program directors, for a response rate of 82%. The results of the Program Directors' Survey are summarized in Table 4. A total of 21% of program directors surveyed felt that the amount of breastfeeding education provided by their program was adequate.

Discussion

Although residents scored slightly above our minimum acceptable score of 70% on the knowledge domain of the survey, there is still significant room for improving pediatric residents' breastfeeding knowledge. Residents' comfort level with assessing and managing breastfeeding difficulties was

Table 3 Unadjusted and Adjusted[a] Linear Regression for Breastfeeding Knowledge Score among Canadian Pediatric Residents ($n = 191$)

	Unadjusted		Adjusted	
	Estimate (95% CI)	P Value	Estimate (95% CI)	P Value
Age		0.28		0.45
< 30	Reference		Reference	
30-50	2.7 (− 2.2-7.6)		−2.23 (− 8.0-3.5)	
Gender		0.05		0.08
Male	Reference		Reference	
Female	6.9 (0.02-13.7)		6.5 (−0.8-13.8)	
Current Year of Residency Training		0.01		0.08
First	Reference		Reference	
Second	0.2 (−5.7-6.1)		−0.8 (−7.1-5.5)	
Third	6.1 (0.3-11.9)		4.4 (−1.8-10.7)	
Fourth	10.1 (3.4-16.8)		7.9 (0.04-15.8)	
Province / Territory of Residency Program		0.06		0.13
Western Provinces (BC, AB, SK, MB)[b]	Reference		Reference	
Ontario	−1.7 (−7.4-4.1)		−0.2 (−5.9-5.5)	
Quebec	2.1 (−4.0-8.2)		3.2 (−3.2-9.6)	
Atlantic Provinces	9.2 (0.8-17.8)		8.8 (0.2-17.4)	
Breastfeeding learning				
Personal experience	4.9 (−0.1-9.9)	0.06	−1.5 (−9.6-6.4)	0.70
Medical school	0.6 (−4.0-5.2)	0.80	4.4 (−0.5-9.4)	0.08
Residency	1.6 (−3.2-6.3)	0.52	−1.4 (−6.7-3.9)	0.60
Course	2.4 (−8.4-13.2)	0.66	−11.3 (−23.2-0.6)	0.06
Self-directed learning	2.6 (−2.1-7.3)	0.28	1.9 (−2.7-6.5)	0.43
Other	−1.8 (−9.8-6.3)	0.66	−0.1 (−8.4-8.2)	0.98
Breastfeeding Education During Residency	6.1 (1.7-10.5)	0.01	4.8 (−0.07-9.7)	0.05
Certification in breastfeeding support	19.5 (−12.7-50.8)	0.24	8.1 (−24.7-41.0)	0.63
Has one or more children	11.6 (6.0-17.2)	< 0.01	12.9 (3.1-22.7)	0.01

[a]Adjusted regression model includes all variables in the table
[b]BC: British Columbia, AB: Alberta, SK: Saskatchewan, MB: Manitoba

suboptimal. Although most residents agree that it is their role to promote and assist with breastfeeding, many have never watched a patient being breastfeed. Our study showed that residents receive very little breastfeeding education. Nearly all residents felt that more breastfeeding education should be incorporated into their residency. This feeling is shared by most program directors, who identified a need for more breastfeeding education in residency.

Our survey identified some specific knowledge gaps among pediatric residents, particularly in the area of latch assessment. Other poorly answered questions related to the pumping and storage of breastmilk, as well as an infant's tongue position while feeding. This suggests that pediatric residents lack knowledge about some of the practical aspects of breastfeeding. These results are in line with those of other studies worldwide [10, 17–19]. In

Canada, a recent study also showed that failing to identify aspects of a successful latch was a significant knowledge gap for family physicians and pediatricians [18].

Given the above results, it is not surprising that very few residents felt comfortable providing parents with assistance in the practical aspects of breastfeeding. Only 8 of our 201 participants felt very comfortable evaluating an infant's latch at the breast, teaching a parent how to position an infant at the breast, and addressing parents' questions about breastfeeding issues. This result is quite different from the results of a recent Canadian study [18], where 75% of physicians in the study reported feeling comfortable addressing breastfeeding difficulties. In that previous study, this number dropped significantly when physicians were asked specifically about their comfort with technical breastfeeding skills, such as latch assessment, milk transfer and teaching mothers how to use a breast pump.

Table 4 Program Director Survey (N = 14)

Question	Answer	Respondents n (%)
How much time does your program devote to educating residents about assessment and management of breastfeeding difficulties (total over 4 years of residency)?	0 h	1 (7.1)
	1-3 h	4 (28.6)
	4-8 h	7 (50.0)
	9-16 h	2 (14.3)
	more than 16 h	0 (0.0)
What modalities are used to educate residents in your program about breastfeeding? (pick all that apply)	None	1 (7.1)
	Didactic teaching	9 (64.3)
	Grand rounds	2 (14.3)
	Computer based tutorials	3 (21.4)
	Interactive workshops with moms	1 (7.1)
	Following lactation consultant	4 (28.6)
	Other	4 (28.6)
To what extent do you agree that the amount of breastfeeding education currently provided to residents in your program is adequate?	Strongly Disagree	1 (7.1)
	Disagree	6 (42.9)
	Neutral	4 (28.6)
	Agree	3 (21.4)

This previous study suggested that perhaps physicians overestimated their overall comfort with breastfeeding as they may not be aware of their deficiencies. The residents in our current study reported significantly lower comfort levels with addressing breastfeeding difficulties, indicating that residents may be more aware of their gaps in breastfeeding knowledge and skills, and may therefore be more receptive to educational interventions.

Not surprisingly, having children, personal experience with breastfeeding, and certification in breastfeeding were all associated with greater comfort level with the practical aspects of breastfeeding and counseling. Interestingly, higher year of residency training was also associated with higher self-reported comfort. However, this increase in comfort was not paralleled by an increase in knowledge, which raises the possibility that residents may feel more confident without necessarily being more proficient.

We found that residents had very limited experience observing their patients being breastfed. This may be due to residents' awareness of their lack of breastfeeding counseling-related knowledge, resulting in residents feeling ill-equipped to help if breastfeeding difficulties arise and therefore avoiding these vulnerable situations. This is particularly concerning since previous studies have established that a lack of physician support negatively impacts breastfeeding duration [20–23]. Nevertheless, we were encouraged to find that despite their discomfort with

assessing and managing some of the practical aspects of breastfeeding, residents have positive perceptions about breastfeeding. Of the pediatric residents who completed our survey, the vast majority agreed that breastfeeding promotion is part of their role as a pediatric resident.

Our results clearly demonstrate that breastfeeding education for pediatric residents in Canada could be greatly improved. The small number of residents who had received breastfeeding education reported that the teaching received was mostly didactic, which corresponds to what the program directors reported. However, when residents were asked about their preferred mode of breastfeeding education, most felt that interactive workshops with breastfeeding mothers or shadowing a lactation consultant would be the best ways to learn. Evidently there is a gap between the breastfeeding education residents are currently receiving and the type of breastfeeding education they perceive would be most beneficial. This shows a significant area for improvement within pediatric residency programs across Canada.

Study limitations include a somewhat low overall response rate, although we expected this for the population surveyed [24]. Given that residents self-selected to complete the survey, this could have resulted in a higher proportion of residents with a breastfeeding interest participating in our study. Such self-selection would be expected to positively skew our results, suggesting that the overall knowledge score of all pediatric residents is actually below the 71% score that we obtained. We specifically designed the survey used in this study and the knowledge items have not been widely used or tested from a psychometric point of view. However, it is important to note that we adapted questions from other studies used to assess physicians' breastfeeding knowledge, confidence, beliefs, and attitudes and as such, we were able to make comparisons between our results and those of the other studies.

This is the largest survey of pediatric residents in Canada assessing breastfeeding knowledge. Moreover, we obtained information from the majority of program directors, giving us a complete view of the state of breastfeeding education among pediatric residents in Canada.

Conclusion

Though the Canadian Pediatric Society, the American Academy of Pediatrics and the World Health Organization all emphasize the important role physicians play in the initiation and continuation of breastfeeding [1, 9, 28], the results of our study show that pediatric residents across Canada are inadequately prepared for this role during their residency. Based on these results, we suggest that a breastfeeding curriculum be implemented in Canadian pediatric residency training programs to ensure that residents are prepared to assess and address breastfeeding difficulties that arise in their patients. We hope that by addressing this education deficit during residency, we can train pediatricians who can provide quality care to breastfeeding infants and mothers and thereby increase the rates and duration of breastfeeding.

Acknowledgements
The authors wish to thank all the residents and program directors who participated in the study.

Funding
This study was funded through a Children's Hospital of Eastern Ontario Research Institute Resident Research Grant. The funding body had no role in the design of the study, in the collection, analysis and interpretation of data, in the writing of the manuscript and in the decision to submit the manuscript for publication.

Authors' contributions
EE participated in the conception and design of the study, data acquisition, and interpretation of the data. She drafted the manuscript, gave final approval of the version to be published, and agreed to be accountable for all aspects of the work. KM participated in the conception and design of the study. She critically revised for important intellectual content, gave final approval of the version to be published, and agreed to be accountable for all aspects of the work. MA analyzed and interpreted the data. She critically revised for important intellectual content, gave final approval of the version to be published, and agreed to be accountable for all aspects of the work. CP supervised EE in all aspects of the study, participated in the conception and design of the study, and interpretation of the data. She helped with drafting of the manuscript, gave final approval of the version to be published, and agreed to be accountable for all aspects of the work. All authors read and approved the final manuscript.

Competing interests
The authors declare that they have no competing interests.

Author details
[1]University of Ottawa, 451 Smyth Road, Ottawa, ON K1H 8M5, Canada. [2]Children's Hospital of Eastern Ontario, 401 Smyth Road, Ottawa, ON K1H 8L1, Canada. [3]Children's Hospital of Eastern Ontario Research Institute, 401 Smyth Road, Ottawa, ON K1H 5B2, Canada.

References
1. American Academy of Pediatrics. Section on breastfeeding. Breastfeeding and the use of human milk. Pediatrics. 2012;129:e827–41.
2. Heinig MJ. Host defense benefits of breastfeeding for the infant. Effect of breastfeeding duration and exclusivity. Pediatr Clin N Am. 2001;48:105–23. ix
3. Duijts L, Jaddoe WV, Hoffman A, Moll HA. Prolonged and exclusive breastfeeding reduces the risk of infectious diseases in infancy. Pediatrics. 2010;126:e18.
4. Horwood LJ, Fergusson DM. Breastfeeding and later cognitive and academic outcomes. Pediatrics. 1998;101:e9.
5. Anderson JW, Johnstone BM, Breastfeeding RDT. Cognitive development: a meta-analysis. Am J Clin Nutr. 1999;70:525–35.
6. Chowdhury R, Sinha B, Sankar MJ, et al. Breastfeeding and maternal health outcomes: a systematic review and meta-analysis. Acta Paediatr. 2015;104: 96–113.
7. Collaborative Group on Hormonal Factors in Breast Cancer. Breast cancer and breastfeeding: collaborative reanalysis of individual data from 47 epidemiological studies in 30 countries, including 50302 women with breast cancer and 96973 women without the disease. Lancet. 2002;360:187–95.
8. American Academy of Pediatrics. Breastfeeding and the use of human milk. Policy statement. Pediatrics. 2005;115:496–506.
9. Pound CM, Unger S. Canadian pediatric society, hospital pediatrics section, nutrition and gastroenterology committee. The baby-friendly initiative: promoting, supporting and protecting breastfeeding. Paediatr Child Health. 2012;17:317–21.
10. Krogstrand K, Parr K. Physicians ask for more problem-solving information to promote and support breastfeeding. J Am Diet Assoc. 2005;105:1943–7.
11. Leavitt G, Martinez S, Ortiz N, Garcia L. Knowledge about breastfeeding among a Group of Primary Care Physicians and Residents in Puerto Rico. J Community Health. 2009;34:1–5.
12. Finneran B, Murphy K. Breast is best for GPs—or is it? Breastfeeding attitudes and practice of general practitioners in the mid-west of Ireland. Ir Med J. 2004;97:269–70.
13. Nakar S, Peretz O, Hoffman R, Kaplan B, Vinker S. Attitudes and knowledge on breastfeeding among paediatricians, family physicians, and gynaecologists in Israel. Acta Paediatr. 2007;96:848–51.
14. Al-Nassaj HH, Al-Ward NJA, Al-Awqati NA. Knowledge, attitudes and sources of information on breastfeeding among medical professionals in Baghdad. East Mediterr Health J. 2004;10:871–8.
15. Brodribb W, Fallon A, Jackson C, Hegney D. Breastfeeding and Australian GP registrars—their knowledge and attitudes. J Hum Lact. 2008;24:422–30.
16. Freed GL, Clark SJ, Sorenson J, Lohr JA, Cefalo R, Curtis P. National assessment of physicians' breast-feeding knowledge, attitudes, training, and experience. JAMA. 1995;273:472–6.
17. Williams EL, Hammer LD. Breastfeeding attitudes and knowledge of pediatricians-in-training. Am J Prev Med. 1995;11:26–33.
18. Pound CM, Williams K, Grenon R, Aglipay M, Plint AC. Breastfeeding knowledge, confidence, beliefs and attitudes of Canadian physicians. J Hum Lact. 2014;30:298–309.
19. Freed GL, Clark SJ, Lohr JA, Sorenson JR. Pediatrician involvement in breast-feeding promotion: a National Study of residents and practitioners. Pediatrics. 1995;96:490–4.
20. Taveras EM, Capra AM, Braveman PS, Jenscold NG, Escobar GJ, Lieu TA. Clinician support and psychosocial risk factors associated with breastfeeding discontinuation. Pediatrics. 2003;112:108–15.
21. Dillaway HE, Douma ME. Are pediatric offices "supportive" of breastfeeding? Discrepancies between mothers' and healthcare professionals' reports. Clin Pediatr (Phila). 2004;43:417–30.
22. Labarere J, Gelbert-Baudino N, Ayral A, Duc C, Berchotteau M, Bouchon N, et al. Efficacy of breastfeeding support provided by trained clinicians during an early, routine, preventive visit: a prospective, randomized, open trial of 226 mother-infant pairs. Pediatrics. 2005;e139:115.
23. Holmes AV, McLeod AY, Thesing C, Kramer S, Howard CR, et al. Physician breastfeeding education leads to practice changes and improved clinical outcomes. Breastfeeding Med. 2012;7:403–8.
24. Asch S, Connor SE, Hamilton EG, Fox SA. Problems in recruiting community-based physicians for health services research. J Gen Intern Med. 2000;15:591–9.
25. American Academy of Pediatrics Breastfeeding Residency Curriculum Pre-test. from https://www.aap.org/en-us/advocacy-and-policy/aap-health-initiatives/Breastfeeding/Documents/Pre_testAnswers.pdf. Accessed Feb 1st 2018.
26. American Academy of Pediatrics Breastfeeding Residency Curriculum Pre-test. from https://www.aap.org/en-us/advocacy-and-policy/aap-health-initiatives/Breastfeeding/Documents/Post_testAnswers.pdf. Accessed Feb 1st 2018
27. Case SM, Swanson DB. Constructing Written Test Questions For the Basic and Clinical Sciences. Third Edition. National Board of Medical Examiners; 1998.
28. UNICEF-WHO. Innocenti declaration. On the protection, promotion and support of breast-feeding. New York: UNICEF; 1990.
29. Ramsay DT, Kent JC, Harmann RA, Hartmann PE. Anatomy of the lactating human breast redefined with ultrasound imaging. J Anat. 2005;206:525–34.

15

Challenges to and opportunities for the adoption and routine use of early warning indicators to monitor pediatric HIV drug resistance in Kenya

Nanlesta A. Pilgrim[1]*(iD), Jerry Okal[2], James Matheka[2], Irene Mukui[3] and Samuel Kalibala[1]

Abstract

Background: Pediatric non-adherence to antiretroviral therapy (ART), loss to follow-up, and HIV drug resistance (HIVDR) are challenges to achieving UNAIDS' targets of 90% of those diagnosed HIV-positive receiving treatment, and 90% of those receiving treatment achieving viral suppression. In Kenya, the pediatric population represents 8% of total HIV infections and pediatric virological failure is estimated at 33%. The monitoring of early warning indicators (EWIs) for HIVDR can help to identify and correct gaps in ART program functioning to improve HIV care and treatment outcomes. However, EWIs have not been integrated into health systems. We assessed challenges to the use of EWIs and solutions to challenges identified by frontline health administrators.

Methods: We conducted key informant interviews with health administrators who were fully knowledgeable of the ART program at 23 pediatric ART sites in 18 counties across Kenya from May to June 2015. Thematic content analysis identified themes for three EWIs: on-time pill pick-up, retention in care, and virological suppression.

Results: Nine themes—six at the facility level and three at the patient level—emerged as major challenges to EWI monitoring. At the facility level, themes centered on system issues (e.g., slow return of viral load results), staff shortages and inadequate adherence counseling skills, lack of effective patient tracking and linkage systems, and lack of support for health personnel. At the patient level, themes focused on stigma, non-disclosure of HIV status to children who are age eligible, and little engagement of guardians in the children's care.
Practical solutions identified included the use of lay health workers (e.g., peer educators, community health workers) to implement a variety of care and treatment tasks, whole facility approaches to adherence counseling, adolescent peer support groups, and working with children directly as soon as they are age eligible.

Discussion: The monitoring of EWIs has not been routine in health facilities in Kenya due to several challenges. However, facilities have implemented novel strategies to address some of these barriers. Future work is needed to assess whether scale-up of some of these approaches can aid in the effective use of EWIs and improving HIV care outcomes among the pediatric population.

* Correspondence: npilgrim@popcouncil.org
[1]Population Council, 4301 Connecticut Avenue NW, Suite 280, Washington, DC 20008, USA
Full list of author information is available at the end of the article

Background

In 2014, UNAIDS launched "90–90–90" targets aimed at ending the HIV epidemic whereby 90% of all people living with HIV are diagnosed, 90% of those diagnosed HIV-positive receive treatment, and 90% of those receiving treatment achieve viral suppression by 2020 [1]. However, there is need for more focused attention on achieving these targets among the pediatric population [2]. Globally, 2.6 million children younger than 15 years of age are living with HIV, 90% of whom reside in sub-Saharan Africa, and only 32% are accessing antiretroviral therapy (ART) [2]. In Kenya, children aged 0 to 14 accounted for 8% of total HIV infections ($n = 120,000$) in 2016, with 45% in need of ART [3]. With such rates, achieving the second and third "90s" among the pediatric population is in danger. It is important that these targets are achieved given that the pediatric population faces lifelong treatment and there are limited treatment options available [2]. The prevention of HIV drug resistance (HIVDR) is therefore critical within the pediatric population.

Existing research finds that the pediatric population living with HIV are at high risk of virological failure of ART and acquiring drug-resistant HIV, with some studies placing drug resistance estimates as high as 60–90% [2, 4, 5]. A 2013 study among 100 Kenyan children, aged 18 months to 12 years, reported 34% of them experienced virological failure and 68% of those with failure had drug-resistant mutations [6]. Similarly, a 2014 Kenyan study of 462 children younger than 5 years in 15 sentinel sites reported 33% of children experienced virological failure with a higher drug resistant mutation rate of 88% [7]. Poor adherence, which is prevalent during early childhood and adolescence, is a significant contributor to failure [8, 9]. One review reported wide adherence estimates, ranging from 49 to 100% among pediatric populations in low and middle income countries [10]. Moreover, loss to follow-up remains a key concern. A recent systematic literature review found that one year retention rates ranged from 71 to 95% among 31,877 African children with 73% of those who were not retained being due to loss to follow-up, and 27% were confirmed to have died [2, 11].

Given the high rates of virologic failure and drug-resistant HIV as well as widely variable rates of adherence and loss to follow-up, there is a need to strengthen health systems to support retention in care and ART adherence among the pediatric population if the ambitious UNAIDS targets are to be realized. The monitoring of early warning indicators (EWIs), developed by the World Health Organization (WHO) in 2004 and refined in 2011, can help to identify and correct gaps in ART program functioning and quality of service delivery to aid in the prevention of HIVDR, improve patient retention in care, and increase adherence [8, 12]. The five EWIs monitor factors that are associated with

HIVDR related to patient care, patient behavior, and clinic management (Table 1). If implemented and monitored consistently, EWIs can provide an evidence base for programmatic change and/or public health action to prevent and address HIVDR or virologic failure among the pediatric population [12].

The positive outcomes that can be realized through the monitoring of the EWIs are dependent on their uptake by clinic and program management as well as their regular use in deciding how to improve program functioning and quality of service delivery. In 2012, the Kenyan National AIDS & STI Control Programme (NASCOP) assessed the use of EWIs in 32 of the approximately 1032 pediatric ART sites across Kenya and found the sites had good prescribing practice (98%) but moderate to poor patient retention in care (69% of patients retained at 12 months), retention on first line therapy (50%), and appointment keeping (29% kept > 80% of appointments) [13]. Results also showed that the routine utilization of EWIs within health facilities was a challenge and their use has not been introduced across the country.

With the need to expand the use of EWIs as a method for reducing HIVDR as well as improving adherence and patient retention in care, the current study was conducted with frontline health administrators to assess the challenges to routine utilization of EWIs and to identify strategies to increase the uptake and utilization of EWIs within pediatric facilities.

Methods
Sample
Key informant interviews (KIIs) were conducted in 23 pediatric ART facilities, between May and June 2015, with the facility official who was fully knowledgeable of the pediatric ART program and procedures. The identified individuals were typically the Officer in Charge or a pediatric provider. The pediatric sites were a subset of the 32 sites, where the 2012 EWI monitoring assessments were conducted by NASCOP [13]. Stratified random sampling by geographic region, facility type (e.g., health center) and administration (e.g., Ministry of Health [MoH], faith-based

Table 1 Early warning indicators for HIV drug resistance

On-time pill pick-up: % of patients with 100% on-time drug pick-up during the first 12 months of ART or during a specified time period

Retention in care: % of patients retained in care 12 months after ART initiation

Drug stockout: % of months with any day(s) of stock out of any routinely dispensed ARV drug

Prescribing practices: % of ART prescriptions congruent with national/ international guidelines

Viral load suppression: % of patients with viral load < 1000 copies/mL 12 months after ART initiation organization [FBO]) were used to select the facilities. Facilities located in the former North Eastern province of Kenya were excluded due to political unrest at the time of the data collection. The facilities included represent 18 of the 47 counties and 7 of the 8 former provinces of Kenya.

Recruitment and interview procedures

Prior to KIIs, the investigators called managers at each facility to explain the purpose of the study and request the support of the Officer in Charge in identifying the most knowledgeable individual to take part in KIIs. A signed letter requesting their support from NASCOP and the MoH was also provided. An appointment was then scheduled for the completion of the KIIs. KIIs were completed with the Officer in Charge of the health facilities. The Officers in Charge were nurses, clinical officers, or doctors.

The KIIs were conducted in English in a private location at each facility and lasted approximately 60 minutes. Trained research assistants with clinical backgrounds conducted all KIIs. Research assistants used a semi-structured interview guide to facilitate the discussion. The KII guide consisted of questions that generated discussion on facility pediatric ART treatment procedures, existing EWI monitoring procedures, and identification of strategies to improve EWI monitoring (Table 2).

Analyses

All KIIs were audio recorded and transcribed verbatim for analysis. Trained research team members verified all transcripts against the original audiotapes to ensure that the transcriptions were accurate. Thematic content analysis, a research method for the subjective interpretation of the content of text data through the systematic classification process of identifying themes or patterns, was used [14]. Themes identifying key factors influencing the routine use and monitoring of EWIs, the challenges and opportunities for EWI monitoring, and strategies facilities have used to overcome challenges were identified by research staff (NP, JO, JM). Identification of themes were an iterative process whereby themes were redefined or merged based on emerging patterns in the data [15]. JO and JM initiated the process by reading and open coding all transcripts and noting all topics raised by the respondents. JO next consolidated topics into major themes, whereby some topics were expanded upon while others were eliminated or merged. Throughout the analytic process, NP reviewed all themes derived from the analyses. The differences in themes by type of clinics were minimal and therefore, we focus on crosscutting findings. Discussions around dispensing practices and pharmacy stock-outs were limited and therefore, the results focus on factors influencing

Table 2 Interview questions asked of health facility officers in charge

1. Please describe the methods this facility uses to monitor HIV drug resistance for the pediatric population.
    a. What challenges, if any, have you experienced using these methods to monitor drug resistance?
    b. What are the positive aspects of using these methods to monitor drug resistance?
2. How effective has any of these drug resistance monitoring systems been in identifying possible drug resistance in the pediatric population?
3. Please describe any standards and procedures regarding conducting pill counts with pediatric ART patients at this facility.
    a. What challenges or barriers does this facility experience regarding conducting pill counts with pediatric ART patients?
    b. How can these barriers or challenges be addressed?
4. Please describe any standards and procedures regarding the conduct of adherence counseling with pediatric ART patients at this facility.
    a. What challenges or barriers does this facility experience regarding conducting adherence counseling with pediatric ART patients?
    b. How can these barriers or challenges be addressed?
5. Please describe any standards and procedures for tracking or tracing pediatric ART patients who miss appointments and drug pickups at this facility.
    a. What challenges or barriers does this facility experience regarding tracking or tracing ART patients? What about among the pediatric ART patients?
    b. How can these barriers or challenges be addressed?
6. Does this facility have the equipment and qualified staff to conduct viral load testing?
    If yes,
    a. Please describe any challenges or barriers to conducting routine viral load testing at this facility.
    b. In your opinion, how can these barriers or challenges be addressed?
    c. What works best in conducting routing viral load testing?
    If no,
    a. Please describe the procedures regarding viral load testing with pediatric patients?
    b. What challenges or barriers does this facility encounter with viral load testing?
    c. In your opinion, how can these barriers or challenges be addressed?
    d. What works best in conducting routing viral load testing?
7. Please describe how the current facility practices regarding pill counts, adherence counseling, and/or patient tracing may affect the quality of records needed for pediatric ART monitoring at this facility.
8. Overall, are the ART medical and pharmaceutical records at this facility well-maintained, or are there some gaps in recording the necessary information?
    a. Please describe any factors or challenges to maintaining complete and up-to-date ART records.
9. What interventions would you recommend to improve routine EWI monitoring at your facility?

on-time medication pick-up, retention on ART and care, and virological suppression.

Ethical approval

This protocol was reviewed and approved by the Population Council Institutional Review Board and the Kenyatta National Hospital/University of Nairobi Ethics & Research Committee. To protect facility Officers in Charge, we did not collect any personal identifying information to ensure that they could not be identified. Facility Officers in Charge provided verbal consent before being interviewed.

Results

KIIs were conducted with participants from five types of facilities: teaching/referral hospital ($n = 2$), provincial hospital ($n = 8$), district hospital ($n = 6$), sub-district hospitals ($n = 3$), and health center/dispensary ($n = 4$). Seventeen facilities were managed by the county government, three by the MoH, and three by FBOs. None of the facilities were currently using EWIs. Table 3 presents the nine themes that emerged across the three EWIs that yielded the most discussion - on-time pill pick-up, retention in care, and virological suppression - and the proportion of transcripts with the theme.

On-time pill pick-up

Five themes emerged that influenced on-time pill pick-up. At the facility level, low human resource capacity and inadequate adherence counseling skills; variable or non-usage of pill count to assess adherence and inappropriate clinical forms to record pediatric information affected providers ability to track medication use. At the patient level, non-disclosure of HIV status to children and stigma hindered adherence to ART and therefore, negatively affected medication pick-up. Within each theme, any associated strategies respondents have used to address the challenges encountered are presented.

Facility level
Inappropriate forms to record pediatric information
Participants explained that there was a lack of space on standard clinical forms to record dosage information

Table 3 Themes and % of transcripts with theme organized by EWI

Theme	%
On-time pill pick-up	
Facility level	
Inappropriate forms to record pediatric information.	39.1
Variable use of pill count to assess adherence.	34.7
Staff shortages and inadequate adherence counseling skills	47.8
Patient level	
Non-disclosure of HIV status to the child hinders adherence	69.6
Stigma hinders adherence	30.4
Retention in care	
Facility level	
Lay providers require support	82.6
A need for a national tracking system and tracking policies	21.7
Patient level	
Guardians pose a challenge to pediatric retention in care	52.2
Viral load suppression	
Facility level	
Systemic issues prohibited viral load measurement	95.7

and other important notes regarding monitoring such as pill counts and adherence counseling. This critical information impeded patient care because there was no way to appropriately and efficiently keep track of pediatric information. While some providers added the information using an extra piece of paper, the process is not standardized and therefore, the next provider seeing the patient might not fill out the information.

> The spaces provided are not adequate. For example, on the space of the drug that I am prescribing for the client, there is no space to prescribe the dosage. It's only the type of drug but the dosage is not there.... [I] wish that it had enough adequate space for us to include the drug dosage. (Provincial hospital, MoH managed)

> For the pediatric population I thought we would have an extra blue card, a different one designed for them because some of the information here is not meant for the pediatrics. (Provincial hospital, County government managed)

Variable use of pill count to assess adherence
Pill count procedures varied across facilities, with some respondents reporting conducting pill counts every visit, some relying on guardians' reports, and others not conducting pill counts at all. Respondents questioned the usefulness of pill counts, especially since the clinician forms did not have a space to record the information. Moreover, they explained that since most pediatric drugs were in liquid formula, it was difficult to get a correct estimate of the remaining drugs if the guardians forgot to bring the bottles. Other times, they could not engage with the pediatric clients themselves because clinic hours occurred during school times. Therefore, they were unable to assess drug usage.

> We don't have anywhere to record those pill counts, we haven't put measures on how to put pill counts on records. (Health center, County government managed)

> Our main challenge as I had told you earlier is most of the population, especially from 5-14 [years old]...is still schooling.... That time for schooling, you only see the caretaker coming or the treatment supporter coming to collect the drugs for the child, while this child was supposed to visit. Yeah, so mainly the challenge we are getting especially where the clients are concerned the failure to visit the clinic in time. (District hospital, FBO managed)

Staff shortages and inadequate adherence counseling skills

Participants recounted a number of factors at their facility that negatively impacted adherence counseling, on-time medication pick-up, and retention in care (EWI 2). Staff shortages resulted in patients receiving shortened and at times, no counseling, due to competing demands among the providers and the increasing volumes of patients. They also noted that providers needed more training to provide specialized counseling and psychosocial support services to their clients. Additionally, high patient volumes resulted in incomplete patient records. While facility staff endeavored at the end of the day to complete all records, they were often overwhelmed, and records remained incomplete. Even with some facilities having electronic medical records (EMR), many only had 1–2 computers. When coupled with unpredictable electricity, they relied on paper-based record keeping systems before entry into the EMR.

> Our facility workload is very large, even though we need more time to counsel, sometimes we shorten our counseling period because we have other patients who are waiting to be seen.... So at least when we deal with the staffing issues we will have dealt with the challenge. (Health center, County government managed)

> We make sure that everything is documented by the end of the day, but sometimes, the workload is too much for us, we find that we have so much to do at the end of the day.... We need more staff, record officers, we are doing work which is not ours, it's for records, filling the files, tracking the clients. (District hospital, County government managed)

Though all participants called for the deployment of more health staff to cope with the high number of clients seeking services, some respondents described strategies they have instituted to combat the challenges faced. One strategy has been to train peer educators, community health workers, and people living with HIV to help with adherence counseling of both adult and pediatric populations. In fact, peer educators also assist with pill count and tracing of clients who miss appointments.

> Okay, the peer educators can show you the record where they capture the adherence counseling and also the patient's file has everything. In the file there is a form for adherence counseling. (Health center, County government managed)

> Respondent: The counseling is done by trained personnel on adherence counseling. We also have PLP taking the clients through adherence counseling.

> Moderator: What is PLP?

> Respondent: That is people living positive.

> Moderator: Okay, they also do the counseling for...

> Respondent: Adherence because we have trained them. (Provincial hospital, MoH managed)

Another strategy has been to take a whole facility approach to adherence counseling. That is, everyone that a client encounters at the facility—from front desk staff to pharmacist to peer educator—has been trained on adherence counseling so that consistent adherence messaging is provided to all clients. While facilities were short-staffed, they endeavored for adherence messaging to be delivered at each point of care. Similarly, a few facilities described regularly (e.g., monthly) bringing together different departments to discuss any clients who might be heading toward drug resistance and implementing steps to address the problem.

> The main adherence counseling is done by the nurse, because we require a professional to do the enrolment as we empower the client with adequate information on care and treatment and everywhere else adherence continues because the clinician will talk about it, the peer educator will talk about it, the records person will talk about it, the pharmacist, the nutritionist the same and the like, it's for each.... Adherence counseling is done on every visit and we reinforce it especially where we identify a gap. (Provincial hospital, County government managed)

To address the inefficient record keeping system, at least one facility hired a records officer dedicated solely to ensuring that all records were kept updated and complete.

> We have our records office being managed by our qualified health information records officer. She has all the registers with her, the daily activity register. She is the one who manages the diary, she manages the ART register and after every activity, she sits down to go through the day's work, identify where the gaps are and they compare their results with the peer educators who have also been asked to monitor all the clients booked for the day's work. Then they bring their data together to see whether there is any data remaining so the records are well kept in the records office. (Provincial hospital, County government managed)

Patient level

Non-disclosure of HIV status to the child hinders adherence

Among the pediatric population, discussions around medication adherence and drug resistance are usually held with guardians, who may or may not be the child's parents. Ideally, participants prefer to start adherence counseling with the pediatric patient as early as possible so that the child understands the importance of taking medication on-time and staying in care. However, many guardians remain reluctant to disclose to their children that they are living with HIV. In return, some children saw no reason to take the medication and stopped, thus affecting on-time pick-up of medications.

> So I think pediatrics is a challenge on adherence. Then the other problem with the pediatrics is disclosure because you question why: "Why am I taking? What are these for?" Most too often than not they won't tell them they are taking drugs for HIV. Like the caregivers, they won't tell them the truth that they are taking them for the HIV disease so they would take and take and sometimes they get tired of taking and say "I won't take again..." till you explain to them why they are taking. We have even had teenagers taking ARVs and don't know they are taking ARVs. (Provincial hospital, County government managed)

Participants explained that they engage in regular adherence counseling with guardians, where a key component is emphasizing early disclosure so that the child is prepared well in advance to transition to adult care. When they have succeeded, they engage the child as early as possible (for some facilities as young as age six) in their care focusing on understanding HIV, the importance of medication adherence, and the importance of keeping appointments. Some participants noted times when children come to the clinic without their parents because of the counseling the child received.

> The issues, especially if they are not disclosed, parents have not disclosed, so it's a problem, they refuse to come back. They are as if they don't want to take the drugs because the parents have not explained to them why they are taking drugs. They say why are they taking drugs and others are not taking. So we get them into groups and explain to them why they are taking drugs and we involve their parents, that is why we are able to retain them in here. (District hospital, County government managed)

> When the child is ten years, we like including them as early as possible. So they are able to understand. Ten years I am imagining it's a child in class four, so this is

a child who is able to understand. So we help them understand the importance of taking the medicine and we assist them in knowing how many they are supposed to take and we involve them in the counting so that they can appreciate how they need to take their drugs and what I expect the next time they come over. (Provincial hospital, County government managed)

Stigma hinders adherence

Participants described that experience of stigma, especially in the school settings, negatively impacted adherence to medications among the pediatric population, especially those in adolescence. Some school-going adolescents live in dormitories and when their status is known, they might be ridiculed or shunned. In response, they would take their medications intermittently, such as when they return home. By the time they see their clinician, they could have developed drug resistance.

> Our adolescents, they experience a lot of challenges when they go to school.... The environment at school may be hostile and he will abandon treatment. How to access the dormitory is a problem. How to take their medication because...it may be during class time is a problem. So you find that they keep the drug until they feel they are free, that is when they take the drugs. So it has led to drug resistance in children. (Provincial hospital, County government managed)

In an attempt to counteract the stigma encountered, some facilities separated clinic days for younger and older pediatric clients, recognizing that each group has their own special needs. Specifically, for older pediatric patients, some facilities formed pediatric support groups.

> For the pediatric patients, we also have some groups, pediatric support group. We have children support groups, when we also follow them and talk to them, so that they can be able to interact together with those who are positive and those who are not. (District hospital, County government managed)

Retention in care

Three themes emerged that influenced retention in care. At the facility level, lack of necessary support for lay health workers and lack of a tracking system and policies, negatively affected the ability to retain the pediatric population in care. At the patient level, challenges with pediatric guardians were the predominant barrier to retention. Within each theme, any associated strategies respondents have used to address the challenges encountered are presented.

Facility level
Lay health workers require support

To facilitate patient retention, participants described relying heavily on lay health workers (e.g., peer educators, volunteers, and community health workers) to conduct tracing of patients who miss appointments. Peer educators initiated outreach via mobile phones and short message services (SMS) to guardians and patients (if old enough) to reschedule missed appointments. If the patient does not have a mobile phone or cannot be reached, their information is given to community health workers to trace them within the community. If the tracing is successful, the clients are brought back to care and intensive counseling is initiated to understand the reasons for missing the appointment and to prevent loss to follow up. If unsuccessful, some facilities mark them as lost to follow-up while others wait until they reappear.

The volunteer who works here is conversant with most of the clients that come from the area that she comes from.... Or she is able to know somebody who comes from an area that is nearer one of the clients so we are able to track them that way. (Sub-district hospital, Country government managed)

If they don't come, we call volunteers or the community health worker to follow them. We also have the SMS system, we send them an SMS daily. (District hospital, County government managed)

However, some participants explained that the ability to trace patients has been hindered by a lack of financial resources to support lay health workers. For example, funds do not exist to purchase airtime to make calls or send SMS to clients nor are there funds for transportation to physically trace clients in the community. Participants describe instances where staff have used their own money to buy airtime to make calls or send SMS. However, staff and volunteers have become increasingly reluctant to use their own money due to the high volume and expense. As a result, little to no effort is made to retain clients in care when they do not show up for appointments.

It all amounts to financial support. For the follow up, we will need financial support. One, they need airtime. Two, in terms of motorcycles or vehicles, they will need fuel. (Teaching/referral hospital, MoH managed)

Some of those patients don't have phone numbers and there is no money provided for physical tracing.

So, when they don't have a phone and don't come, we just wait for them. We don't trace them physically. (Sub-district hospital, County government managed)

A need for a national tracking system and tracking policies

Closely linked to the ability to trace clients is the need for tracking policies and a national tracking system. A few respondents noted that guidelines on how to track clients did not exist. For staff safety, guidelines should be created and distributed to facilities.

How do I do a follow up? How am I covered with the policy, in case anything happens to me there? Is this policy designed in a way to protect me? ...you could go somewhere you find [gangs], you find them armed with knives, so is there anything to show if I go there and anything happens? So the guidelines [would] really assist, ...the guidelines should come officially in this manner so that you can just put it there... even when clients come you can point out to the client and say, you see what the government says in this and this. (Health center, Country government managed)

For both pediatric and adult populations, participants expressed frustration over patients moving between health care facilities and not being able to adequately track them or record the information within their records. That is, if a patient moves away for a short while, they might register at a different clinic and receive medications from that facility. When they return, they come back to their original health facility. While some providers call the other facilities to fill in the necessary information to have complete records, there is no standardized process of doing this. Additionally, they must rely on patient self-report that they were under the care of another provider when they were absent from the facility.

Clients on transit are a challenge and those are the things we experience as a facility, if NASCOP had a mechanism like a national ID card such that all clients who are enrolled to care and treatment are able to be tracked at one point, it will help us. (Provincial hospital, County government managed)

Patient level
Guardians pose a challenge to pediatric retention in care

Participants explained that retention in care for their pediatric populations is a major problem primarily due to challenges with caregivers. In addition to the non-disclosure previously noted, participants explained that some caregivers had little or no interest in being engaged in their children's/ward's health care and therefore, neither brought the child to their appointment nor made sure they took their medications. Some children, especially those who are orphans, switched caregivers frequently with the new caregivers often unaware of the child's HIV status. Therefore, the continuity of the child's care is compromised.

> Getting the relative's contact becomes hard because whoever has been the treatment support sometimes when you call back they say they do not know the child, or the child went with other relatives. They do not know how the child is fairing on, so it becomes hard because they hand over from one person to another. (Provincial hospital, County government managed)

> The father is there but he is not cooperative because when I asked the child to be accompanied by him, he doesn't come. I have never seen him.... The other relatives are not near. He only stays with the father and the mother is not there. She passed on. (District hospital, FBO managed)

In light of the challenges posed by guardians, some facilities instituted practices to help increase retention among the pediatric population. These practices included a community approach to pediatric care, whereby providers identify multiple individuals within the child's social circle, including relatives and teachers, who can support the child in their care and treatment. They also collected multiple forms of contact information from the child's current guardians of all relatives the child could potentially live with. As stated previously, where possible, they engage the children early so they understand the importance of visiting the facility regularly.

> For the pediatric, we try to have several phone numbers on how we can reach them. If we can have two or three caregivers who stay with the child, if at all we are not able to reach one, we can try the other one. (Sub-district hospital, County government managed)

> Maybe community—identifying other people who can be able to support the child outside that person who comes with the child. Addressing the family as a whole so that when one person is not there, the others can be able to sit in for the main one, and also involving the child quite early and making the child understand the importance of drug adherence. (Provincial hospital, County government managed)

Viral load suppression
One theme at the facility level emerged as a challenge to monitoring potential virological failure.

Systemic issues prohibited viral load measurement
Participants stated that they relied mainly on CD4 counts and clinical staging of patients to aid in the assessment of drug resistance as there were several systemic issues that prohibited the measurement of viral loads. Although all participants noted they had access to viral load testing, either by having viral load machines on site or sending specimens to a neighboring facility, many identified several issues prohibiting the on-time measurement of viral loads: constant stock-out of dry blood spot filter paper and reagents, machine breakdown, long turnaround time (e.g., 2–3 months) to receive testing results, rejection of samples due to poor packaging, and samples getting spoiled during transportation. Some facilities were located far from a testing site and lacked adequate transport, making it difficult to transport specimen in a timely manner.

> CD4 we did not have that much of the challenge. The turnaround time was short, we would get the results even in a week's time. But for viral load the turnaround time is very long. The thing is that by the time I bleed until I get my results, even 2/3 months can go by. So that is not appropriate because you need to have results as soon as possible so that we can make decisions as soon as we wish to. (Provincial hospital, County government managed)

Participants emphasized the need for timely replenishment of the necessary supplies to conduct appropriate tests because the current system negatively impacts the quality of care provided to patients and the degree to which patients engage in their care. Participants explained that patients stop coming for care after being repeatedly informed that the facility did not have the appropriate supplies to test them or have not yet received their test results. Thus, it is closely linked to retention in care.

> Provide a viral load machine...and also have continuous supply of filter papers or what is required for the viral loads to be done so that we can be able to meet our targets. (Provincial hospital, MoH managed)

> Yes, erratic supply also demotivates the client actually. You come today and you are told it's not there; you come next time you are told it's not there, so you will not bother again and just forget about it. (Provincial hospital, MoH managed)

Discussion

In this study, we conducted KIIs with frontline heads of facilities to assess the challenges to routine utilization of the EWIs and to identify strategies to increase the uptake and utilization of EWIs within pediatric facilities. We identified challenges at the facility level as well as the patient level associated with the monitoring of EWIs.

For EWI monitoring to be used routinely in the provision of care and treatment to pediatric patients, there is a need to address staff shortage. In our study, some facilities filled the gap by using lay health workers to provide several services, including adherence counseling, pill counting, and client tracking. Task shifting and sharing within the health system has been a key HIV care and treatment implementation strategy and the use of lay health workers can aid in ensuring high quality care is provided [16]. For EWI to become more routinized, capitalizing on the strengths of lay health workers would contribute to alleviating the concerns of overburdened and short-staffed health system. However, they will require the necessary resources, support, and training to be effective. For example, if trained appropriately, a dedicated lay health worker at each facility can be used to regularly abstract the information from clinical records to calculate the EWIs. Additionally, the rapid initiation of EMR systems in facilities can facilitate the process. This can allow for timely retrieval of EWI results and the implementation of steps to address barriers hindering optimal performance. Additionally, there is need to conduct studies to project how the use of lay health workers can aid the health system on a larger scale.

The monitoring of EWIs is insufficient without equipping health professionals with the necessary skills to combat the barriers linked to on-time medication pick-up or retention in care. Training in the provision of psychosocial support, especially adherence counseling, is urgently needed. In a few facilities, a paradigm shift to training has occurred whereby everyone the patient encounters during their visit has received adherence counseling training, and this could be implemented on a larger scale. This paradigm of operation serves to reinforce positive messages at all levels. It also ensures that the patient receives the messaging even when the clinician does not have the time to provide counseling. Further study is needed to assess whether this approach is linked to increased adherence and retention in care.

There is also a need to establish and expand psychosocial and peer support groups for both pediatric patients and their caregivers. Early childhood and adolescence is a time of opportunity but it is also a time when children begin to form their identities [17]. As such, they are particularly susceptible to stigma, which can play a detrimental role in their physical, mental and sexual health and development [18, 19]. Therefore, it is critical that the necessary youth-sensitive, age-specific psychosocial and peer support groups are available for this population at health care facilities or within their communities. Peer support groups have been shown to be successful in improving adolescents' emotional well-being and positively influencing medical outcomes, including medication adherence [20, 21]. These types of groups are also needed for caregivers, who are often reluctant to disclose to their children their HIV status or who are not as engaged in their children's care and treatment. This type of reaction by caregivers is often driven by stigma and discrimination, whereby they try to preserve their children's 'normal' childhood by protecting them from the potential stigma or discrimination they might encounter as a result of being known to be living with HIV [22, 23]. However, the WHO recommends that children of school age, six years and above, should be told their HIV status and younger children be told their status incrementally in preparation for full disclosure because there is evidence of health benefits and little evidence of psychological or emotional harm from disclosure of HIV status to HIV-positive children [24]. As such, there is a need for guardians to receive ongoing support as they prepare children for the adjustment process of living with HIV, addressing the associated life challenges, and becoming self-sufficient and independent [22–24]. Standardized protocols are also needed across facilities to help track children receiving HIV care. These could include the provision of forms to allow for the collection of multiple options of contact information for different potential caregivers of children.

Investments are needed to develop and improve facility systems to make the routine monitoring and use of EWIs a reality. The use of mobile technologies to support the achievement of health objectives has the potential to transform health service delivery, including health promotion, information access, health awareness raising, and decision support systems as well as enable behavior change and improve health outcomes in resource-limited settings [25–28]. For example, two randomized controlled trials in Kenya demonstrated improvements in ART adherence using mobile health platforms [26, 27]. Capitalizing on the proliferation of mobile technology across sub-Saharan Africa provides opportunities for improving EWIs. It can also be used in the design and implementation of a referral and linkage system to reduce loss to follow-up and ensure continuity of care among the pediatric population [29]. For example, one pilot study in Kenya utilized both internet-based coordination and text messaging to address barriers and improve the provision of early infant diagnosis of HIV [29]. The procurement system for medical supplies should also be regularly evaluated to prevent the stock-out of necessary supplies.

Limitations

This study had limitations. The data for this study were self-reported. As such, the data generated should be assessed being mindful of the likely impact of social desirability bias, comprehension, and limitations of recall accuracy. However, qualitative interviews provided detailed insights into the key challenges faced by facilities in monitoring and using EWIs and possible strategies that can be expanded to facilitate their regular use. Only one person per facility was interviewed which increases the risk of bias but the interviewee was the Officer in Charge, whose responsibilities included having a wide breath of knowledge of the facilities processes. Thematic content analysis uses subjective interpretation of data. However, the credibility of the themes derived was checked through an external process whereby a data interpretation meeting was conducted with key stakeholders in Kenya, including health care providers [30]. The results were presented, and the key stakeholders confirmed the accuracy of the themes. We did not directly interview family caregivers of the children and might have missed other salient issues concerning challenges to retention and on time pill pick up. The paper does not present results on dispensing practices and pharmacy stock-outs as limited discussions emerged on these two EWIs.

Conclusion

The routine monitoring and use of EWIs has the potential to significantly contribute toward achieving the UNAIDs' targets of 90% retention on ART with 90% viral suppression rates on first-line therapy. The usefulness of EWIs is negatively impacted by weaknesses within the health system (e.g., staff shortages, long turnaround times for viral load results, lack of filter paper) as well as patient-level factors (e.g., guardian challenges and stigma). However, facilities have implemented strategies (e.g., use of lay health workers) to address some of these barriers. Future work is needed to assess whether scale-up of some of these approaches can aid in the effective use of EWIs as well as improving HIV care outcomes among the pediatric population.

Abbreviations

ART: Antiretoviral therapy; EMR: Electronic medical records; EWI: Early warning indicators; FBO: Faith-based organization; HIV: Human immunodeficiency virus; HIVDR: HIV drug resistance; KII: Key informant interviews; MOH: Ministry of Health; NASCOP: Kenyan National AIDS & STI Control Programme; SMS: Short message services; UNAIDS: Joint United Nations Programme on HIV/AIDS

Funding

This study and manuscript were made possible through support provided by the US President's Emergency Plan for AIDS Relief and the US Agency for International Development (USAID) via HIVCore, a Task Order funded by USAID under the Project SEARCH indefinite quantity contract (contract no. AID-OAA-TO-11-00060); and Project SOAR (Supporting Operational AIDS Research), Cooperative Agreement number AID-OAA-14-00060, respectively. The Task Order was led by the Population Council in partnership with the Elizabeth Glaser Pediatric AIDS Foundation, Palladium and the University of Washington. Project SOAR is led by the Population Council in partnership with Avenir Health, Elizabeth Glaser Pediatric AIDS Foundation, Johns Hopkins University, Palladium, and The University of North Carolina.

Authors' contributions

Conceptualization of manuscript: NP, SK, JO. Drafted manuscript: NP, SK, JO, IM. Data Collection: JO, JM, IM. Analyzed the data: JO, JM, NP. Contributed to study instrument development: NP, JO, JM, SK. All co-authors reviewed and provided input on the manuscript. All authors read and approved the final manuscript.

Competing interests

The authors declare that they have no conflict of interest.

Author details

Population Council, 4301 Connecticut Avenue NW, Suite 280, Washington, DC 20008, USA. ²Population Council, Nairobi, Kenya. ³National AIDS & STI Control Programme, Nairobi, Kenya.

References

1. UNAIDS. 90–90–90: an ambitious treatment target to help end the AIDS epidemic. Geneva: UNAIDS; 2014.
2. Davies M-A, Pinto J. Targeting 90–90–90–don't leave children and adolescents behind. J Int AIDS Soc 2015;18(7Suppl 6).
3. UNAIDS. Country factsheets: Kenya 2016. Geneva: UNAIDS; 2017.
4. Kityo C, Sigaloff KCE, Boender TS, Kaudha E, Kayiwa J, Musiime V, et al. HIV drug resistance among children initiating first-line antiretroviral treatment in Uganda. AIDS Res Hum Retrovir. 2016;32(7):628–35.
5. Hamers RL, Sigaloff KC, Kityo C, Mugyenyi P, de Wit TFR. Emerging HIV-1 drug resistance after roll-out of antiretroviral therapy in sub-Saharan Africa. Curr Opin HIV AIDS. 2013;8(1):19–26.
6. Wamalwa D, Lehman DA, Benki-Nugent S, Gasper M, Gichohi R, Maleche-Obimbo E, et al. Long-term virologic response and genotypic resistance mutations in HIV-1 infected Kenyan children on combination antiretroviral therapy. J Acquir Immune Defic Syndr. 2013;62(3):267.
7. Ngugi E, Nge'no B, Odhiambo F, Ojoo S, Masyuko S. Virologic response and genotypic resistance mutations in HIV infected children on combination antiretroviral therapy in Kenya. Poster presentation presented at 20th International AIDS Conference, Melbourne. vol. Abstract MOPE048. 2014;
8. El-Khatib Z, Katzenstein D, Marrone G, Laher F, Mohapi L, Petzold M, et al. Adherence to drug-refill is a useful early warning indicator of virologic and immunologic failure among HIV patients on first-line ART in South Africa. PLoS One. 2011;6(3):e17518.
9. Haberer J, Mellins C. Pediatric adherence to HIV antiretroviral therapy. Curr HIV/AIDS Rep. 2009;6(4):194–200.
10. Vreeman RC, Wiehe SE, Pearce EC, Nyandiko WM. A systematic review of pediatric adherence to antiretroviral therapy in low-and middle-income countries. Pediatr Infect Dis J. 2008;27(8):686–91.
11. Abuogi LL, Smith C, McFarland EJ. Retention of HIV-infected children in the first 12 months of anti-retroviral therapy and predictors of attrition in resource limited settings: a systematic review. PLoS One. 2016;11(6): e0156506.
12. World Health Organization. Global report on early warning indicators of HIV drug resistance: technical report. Geneva: World Health Organization; 2016.
13. Ngugi E, Masyuko, S., Mukui, I., Katana, A., Waruru, A., Gichangi, A. Early warning indicators for HIV drug resistance in adult and pediatric antiretroviral therapy sites in Kenya: results of a national survey. Poster presentation presented at 7th conference on HIV pathogenesis, treatment, and prevention, Kuala Lumpur. Abstract MOPE184; 2013.
14. Hsieh HF, Shannon SE. Three approaches to qualitative content analysis. Qual Health Res. 2005;15(9):1277–88.
15. Brown NA, Smith KC, Thornton RL, Bowie JV, Surkan PJ, Thompson DA, et al. Gathering perspectives on extended family influence on African American children's physical activity. J Health Dispar Res Pract. 2015;8(1):10.

16. Callaghan M, Ford N. Schneider H. A systematic review of task-shifting for HIV treatment and care in Africa. Hum Resour Health. 2010;8(1):8.

17. Pilgrim NA, Blum RW. Protective and risk factors associated with adolescent sexual and reproductive health in the English-speaking Caribbean: a literature review. J Adolesc Health. 2012;50(1):5–23.

18. Ayres JR, Paiva V, Franca I Jr, Gravato N, Lacerda R, Della Negra M, et al. Vulnerability, human rights, and comprehensive health care needs of young people living with HIV/AIDS. Am J Public Health. 2006;96(6):1001–6.

19. Rao D, Kekwaletswe T, Hosek S, Martinez J, Rodriguez F. Stigma and social barriers to medication adherence with urban youth living with HIV. AIDS Care. 2007;19(1):28–33.

20. Funck-Brentano I, Dalban C, Veber F, Quartier P, Hefez S, Costagliola D, et al. Evaluation of a peer support group therapy for HIV-infected adolescents. AIDS. 2005;19(14):1501–8.

21. Hodgson I, Ross J, Haamujompa C, Gitau-Mburu D. Living as an adolescent with HIV in Zambia—lived experiences, sexual health and reproductive needs. AIDS Care. 2012;24(10):1204–10.

22. Bikaako-Kajura W, Luyirika E, Purcell DW, Downing J, Kaharuza F, Mermin J, et al. Disclosure of HIV status and adherence to daily drug regimens among HIV-infected children in Uganda. AIDS Behav. 2006;10(4 Suppl):S85–93.

23. DeMatteo D, Wells LM, Goldie RS, King SM. The'family'context of HIV: a need for comprehensive health and social policies. AIDS Care. 2002;14(2):261–78.

24. World Health Organization. Guideline on HIV disclosure counselling for children up to 12 years of age. Geneva: World Health Organization; 2011.

25. Catalani C, Philbrick W, Fraser H, Mechael P, Israelski DM. mHealth for HIV treatment & prevention: a systematic review of the literature. Open AIDS J. 2013;7:17–41.

26. Lester RT, Ritvo P, Mills EJ, Kariri A, Karanja S, Chung MH, et al. Effects of a mobile phone short message service on antiretroviral treatment adherence in Kenya (WelTel Kenya1): a randomised trial. Lancet. 2010;376(9755):1838–45.

27. Pop-Eleches C, Thirumurthy H, Habyarimana JP, Zivin JG, Goldstein MP, De Walque D, et al. Mobile phone technologies improve adherence to antiretroviral treatment in a resource-limited setting: a randomized controlled trial of text message reminders. AIDS. 2011;25(6):825.

28. Aranda-Jan CB, Mohutsiwa-Dibe N, Loukanova S. Systematic review on what works, what does not work and why of implementation of mobile health (mHealth) projects in Africa. BMC Public Health. 2014;14(1):1.

29. Finocchario-Kessler S, Goggin K, Khamadi S, Gautney B, Dariotis JK, Bawcom C, et al. Improving early infant HIV diagnosis in Kenya: study protocol of a cluster-randomized efficacy trial of the HITSystem. Implement Sci. 2015;10(1):96.

30. Nowell LS, Norris JM, White DE, Moules NJ. Thematic Analysis: Striving to meet the trustworthiness criteria. Int J Qual Methods. 2017;16:1–13.

16

Developing "My Asthma Diary": a process exemplar of a patient-driven arts-based knowledge translation tool

Mandy M. Archibald[1]*⬡, Lisa Hartling[2], Samina Ali[2], Vera Caine[3] and Shannon D. Scott[3]

Abstract

Background: Although it is well established that family-centered education is critical to managing childhood asthma, the information needs of parents of children with asthma are not being met through current educational approaches. Patient-driven educational materials that leverage the power of the storytelling and the arts show promise in communicating health information and assisting in illness self-management. However, such arts-based knowledge translation approaches are in their infancy, and little is known about how to develop such tools for parents. This paper reports on the development of "My Asthma Diary" – an innovative knowledge translation tool based on rigorous research evidence and tailored to parents' asthma-related information needs.

Methods: We used a multi-stage process to develop four eBook prototypes of "My Asthma Diary." We conducted formative research on parents' information needs and identified high quality research evidence on childhood asthma, and used these data to inform the development of the asthma eBooks. We established interdisciplinary consulting teams with health researchers, practitioners, and artists to help iteratively create the knowledge translation tools.

Results: We describe the iterative, transdisciplinary process of developing asthma eBooks which incorporates: (I) parents' preferences and information needs on childhood asthma, (II) quality evidence on childhood asthma and its management, and (III) the engaging and informative powers of storytelling and visual art as methods to communicate complex health information to parents. We identified four dominant methodological and procedural challenges encountered during this process: (I) working within an inter-disciplinary team, (II) quantity and ordering of information, (III) creating a composite narrative, and (IV) balancing actual and ideal management scenarios.

Conclusions: We describe a replicable and rigorous multi-staged approach to developing a patient-driven, creative knowledge translation tool, which can be adapted for use with different populations and contexts. We identified specific procedural and methodological challenges that others conducting comparable work should consider, particularly as creative, patient-driven knowledge translation strategies continue to emerge across health disciplines.

Keywords: Asthma, Knowledge translation, Parents, Children, Family-centered, Arts-based knowledge translation, Storytelling, Intervention development

* Correspondence: mandy.archibald@flinders.edu.au
[1]College of Nursing and Health Sciences, Flinders University, Sturt Road, Bedford Park, Adelaide, SA 5042, Australia
Full list of author information is available at the end of the article

Background

Educating parents about the complexities of childhood asthma is foundational to effective asthma management [1]. However, parents continue to struggle with fear and uncertainty about childhood asthma care, a problem compounded by inconsistent and often ineffective provision of asthma education [2, 3]. The paradoxical existence of high quality research evidence about asthma and continued deficiencies in parental knowledge, self-efficacy and suboptimal at-home asthma management is a knowledge translation (KT) problem. As such, finding effective ways to deliver asthma education to parents is essential given that asthma prevalence and childhood asthma morbidity continue to rise globally [4].

KT is an iterative process of synthesizing, disseminating and ethically applying knowledge to improve health, health services, and health systems globally [5]. Yet, mobilizing knowledge for use by health care professionals alone is insufficient to affecting change in real-life settings [6]. KT strategies targeting the wide-range of stakeholders (e.g., parents, non-health care professionals) are necessary, particularly in light of the growing emphasis on patient-centeredness, shared-decision-making, and community-based health management of chronic illnesses, including childhood asthma.

Arts-based approaches to KT offer viable ways of engaging key knowledge-users, such as parents, in a meaningful manner. Arts-based KT, defined here as the use of any art form to communicate knowledge (e.g., research from various sources), re-present and re-construct data, and promote empathetic understanding to affect attitudinal, knowledge or behavioural change, is gaining momentum across health disciplines concerned with mobilizing evidence to improve health outcomes [7, 8]. Arts-based approaches enable a human relationship to form with otherwise impersonal information by using artistic techniques, such as plot, characters, and specific vernacular [9, 10].

Although arts-based KT shows promise, the field is in an early developmental stage for healthcare professionals and data pertaining to the development, application, and evaluation of arts-based KT is generally lacking. As such, few examples of how to create arts-based KT strategies exist in the literature [11]. We address this gap by offering an account of how a visual art and story-based KT tool for parents of children with asthma was developed, while highlighting challenges encountered during this process. Although we developed this tool for parents of children with asthma, we believe our process can serve as a guide for others conducting similar work with different populations, including those interested in science communication (i.e., SciComm) more generally. Through describing this process we also explore general tensions related to the broader field of arts-based KT.

Arts-based knowledge translation

Different artistic representations convey various expressive qualities and as such, foreseeably impact viewers in distinct ways [9]. Visual representations may foster more emotive than rational responses compared with text [12]. Music ignites the imagination and fosters the development of mental models to help make sense of the world [13]. Theatre promotes engagement and renders abstract concepts, concrete [14]. The selection of an arts-based approach should be informed by an understanding of the form; population, context, and location of use; desired outcome of interest (e.g., attitude change); and the degree of precision in key messages and extent of participation enabled through each form of representation [7].

Considering how to faithfully represent health research data and how to precisely convey key messages are paramount considerations in arts-based KT. Precision and communication accuracy may account for the absence of exclusively visual KT tools in the literature [15, 16]; text is a necessary accompaniment to the visual form if precision in information delivery, a critical aim of much KT, is to be attained [7]. These considerations should occur in tandem with the extent of participation enabled through the selected strategy; for instance, whether a knowledge user can help shape the outcome of a narrative, as is the case with forum theatre or classical "choose-your-own adventure" stories. Generally, health information interwoven into a printed story has less variability in its delivery; the precision in its key messages and the extent of participation with the art form are more consistent [7]. Although visual and text-based strategies tend to have limited interactivity, they are often portable and accessible, particularly when digitized. Artistic form and method of delivery thereby constrain and liberate aesthetic effects and foreseeably impact usability and effectiveness.

Information literacy theory supports combining textual and visual forms to depict information emotively and rationally [17]. However, the paucity of accompanying literature on developing these complex tools limits current understanding [12]. Specifically, visual and text can be combined in endless ways across artistic styles, methods of delivery, degrees of abstraction, precision of key messages and extents of participation (e.g., cartoons, poetry, interactive web-platforms) [7]. As such, identifying arts-based KT strategies with comparable attributes and purposes is particularly challenging.

Examples of visual and text-based tools for non-health care provider stakeholder groups can be found in the literature, yet reporting of tool characteristics are generally lacking (Archibald & Scott, unpublished observations).

Lafreniere and colleagues [12] combined text and web--based cartoons to disseminate findings from nutrigenomics/nutrigenetics research. Each cartoon illustrated a research theme and was reinforced through text. The authors report that the approach was effective in conveying findings from the larger study, highlight pertinent procedural challenges to KT intervention development, and consider the impact of these challenges on effectiveness (e.g., simplification, aesthetics). Hartling and colleagues developed [11] paper-based storybooks for parents to communicate health information about childhood croup. Qualitative data from parents was used to revise the KT tools, led the authors to conclude that "the storybook format is a useful KT device" [18] (p. 162), and provided support for a user-centered development process. For our reported research, we learned from these examples, and designed a visual and text-based tool for parents, guided by parental information needs, preferences, and user-centered design principles.

Methods

We used a four stage, iterative process to develop the asthma eBooks (Fig. 1). We have detailed stage one and the interpretive description component of stage two in previous manuscripts [3, 4] and therefore only briefly describe these stages here. We then focus on stage three—the process of developing the arts-based KT tool. Stage four involves usability testing of the arts-based KT tool and will be discussed in a forthcoming manuscript.

Stage 1: Literature review

We conducted a state-of-the-science literature review of the information needs of parents of children with asthma [3]. This review illustrated a need to explicitly assess the information needs of parents of children with asthma. Based on findings from the 11 included articles, we constructed a parental information needs taxonomy, which included (i) asthma basics (e.g., basic pathophysiology), (ii) treatment modalities, (iii) coping, and (iv) medical expectations. We then used this to inform the development of a semi-structured interview guide for use in a qualitative study.

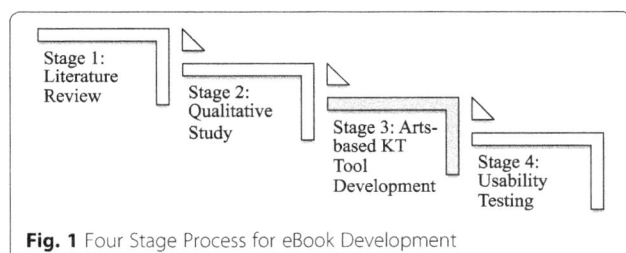

Fig. 1 Four Stage Process for eBook Development

Stage 2: Qualitative study

Interpretive description of information needs

We conducted an interpretive descriptive study [3, 19] of the information needs of 21 parents of children with asthma from diverse backgrounds and stages of asthma illness in an urban pediatrics centre in Western Canada [3]. Our research questions focused on parents' information needs and the general experiences of having a child with asthma. These data were foundational to developing the arts-based KT tool. For instance, parental uncertainty surrounding day-to-day asthma management enabled integration of "real-life" examples into the tool.

Through thematic analysis we identified four core themes: (I) recognizing severity, (II) acute management and inhaler use, (III) prevention versus crisis orientation to asthma management, and (IV) knowing about asthma [3]. We identified interactions with health care providers (HCPs) (e.g., how education was provided) and beliefs about asthma (e.g., acute or chronic) as two factors influencing these themes. These themes formed an information needs hierarchy and influenced which information to include in the KT tool (Fig. 2).

Stage 3: Arts-based KT tool development

We combined storytelling and visual art in an online format to deliver asthma education to parents. This decision was influenced by the stage two findings and the degree of ambiguity in key-message delivery permissible in this context of illness management [7]. For example, managing childhood asthma is a complex process involving viewing asthma as a chronic illness while responding appropriately during acute exacerbation periods. Integrating asthma management into family life, identifying and monitoring symptoms, and employing preventative measures are integral to positive outcomes. Factual and procedural knowledge related to asthma care are needed, which requires that information be clearly provided. Yet, changes in attitudes and beliefs about the nature of asthma are also necessary and may be less responsive to non-arts based information provision given the capacity of the arts to challenge entrenched assumptions [7]. The need to attend to knowledge, beliefs and attitudes reinforces the potential merits of using a story and visual arts-based KT approach. Using the Archibald Classification Schema of Arts-Based Knowledge Translation Strategies [7] (Fig. 3), we therefore categorized this strategy as a multimodal quadrant one approach due to the presence of precise key messaging and relative passive involvement with its use.

Determining the voice and presentation format for the tool were key considerations. A first-person, diary-format was selected for many reasons. First, participants emphasized the importance of personalized and compassionate

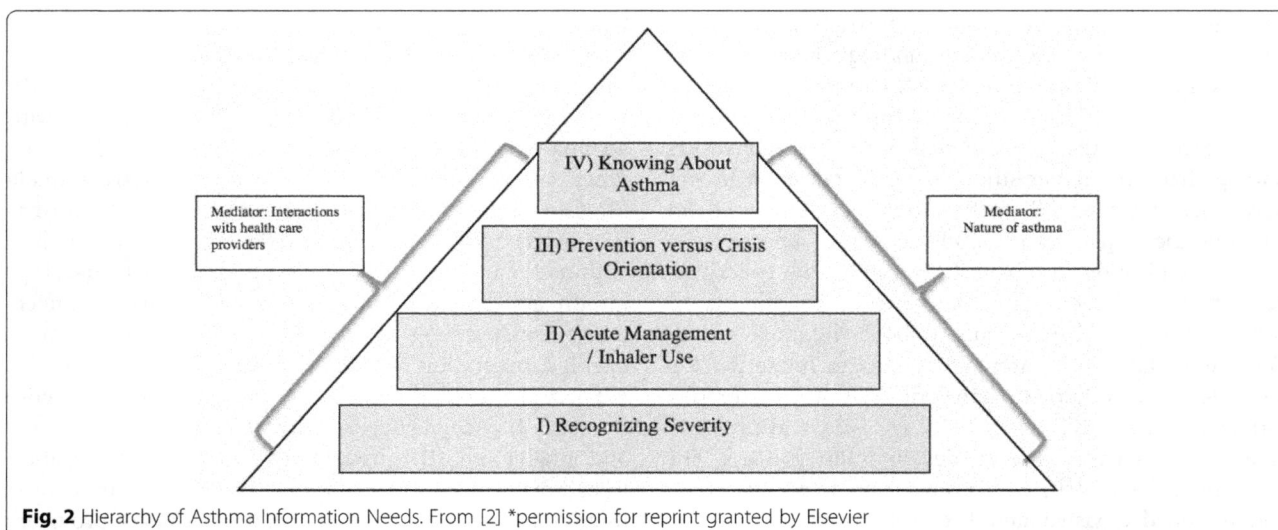

Fig. 2 Hierarchy of Asthma Information Needs. From [2] *permission for reprint granted by Elsevier

education during the stage two interviews. A first-person narrative promotes resonance and authenticity in the reader, and is more personalized than a third-person approach. Second, in previous research, parents expressed a preference for the first-person over the third-person narrative [18, 20]. Third, the diary-format is aligned with the rise of the "reality phenomenon" prevalent in social cultures which leverages the concept of connectedness between viewers and characters [21]. A diary-format provides an insider's perspective into the life of another family living with asthma.

Constructing interdisciplinary teams

We constructed two interdisciplinary teams to assist with developing the arts-based KT tool: (I) a review committee, and (II) a creative consulting team. The review committee consisted of five individuals with expertise in arts-based KT, visual arts, KT science, narrative methods, pediatrics, and emergency medicine. The team provided written or verbal feedback at various time points on versions of the illustrations and narrative. The in-person meetings indicated support for the KT approach and although conflicting perspectives arose, they resulted in important considerations about individual aesthetic preferences. In addition to the core review committee, a registered nurse at a participating pediatric asthma clinic provided clinical feedback when needed.

The creative consulting team was assembled to enable a mosaic of innovative ideas, capitalize on expertise in different styles of visual and narrative arts, and allow enough distance from the research team so that objective feedback could be provided. The first author advertised for a creative writer and illustrator on two freelancer forums, screened applications, and invited five visual artists to provide artistic samples based on an

asthma-case scenario. One visual artist with experience in character development and diverse illustration styles was contracted. Similarly, the first author reviewed the curriculum vitae and writing samples of the creative writers; one writer was hired based on her extensive experience, enthusiasm for the topic, and perceived fit with the project and team. Confidentiality, work agreements, and terms-of-payment were agreed upon and signed. A digital media company was hired to digitize the KT tool for web hosting.

Developing the KT tools

The first author developed an outline of significant and common events in the experience of having a child with asthma, based on the frequency or impact of their occurrence during the stage two interviews. For instance, because receiving an asthma diagnosis was a noteworthy and anxiety-provoking event for most participants, these events were noted for the creative writer to include. "Illustration ideas" were included in the outline when appropriate but prescriptively directing the illustrator was deliberately avoided, as this would be antithetical to the creative generation possible through such a partnership.

The outline also included an "evidence insertion opportunities" column which listed information identified as important to parents and to the successful management of childhood asthma (Table 1). For instance, participants had concerns surrounding diagnosis. Similarly, parents had information deficits regarding the signs of asthma exacerbation [3]. Such incidences were classified as important educational opportunities based on their relevance to asthma management and the child's well-being.

The creative writer then crafted story entries to align with the outline and the first author ensured that

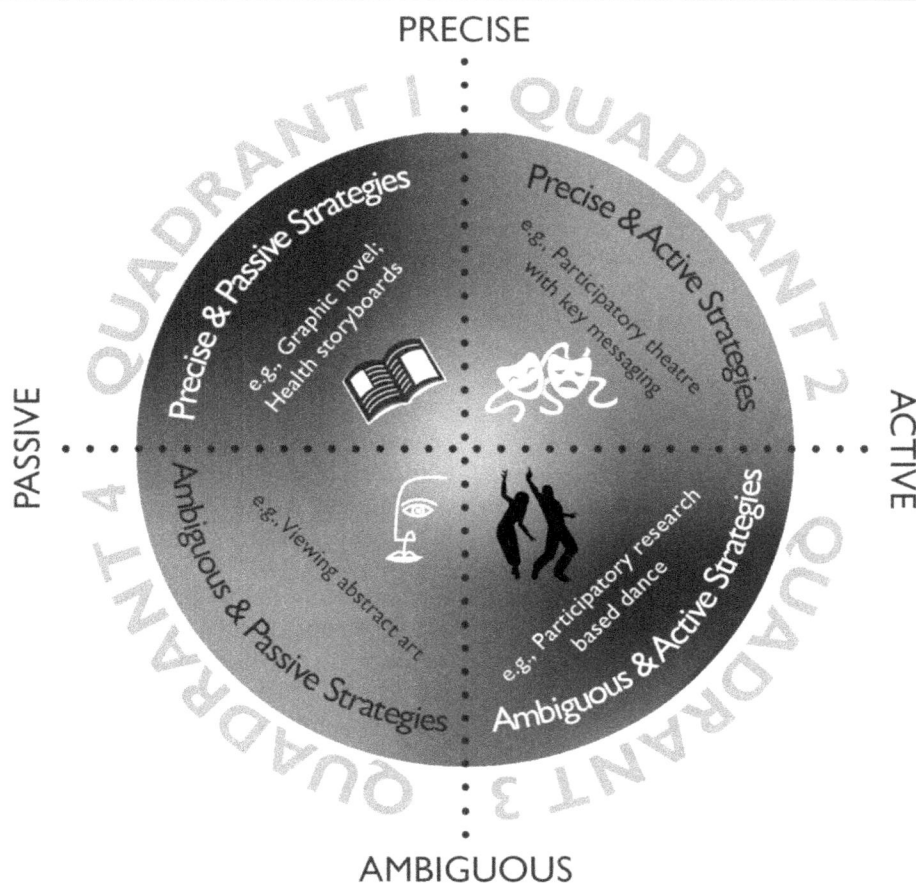

Fig. 3 Classification Schema of Arts-Based Knowledge Translation Strategies. From [7] * permission for reprint granted by WILEY

evidence was included. The process of evidence insertion involved iteratively synthesizing and compiling diverse research (e.g., systematic reviews, qualitative studies, reputable websites, asthma guidelines) into a readable format to correspond with the emerging story framework. The "key items for narrative" column was refined and the creative writer drafted story segments that were reviewed to ensure the events, tone, and spirit of the participants' experiences was reflected. Consulting with the review committee assisted when specific clinical questions arose.

In addition to synthesizing information, five links to existing educational online and community resources were provided. The host organizations were contacted in August 2014, and processes for requesting permission of content were completed. Linking to resources was important because locating and assessing information reputability is challenging [3, 22]. Additionally, parents felt that a list of resources would be useful during the previous information needs study and qualitative evaluation of croup storybooks [3, 11].

Although the research team and creative writer did not pre-determine the number of story entries, we did attempt to limit these to fewer than 25 for time and usability considerations. We felt that limiting the number of story entries prematurely could restrict the creative process. By entry number 18 we could foresee a natural end to the story and began tying together extraneous details. Once complete, the review committee

Table 1 Example of Asthma Diary Outline

Page #	Key Items for Narrative	Evidence Insertion Opportunities	Illustration Ideas
2	• Child showing asthma symptoms • Mother reflects on child's frequent illness, including Emergency Department (ED) visits • Visits ED for respiratory illness • Multiple diagnostic procedures; experiences uncertainty • Receives asthma diagnosis	Asthma symptoms Incidence of viral infections Process of asthma diagnosis	Child in respiratory distress Child visiting ED with mother

ensured all textual information was clinically accurate, relevant, and readable.

The story segments were then provided to the illustrator who constructed visuals through a multi-stage process. First, she drafted an illustration to align with each story entry. These drafts were reviewed and suggested revisions were discussed with the review committee as needed. The illustrator revised all illustrations once the composition, feeling, and scene were agreed upon. The first author compared all illustrations to ensure internal consistency and requested further revisions. An average of three to four revisions per illustration was required before the final output was achieved. An example of the illustration iterations is provided in Fig. 4.

We were interested in differences in parents' responses to diverse illustration styles. As such, four distinct illustration styles were requested from the illustrator. The illustration styles differed by color and line; all other illustration components were unchanged across the prototypes (e.g., composition) (Fig. 5).

Results

Although we previously reported on parents' information needs from Stage Two, here we provide additional, previously unpublished data from the qualitative study on parent's information preferences and then explore in the discussion how this helped inform the development of the KT tool.

Topical survey of information preferences

Information about the format and perceived relevance of asthma education was essential to developing the KT tool. Although we depicted findings from the interpretive descriptive study largely at the level of thematic description (e.g., reflecting latent patterns), here we augment those results and provide previously unpublished findings to discuss the informational preferences of parents in a more concrete manner through topical survey

[19]. During the interviews, we inquired about the information parents received, its effectiveness, and how they would like to receive information in the future. Parents generally felt they received insufficient information about asthma. Parents had difficulty identifying their information needs and numerous information deficits were present. For instance, when asked open-ended questions about asthma knowledge (e.g., What areas, if any, do you need more information about asthma?) parents infrequently identified areas of deficient knowledge about asthma or its management. The inability to identify specific learning needs limited parents' information seeking behaviors at home and during interactions with HCPs. Further, many parents were overwhelmed by the abundant asthma information available online, and had difficulty determining its reputability [3].

When discussing their preferences about formats of information delivery, parents identified web-based information (44%) followed by pamphlets (33%) and face-to-face or verbal information (33%) as most desirable. Parents valued personalized information and reassurance provided by HCPs. Approximately 25% of participants commented that visuals, illustrations, or animation would be helpful ways of receiving information. Illustrating how an inhaler "works" on respiratory muscles or animating inhaler technique were examples of potentially useful visuals.

Emotionally sensitive information delivery was important to parents. Parents used the words "supportive," "compassionate," and "validation" to reference these emotions and at times desired more emotional support than they currently were receiving. As one parent stated "one thing I'd like. .. I don't think I got much support. .. for the emotional side of it" (participant 18). Other participants emphasized the emotionally laden nature of having a child with asthma. As one mother stated, "it's the emotional part that is the worst of it —it really is" (participant 7). Based on this, as well as the pervasive uncertainty, fear and anxiety expressed by parents

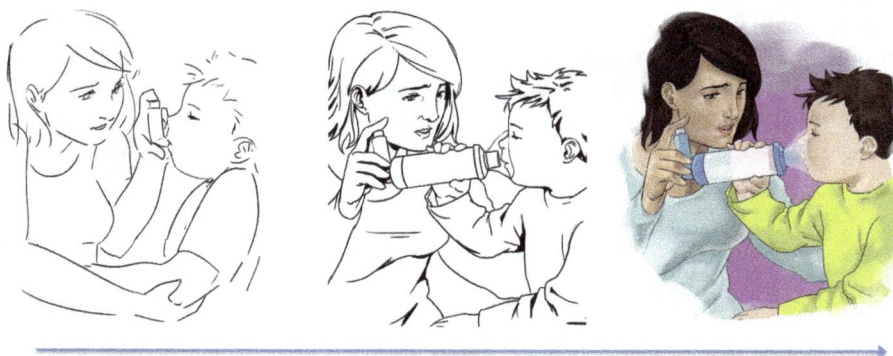

Fig. 4 Iterations of Illustrations

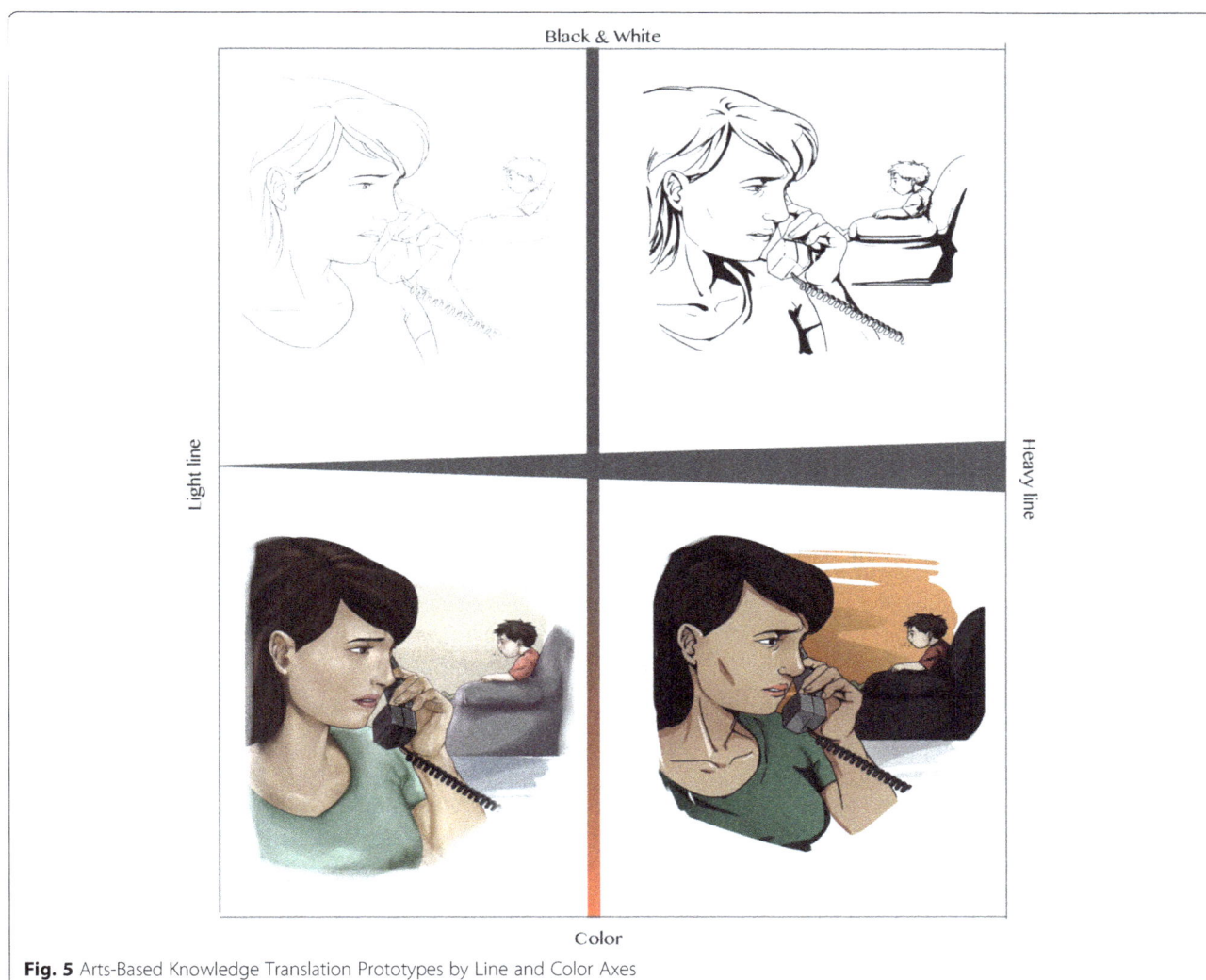

Fig. 5 Arts-Based Knowledge Translation Prototypes by Line and Color Axes

during the interviews, we were attentive to the emotional sensitivity of the KT messaging. The emphasis on the emotional aspects of having a child with asthma, the desire for reputable web-based written information with visual components and the value placed on personalized information reinforced that an arts-based approach to KT may be a useful and effective method of delivering asthma education to parents.

We faced numerous challenges when developing the arts-based KT tool that may likely be encountered in future efforts. We summarize four of these considerations, including: (I) working within an inter-professional team; (II) quantity and ordering of information; (III) creating a composite narrative, and (IV) balancing the actual with the ideal, and later discuss approaches to mitigating these challenges. These challenges as experienced by the first author and KT development leader were documented as reflective memos throughout the process of tool development. Challenges were

shared and discussed with members of the inter-professional team during face-to-face meetings, with particular debriefing and consultation occurring between the first and fifth authors.

(I) Working within an inter-professional team
An unanticipated challenge we encountered was the perceived appropriateness of feedback. Researchers may be accustomed to a high volume of feedback because of the culture surrounding grantsmanship, co-authorship, and peer-review. Artists may be less accustomed to this type of exchange. During our process, a collaborating artist expressed that her creative process was hampered by the detailed feedback received.

(II) Quantity and ordering of information
Information sequencing was an ongoing challenge. At times a concept (e.g., asthma action plan) was introduced in one diary entry but was not explained until

later. Explaining each concept as it was introduced was not always feasible, particularly for recurring concepts (e.g., triggers) because other concepts (e.g., emergency asthma kits) were only present in one story segment and therefore took precedence. The challenge of information ordering raised potential issues for parents navigating the KT tool; the table of contents created did not align seamlessly with the information provided. Information was matched to the diary-entries wherever possible.

(III) Creating a composite narrative

Amalgamating the experiences of multiple participants into a composite narrative while maintaining resonance, appeal, and authenticity for the reader was one of the most profound challenges encountered. Commonalities between the experiences of multiple participants were easier to integrate into the overall storyline. Participant cases that were considered "outliers" were not directly included; rather, language reflecting the individual nature of children's asthma trajectories was at times selected.

Terminology considerations were also ongoing when developing the composite narrative. We strived for relatability and aimed to use parents' words whenever possible; however, parents used various terms to refer to health related concepts. For instance, parents referred to the emergency department as the emergency, emergency room/ department/ clinic/ facility/ ward and "ER," with "emergency" being the most common term. The reviewing paediatrician (S.A) advocated for the more formal term "emergency department"; as such, we to had to balance parents' terminology with that of practitioners who may be endorsing the tool.

Parents also used different terms to describe HCPs. The vast majority (86%) referred generically to "doctor" multiple times during an interview. Nurses were referred to less frequently (38%). No parent mentioned nurse practitioners or health care professionals. Emergency professional and HCPs were referenced by 5% of participants. We were alerted to the merits of specificity and consistency in terminology when the same parent would use multiple terms to describe the same concept.

(IV) Balancing the actual with the ideal

We grappled with authentically portraying parents' experiences of care when they did not reflect ideal medical practices. For instance, some parents reported that HCPs reinforced the notion of growing out of asthma [3]. This reinforced beliefs about asthma as an acute condition and undermined the importance of prevention and day-to-day management. To address this, characters in the KT tool discussed their hopes about growing out of asthma but chronicity was reinforced.

As another example, mothers represented 95% of parents presenting for asthma related care in this sample. We reflected this in the storyline but not without hesitancy. We recognized that our sample might not represent the wider population of parents of children with asthma. Further, one parent found the overrepresentation of mothers in the croup storybooks to be an inaccurate depiction of real-life management scenarios [11]. We decided to portray a mother as the primary character in our story and included the father in the text and illustrations.

Balancing the ideal and the actual also related to the emotions of parents. Parents in Stage Two commonly experienced panic, anxiety, fear, and uncertainty. We needed to convey these experiences to enhance relatability but did not want to reinforce that parents should panic during asthma exacerbations. We were cognizant that doing so may contradict messages conveyed in the KT tool. This tension was captured in the comments of one expert reviewer: "*ran suggests urgency and panic... I would like to relay some comfort and decrease the panic... if the point is to mirror what a 'real parent' might feel at home, then the word is exactly right!*" Recognizing that different terminology serves different purposes, we felt compelled to stay true to the data in our narrative; parents in the qualitative study expressed urgency and we mirrored this through our selected terminology.

Discussion

Our unique inter-professional team assembled in this study consisted of a nurse academic and artist, a creative writer, an illustrator, a digital media company, and an interdisciplinary review committee representing nursing, pediatrics, emergency medicine, and KT science. Through this study, we discovered the potential of collaboration to foster innovation and enable creative approaches to research problems, yet found that its success is greatly influenced by communication dynamics, mutual understanding, and the characteristics of individual collaborators [23, 24]. Challenges such as communicating across disciplines may be proportionate to the diversity of collaborating professionals [25]. Communicative openness and a willingness to receive feedback were imperative to overcoming these challenges. To overcome challenges faced by the quantity of feedback received by team members, the research team provided the artists only with feedback of a substantive nature and the first author (M.A) made editorial adjustments independently. Challenges with the quantity of feedback received were not encountered between the researchers and the digital media company.

Balancing information comprehensiveness with length was an ongoing consideration. Hartling and colleagues [11] encountered similar struggles; parents generally desired abundant information about croup (an acute respiratory illness) but some found the storybooks to be too lengthy. This challenge extends beyond the technical into the realm of aesthetics, highlighting a fundamental tension of using arts-based approaches for KT. Specifically, any extraneous inclusion detracts from the concision of the artistic rendering, which potentially reduces its aesthetic appeal, and foreseeably hinders its effectiveness [9, 10]. We mitigated this by limiting each diary-entry to approximately 90 words (a common length for a short paragraph), providing information in point-form when possible, externally linking to supplemental content, and eliminating content not immediately reflective of asthma priorities, parents' information needs, and information deficits as identified in our previous research.

Participants' ability to relate to characters was a recurring theme [11, 18]. We contend that this challenge of verisimilitude [10] is not unique to arts-based representations but reflects issues of representation more generally; there is a longstanding tension between representing individual cases alongside a shared reality. The tension between general knowledge and shared experience and between the individual experience and experience *applied* to the individual has also been illuminated by others exploring research methods [21, 26]. We recognized that we could not resolve this tension, yet we strived to create a narrative that reflected some aspect of the majority of parent's experiences. To assist with this, we examined our data for negative cases/outliers. We determined that narrative examples from these outliers were less likely to resonate with the majority of parents and as such, were not directly communicated in the composite. To honor individual narratives, we selected examples from the lives of our participants and used their own words to convey these experiences. This reflects Denzin's (2012) perspective that "our texts must always return to and reflect the words persons speak as they attempt to give meaning and shape the lives they lead" [26] (p. 5).

We grappled with using specific, consistent terminology that is valued in research or the diverse and often, nonspecific terms used by parents. Unfamiliar terms may lack appeal and alienate parents from diverse backgrounds. Specificity may be undesirable when parents possess low baseline knowledge about asthma. For example, parents generically referred to "pulmonary tests." The reviewing paediatrician (S.A) questioned how specific terminology should be when providing information about this content area: *"there are pulmonary function tests. ... there are peak flow tests. ... do you want to label it more specifically, or are you being purposefully vague?"* In these instances we referred back to the participant interviews to address this question and found that 29% of participants referred to "pulmonary tests" in any capacity. Participants most often referred to "a test," or, a "breathing" or "capacity" test. Only 10% of participants

referred to a pulmonary function test and never to peak flow. Given this, the decision was made to use general terminology.

The issue of voice extended beyond using parents' terminology in the diary entries. We questioned whether to present evidence as personal (e.g., "your child may. ..") or impersonal (e.g., "common symptoms include. .."). This was a challenge of evocation; that is, ensuring the work can reach the reader to arouse feeling, and therefore meaning [9]. A personal presentation of evidence was generally adopted for this reason.

Conclusions

There is a need to learn about the processes and potential challenges associated with developing patient-driven arts-based KT tools, particularly as these strategies continue to emerge. Data is lacking on how arts-based KT resources have been developed, the process of integrating research evidence with artistic form, and associated challenges encountered. Working with stakeholder groups (e.g., through qualitative research) is necessary to identify the need for, and appropriateness of, an arts-based strategy. Foundational research can help identify which knowledge sources the target audience uses; preferences held about information delivery, and pervasive information and emotional needs. Fluency with the artistic form(s) and information literacy within the creative team are required to construct a meaningful and aesthetic artistic output with merit as a KT strategy. Establishing a review committee of individuals with clinical, content and methodological expertise is recommended to ensure accuracy and relevancy of the KT approach. We believe that collaboration within a diverse inter-professional team, considerations related to the quantity and ordering of information, representation issues encountered through creating a composite narrative, and harmonizing actual and ideal management scenarios are likely to be encountered when developing patient-driven arts-based KT tools.

Abbreviations
ED: Emergency department; HCP: Health care provider; KT: Knowledge translation

Acknowledgements
MA acknowledges the generous support of the Canadian Child Health Clinician Scientist Program and the Women and Children's Health Research Institute for her PhD research. LH and VC are supported through a New Investigator Salary Award from the Canadian Institutes of Health Research. SS acknowledges her research personnel funding from the Canada Research Chair program. The authors acknowledge Tina Marie-Powell (creative writer) and Lea Ragos Segarra (illustrator) who contributed their outstanding creative skills to this project.

Funding
The Canadian Child Health Clinician Scientist Program and the Women and Children's Health Research Institute provided salary support for MA's PhD research.

Declarations

This work was a component of the first author's PhD thesis. The appropriate permissions have been granted to present the information contained in the thesis for use in the current manuscript.

Authors' contributions

MA carried out all stages of the multiphase study including leading the development of "My Asthma Diary", with guidance from SS, LH, VC and SA. MA drafted the manuscript. SS, LH, VC and SA contributed intellectually to the manuscript draft and helped edit the manuscript. All authors read and approved the final manuscript.

Authors' information

MA is a visual artist, and Registered Nurse (RN) with a PhD in Nursing, a Canadian Institutes of Health Research (CIHR) funded Postdoctoral Research Fellow, and a National Health and Medical Research Council (NHMRC) Postdoctoral Research Officer. SS, RN, PhD is a Professor in the Faculty of Nursing, University of Alberta, and holds a Tier II Canada Research Chair in Knowledge Translation for Child Health. VC, RN, PhD is a Professor in the Faculty of Nursing, University of Alberta, and a CIHR New Investigator. LH, PhD is a Professor and is the Director for the Alberta Research Center for Health Evidence. SA is a MD and Professor in the Departments of Pediatrics and Emergency Medicine at the University of Alberta.

Competing interests

The authors declare that they have no competing interests.

Author details

[1]College of Nursing and Health Sciences, Flinders University, Sturt Road, Bedford Park, Adelaide, SA 5042, Australia. [2]Department of Pediatrics, Faculty of Medicine & Dentistry, University of Alberta, Edmonton Clinic Health Academy, 11405-87 Avenue, Alberta T6G 1C9, Canada. [3]Faculty of Nursing, University of Alberta, Level 3, Edmonton Clinic Health Academy, 11405-87 Avenue, Alberta T6G 1C9, Canada.

References

1. Boyd M, Lasserson T, McKean M, Gibson P, Ducharme F, Haby M. Interventions for educating children who are at risk of asthma-related emergency department attendance. Cochrane Database Syst Rev. 2010;2: CD001290.
2. Archibald MM, Caine V, Ali S, Hartling L, Scott SD. What is left unsaid: an interpretive description of the information needs of parents of children with asthma. Res Nurs Health. 2015;38:19–28.
3. Archibald MM, Scott SD. The information needs of north-American parents of children with asthma: a state-of-the-science review of the literature. J Pediatr Health Care. 2014;2014(12):5–13.
4. Garner R, Kohen D. 2008. Changes in the prevalence of asthma among Canadian children. Statistics Canada. Retrieved from http://www.statcan.gc.ca/pub/82-003-x/2008002/article/10551-eng.pdf.
5. Canadian Institutes of Health Research. Knowledge Translation. [http://cihr-irsc.gc.ca].
6. Kontos P, Poland B. Mapping new theoretical and methodological terrain for knowledge translation: contributions from critical realism and the arts. Implement Sci. 2009;4:1–10.
7. Archibald MM, Caine V, Scott SD. The development of a classification schema for arts-based approaches to knowledge translation. Worldviews Evid Based Nurs. 2014;11:316–24.
8. Parsons J, Boydell K. Arts-based research and knowledge translation: some key concerns for health-care professionals. J Interprof Care. 2012;26:170–2.
9. Barone T, Eisner E. Arts based research. Los Angeles: SAGE; 2012.
10. Leavy P. Fiction as research practice: Short stories, novellas, and novels. Walnut Creek, CA: Left Coast Press; 2013.
11. Hartling L, Scott SD, Pandya R, Johnson D, Bishop T, Klassen T. Storytelling as a communication tool for health consumers: development of an intervention for parents of a child with croup. Stories to communicate health information. BMC Pediatr. 2010;10:64.
12. Lafreniere D, Hurlimann T, Menuz V, Godard V. Evaluation of a cartoon-based knowledge dissemination intervention on scientific and ethical challenges raised by nutrigenomics/nutrigenetics research. Eval Program Plann. 2014;46:103–14.
13. Perlovsky L. The cognitive function of music part II. Interdiscip Sci Rev. 2013;39:162–86.
14. Mason S. The healthy balance research program: theatre as a means of knowledge translation. Can J Nurs Res. 2008;40:126–31.
15. Archibald MM, Scott SD, Hartling L. Mapping the waters: a scoping review of the use of visual arts in pediatric populations with health conditions. Arts Health. 2014;6:5–23.
16. Fraser KD, al Sayah F. Arts-based methods in health research: a systematic review of the literature. Arts Health. 2011;3:110–45.
17. Hoover S. The case for graphic novels. Commun Inf Literacy. 2012;5:174–86.
18. Scott SD, Hartling L, O'Leary K, Archibald MM, Klassen T. Stories - A novel approach to transfer complex health information to parents: A qualitative study. Arts Health. 2012;42:162–73.
19. Thorne S. Interpretive description. Walnut Creek, CA: Left Coast Press; 2008.
20. Hartling L, Scott SD, Johnson D, Bishop T, Klassen T. A randomized controlled trial of storytelling as a communication tool. PLoS One. 2013;8:e77800.
21. Tran G, Strutton D. Has reality television come of age as a promotional platform? Modeling the endorsement effectiveness of celebreality and reality starts. Psychol Mark. 2014;31:294–305.
22. Harrison S. Health communication design: an innovative MA at Coventry University. J Vis Commun Med. 2007;30:119–24.
23. Archibald MM. Investigator triangulation: a collaborative strategy with potential for mixed methods research. J Mixed Methods Res. 2016;10:228–50.
24. Lunde A, Heggen K, Strand R. Knowledge and power: exploring unproductive interplay between quantitative and qualitative researchers. J Mixed Methods Res. 2013;7:197–210.
25. Archibald M, Lawless M, Harvey G, Kitson A. Transdisciplinary research for impact: Protocol for a realist evaluation of the relationship between transdisciplinary research collaboration and knowledge translation. BMJ Open. 2018;8(4):e021775.
26. Denzin N. Interpretive autoethnography. 2nd ed. Thousand Oaks, CA: Sage; 2014.

17

Active case finding: comparison of the acceptability, feasibility and effectiveness of targeted versus blanket provider-initiated-testing and counseling of HIV among children and adolescents in Cameroon

Habakkuk Azinyui Yumo[1,2]* [iD], Christopher Kuaban[3], Rogers Awoh Ajeh[1], Akindeh Mbuh Nji[1,4], Denis Nash[5], Anastos Kathryn[6,7], Marcus Beissner[2] and Thomas Loescher[2]

Abstract

Background: Children and adolescents still lag behind adults in accessing antiretroviral therapy (ART), which is largely due to their limited access to HIV testing services. This study compares the acceptability, feasibility and effectiveness of targeted versus blanket provider-initiated testing and counseling (PITC) among children and adolescents in Cameroon.

Methods: During a 6-month period in three hospitals in Cameroon, we invited HIV-positive parents to have their biological children (6 weeks-19 years) tested for HIV (targeted PITC). During that same period and in the same hospitals, we also systematically offered HIV testing to all children evaluated at the outpatient department (blanket PITC). Children of consenting parents were tested for HIV, and positive cases were enrolled on ART. We compared the acceptability, feasibility and effectiveness of targeted and blanket PITC using Chi-square test at 5% significant level.

Results: We enrolled 1240 and 2459 eligible parents in the targeted PITC (tPITC) and blanket PITC (bPITC) group, and 99.7% and 98.8% of these parents accepted the offer to have their children tested for HIV, respectively. Out of the 1990 and 2729 children enrolled in the tPITC and bPITC group, 56.7% and 90.3% were tested for HIV ($p < 0.0001$), respectively. The HIV positivity rate was 3.5% (CI:2.4–4.5) and 1.6% (CI:1.1–2.1) in the tPITC and bPITC ($p = 0.0008$), respectively. This finding suggests that the case detection was two times higher in tPITC compared to bPITC, or alternatively, 29 and 63 children have to be tested to identify one HIV case with the implementation of tPITC and bPITC, respectively. The majority (84.8%) of HIV-positive children in the tPITC group were diagnosed earlier at WHO stage 1, and cases were mostly diagnosed at WHO stage 3 (39.1%) ($p < 0.0001$) in the bPITC group. Among the children who tested HIV-positive, 85.0% and 52.5% from the tPITC and bPITC group respectively, were enrolled on ART ($p = 0.0018$).

Conclusions: The tPITC and bPITC strategies demonstrated notable high HIV testing acceptance. tPITC was superior to bPITC in terms of case detection, case detection earliness and linkage to care. These findings indicate that tPITC is effective in case detection and linkage of children and adolescents to ART.

Keywords: HIV, Identification, Children, Adolescents, Case detection, Linkage, Targeted PITC, Blanket PITC

* Correspondence: ha.yumo12@gmail.com
[1]R4D International Foundation, Yaounde, Cameroon
[2]Center for International Health (CIH), Ludwig-Maximilians-Universität, München, Germany
Full list of author information is available at the end of the article

Background

Human immunodeficiency virus (HIV) case identification has been and remains a major obstacle to the expansion of antiretroviral therapy (ART) among infants, children and adolescents in sub-Saharan Africa due to multifaceted barriers at the patient, provider, community and national policy levels [1]. The uptake of early infant diagnosis (EID) using deoxyribonucleic acid-polymerase chain reaction (DNA-PCR) techniques for infants younger than 18 months of age is sub-optimal with a global coverage of 50% [2]. This gap is due to numerous barriers, including low antenatal consultation (ANC) attendance, weak supply chain management of pediatric HIV commodities, low retention, delayed test results, weak follow-up after delivery and poor linkage to treatment [3]. Implementation of the routine or blanket provider-initiated-testing and counseling (PITC), a strategy recommended by the World Health Organization (WHO) for HIV case finding among older children (≥18 months) is fragmentary. This situation is attributable to many factors, including fear of stigma, lack of staff training, lack of HIV testing kits, poor commitment from facility leadership, and missed parental consent to test children [4, 5].

As a result of these programmatic gaps, only approximately 10% and 15% of HIV-infected young (15–24 years) males and females, respectively, in Sub-Saharan Africa are aware of their HIV status [6]. As the gateway to HIV treatment and care, this low HIV testing uptake among children and adolescents translates to the current low pediatric ART coverage with only 43% of eligible children being on treatment compared to 54% of adults [7].

In Cameroon, the pediatric ART coverage gap is even wider, with only 18% of eligible children being on ART compared with 38% of adults [8]. This is happening despite the availability of HIV commodities (testing kits and antiretroviral drugs) provided free of charge for children by the government of Cameroon with the support of external funding agencies, most notably the Global Fund to fight HIV/AIDS, Tuberculosis and Malaria (GFATM) and the United States President's Emergency Plan for AIDS Relief (PEPFAR). This gap indicates the need for alternative and/or innovative approaches to increase pediatric and adolescent HIV case identification and linkage to care in Cameroon and globally.

Given that over 90% [9] of pediatric HIV infections result from mother to child transmission, targeting with HIV testing, children of parents living with HIV/AIDS is a plausible high-yield case finding strategy as indicated by a study conducted in 2006 in Cameroon [10]. Though recommended by WHO since 2010 [11], implementation of this targeted PITC (tPITC) strategy is still sub-optimal in Cameroon and in other sub-Saharan African countries. Currently, there is a dearth of literature on the implementation outcome of tPITC, and most importantly, there is a lack of knowledge on its comparative advantage over the blanket PITC (bPITC). This study aimed to bridge this evidence gap and to contribute to the expansion of HIV treatment and care among children and adolescents.

Methods

Design

We conducted an interventional study in which we invited all parents living with HIV/AIDS receiving HIV care in three hospitals in Cameroon to have their children of unknown HIV status aged 6 weeks to 19 years to be tested for HIV (tPITC group). In the same hospitals, all parents/guardians who accompanied their sick children of the same age group for consultation at the outpatient departments were also counseled, and these children were invited to test for HIV irrespective of the presenting complaint (bPITC group).

Setting

The study was conducted in the Limbe Regional Hospital (LRH), Ndop District Hospital (NDH) and Abong-Mbang District Hospital (ADH). These hospitals provide comprehensive health care services to the catchment population, including the management of HIV/AIDS. The study was conducted within the Active Search for Pediatric HIV/AIDS (ASPA) project, an initiative of Research for Development (R4D) International Foundation, a Cameroon-based global health research non-governmental organization. The ASPA project aimed to promote pediatric HIV service delivery through a range of activities, including capacity building of health personnel, services delivery both at facility and community level, nutritional support, monitoring and evaluation.

Study period and population

Data were collected in the LRH from July to December 2015, and in ADH and NDH from June to November 2016. The study population in the tPITC group consisted of parents living with HIV/AIDS receiving care in the hospital and their children of unknown HIV status, aged 6 weeks to 19 years. Similarly, in the bPITC group, the study population consisted of parents/guardians and their sick children of the same age group who attended the hospital outpatient department for any reason. Children or parents critically ill (in vital distress) were excluded from the study.

Study procedures

Site preparation

Prior to the study, input and support provided by the project to the respective hospitals included the following: staff training on both tPITC and bPITC activities, provision of HIV testing kits, and human resource support (dedicated staff to support project implementation).

Enrollment of participants and data collection

In the tPITC group, HIV-positive parents in care at the HIV treatment center (ART clinic) were counseled and invited by a trained counselor to participate in the study together with their children with unknown HIV status. These parents were offered a testing opportunity for their biological children in either the hospital or at home (community testing). In the bPITC group, parents/guardians were also counseled and invited to have their sick children tested for HIV irrespective of the reason of consultation.

In both groups, all parents/guardians who consented to participate in the study were enrolled together with their children. Pre-tested and structured questionnaires (Additional file 1: Questionaires 1–4) were used by a trained data clerk to collect socio-demographic information and the HIV/AIDS history of parents and children (Fig. 1). In the tPITC group, a sub-population of parents who initially agreed to bring their children for HIV testing, but subsequently did not, were interviewed using a structured questionnaire (Additional file 2: Questionaire 5) and this to determine the reason of their failure to bring children for testing.

HIV testing, linkage and ART enrolment

For children younger than 18 months of age, HIV testing was performed using DNA-PCR techniques. For children older than 18 months, HIV testing was performed using two HIV antibody rapid tests according to the Cameroon national guidelines. The WHO test and treat policy was not effective at the site level at the time of the study. Thus, children who tested positive for HIV were assessed for ART eligibility using WHO clinical staging

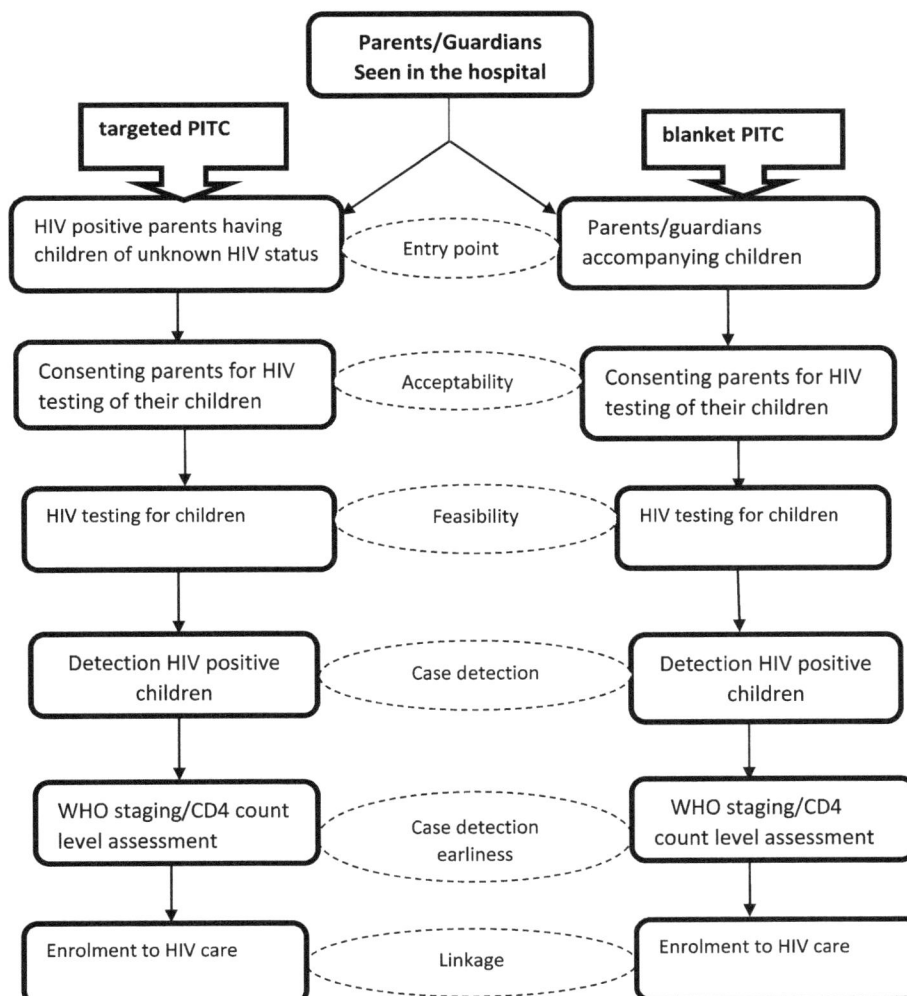

Fig. 1 Enrollment, HIV testing and linkage to care and treatment of children and adolescents, ASPA Study, July–November 2016, Cameroon

and/or baseline biological analysis, including CD4 count. Eligible children were initiated on ART and monitored according to the Cameroon national guidelines.

Sample size

We used the following formula to calculate the sample size for 2 proportions with dichotomous outcome [12]:

$$N = (Z_{\alpha/2} + Z_{\beta})^2 * (p_1(1-p_1) + p_2(1-p_2))/(p_1-p_2)^2,$$

Where: $\alpha = 5\%$, $\beta = 20\%$, $p_1 = 10\%$, $p_2 = 5\%$. We found $N = 432$ children and adolescents per group and per hospital or 1296 per group for the three hospitals. Thus, a total of $n = 1296 \times 2 = 2592$ children and adolescents for the two groups and three hospitals.

Data management and analysis

Anonymous data from the questionnaires were entered into a database and analyzed using STATA 2013 (College Station, TX: StataCorp LP). The study outcomes were determined by computing the proportions and comparing the values using Chi-square test (X2) at 5% significant level.

Definitions of terms

The study outcomes were defined and calculated as follows:

i) *Acceptability (acceptance rate):* proportion of parents who accepted to have their children tested among all eligible parents enrolled in the study
ii) *Feasibility (HIV testing uptake rate):* proportion of children who tested for HIV among all eligible children identified by the study

iii) *Effectiveness:* It was defined and measured as follows:
   a) *HIV case detection/positivity rate:* proportion of HIV cases detected among children and adolescents tested for HIV
   b) *HIV case detection earliness:* proportion of cases detected at WHO stage 1
   c) *ART linkage rate:* proportion of cases linked to care or enrolled on ART

Results

Acceptability of tPITC and bPITC

The study offered enrolment to 3699 parents, including 1240 and 2459 in the tPITC and bPITC groups, respectively. In both groups, parents were predominantly from Ndop District Hospital (38.6%), followed by Limbe Regional Hospital (36.4%) and Abong-Mbang District Hospital (25.0%). Among these parents, 99.7% (1236/1240) and 98.8% (2430/2459) in the tPITC and bPITC, respectively, accepted to have their children tested for HIV.

Feasibility of tPITC and bPITC

Through parents, 4719 eligible children were enrolled for HIV testing, including 1990 and 2729 in the tPITC and bPITC groups, respectively. In both groups, the children were predominantly from Ndop District Hospital Hospital (41.1%), followed by Limbe Regional Hospital (37.2%) and Abong-Mbang District Hospital (21.7%) (Table 1). None of the children enrolled had refused to be tested for HIV. Among the participating children, 56.7% (1129/1990) and 90.3% (2465/2729) ($p < 0.0001$) tested for HIV, respectively, in the tPITC and bPITC groups (Table 2). Among children ≤12 years, the HIV

Table 1 Uptake of HIV services among children and adolescents in three hospitals in Cameroon, ASPA study, July 2015–November 2016

HIV services	tPITC				bPITC			
	Limbe	Abong-Mbang	Ndop	Total	Limbe	Abong-Mbang	Ndop	Total
	n (%)	n (%)	n (%)	n	n (%)	n (%)	n (%)	n
Children and adolescents enrolled	552 (27.7)	400 (20.1)	1038 (52.1)	1990	1205 (44.1)	623 (22.8)	901 (33.0)	2729
Children and adolescents tested for HIV in the hospital	257 (27.6)	212 (22.7)	462 (49.6)	931	951 (38.5)	619 (25.1)	895 (36.3)	2465
Children and adolescents tested for HIV in the community (only tPITC)	43 (21.7)	140 (70.7)	15 (7.5)	198	N/A	N/A	N/A	N/A
Children tested for HIV (both community and hospital)	300 (26.5)	352 (31.1)	477 (42.2)	1129	951 (38.5)	619 (25.1)	895 (36.3)	2465
Children and adolescents tested HIV+ in the community	0 (0.0)	1 (100)	0 (0.0)	1	N/A	N/A	N/A	N/A
Children and adolescents tested HIV+ in the hospital	5 (12.8)	13 (33.3)	21 (53.8)	39	14 (35.0)	21 (52.5)	5 (12.5)	40
Children and adolescents tested HIV+ (both hospital and community)	5 (12.5)	14 (35.0)	21 (52.5)	40	14 (35.0)	21 (52.5)	5 (12.5)	40
Children and adolescents initiated on ART	1 (2.9)	13 (38.2)	20 (58.8)	34	3 (14.2)	16 (76.1)	2 (9.5)	21

N/A Not applicable

Table 2 Acceptability and effectiveness of targeted versus blanket PITC in three hospitals in Cameroon, ASPA study, July 2015–November 2016

Outcome	tPITC				bPITC				P*
	Limbe	Abong-Mbang	Ndop	Total	Limbe	Abong-Mbang	Ndop	Total	
	% (n)	% (n)	% (n)	% (n)	% (n)	% (n)	% (n)	% (n)	
Acceptability rate	100.0 (327/327)	99.7 (344/345)	99.6 (566/568)	99.8 (1616/1619)	99.2 (1013/1021)	99.3 (575/579)	98.0 (842/859)	98.8 (2430/2459)	0.0005
Feasibility rate	54.3 (300/552)	88.0 (352/400)	46.0 (477/1038)	56.7 (1129/1990)	78.9 (951/1205)	99.4 (619/623)	99.3 (895/901)	90.3 (2465/2729)	< 0.0001
HIV positivity rate	1.7 (5/300)	4.0 (14/352)	4.4 (21/477)	3.5 (40/1129)	1.5 (14/951)	3.4 (21/619)	0.6 (5/895)	1.6 (40/2465)	0.0008
Linkage rate	20.0 (1/5)	92.9 (12/14)	95.2 (20/21)	85.0 (33/40)	21.4 (3/14)	76.2 (16/21)	40.0 (2/5)	52.5 (21/40)	0.0018

*p value comparing the outcome (total) of tPITC vs. bPITC in the 3 study sites

testing uptake (feasibility) rate was 60.5% compared to 91.2% ($p < 0.0001$), respectively, in the tPITC and bPITC groups. In comparison, among children older than 12 years of age, this rate was 43.8% vs 86.7% ($p < 0.0001$).

The lack of transport fare (38.4%), children not living with biological parents (25.6%) and lack of time (10.5%) were the three primary reasons affecting the feasibility of tPITC strategy. These reasons were provided by a subgroup of 86 parents who initially accepted to have their children tested, but subsequently did not return to the hospital with their children for HIV testing (Fig. 2).

HIV positivity/case detection

A total of 3594 children and adolescents were tested for HIV during the recruitment period; 1129 and 2465 in the tPITC and bPITC group, respectively (Table 1). The HIV positivity rate (case detection) was 3.5% (95% CI: 2.4–4.5) in tPITC group compared to 1.6% (95CI: 1.1–2.1) in the bPITC group ($p = 0.0008$) (Table 2). Among children ≤12 years, the HIV positivity rate was 3.3% vs

1.4% ($p = 0.0006$), respectively, in the tPITC and bPITC groups. In comparison, among children older than 12, this rate was 4.6% vs. 2.5% ($p = 0.1621$).

In the tPITC group, 17.of children were tested in the community and the hospital, respectively. The HIV positivity rate was 0.5% (1/198) in children tested in the community compared 4.2% (39/931) ($p = 0.0107$) among those tested in the hospital.

Early detection of HIV cases

The proportion of HIV infected children diagnosed at WHO stage 1 and WHO stage 3 were 84.8% (28/33) and 15.2% (5/33) in the tPITC group, respectively, compared to 21.7% (5/23) and 39.1% (9/23) in the bPITC ($p = 0.0001$), respectively.

Linkage to HIV care and treatment

In the tPITC group, 85.0% (34/40) of children tested HIV+ were linked to HIV treatment compared to 52.5% (21/40) of the cases in the bPITC ($p = 0.0018$) (Table 2).

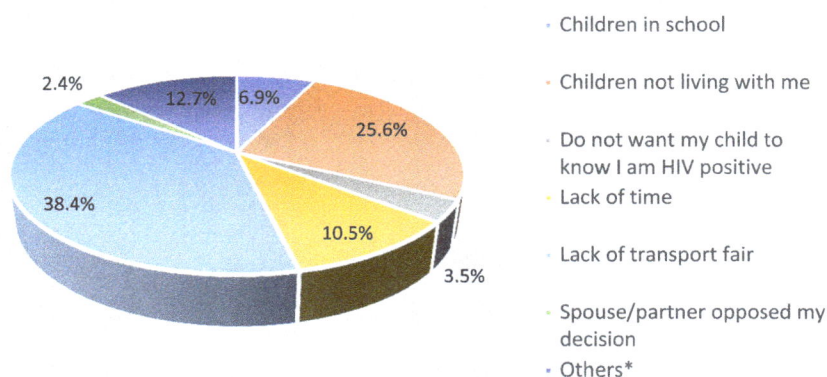

Fig. 2 Reasons of PLHIV for not returning with children for HIV testing, ASPA study, July 2015–November 2016, Cameroon

Among children ≤12 years, the linkage rate was 90.3% vs 58.6% ($p = 0.005$) in the tPITC and bPITC groups, respectively. Among children older than 12 years, this rate was 66.7% vs. 36.4% ($p = 0.3698$) in the tPITC and bPITC groups, respectively.

Discussion

Applying the ambitious 90–90-90 target of the UNAIDS [13] to pediatrics would require global identification of 3.7 million infants, children and adolescents with HIV infection, treatment of 3.3 million, and achieving viral suppression among 3 million within the next four years [14]. Pediatric HIV case finding represents a major challenge in meeting these targets. The findings of this study add to the growing evidence that targeted strategies may increase HIV testing uptake, yield and linkage to treatment.

In the tPITC group, we found an HIV positivity rate (case detection rate/yield) of 3.5%, which was closer to the 4.0% but lower than the 7.4% reported by Saeed et al. in Malawi [15] and Wagner et al.in Kenya [16], respectively. The HIV prevalence (4.3%) in the general population in Cameroon (4.3%) [17] is lower compared to Malawi (9.2%) and Kenya (5.4%) [8] and this may explain the lower HIV positivity rate observed among the pediatric and adolescent population in our study compared to Malawi and Kenya as reported in the aforementioned studies. In the bPITC group, we found a prevalence of 1.6%, which was similar to the 1.8% reported by Zoufaly et al. in rural Cameroon [18] and closer to the 2.7% reported by Cohn et al. in a meta-analysis [19].

The HIV positivity rates reported by this study imply that the yield of newly identified HIV cases among children was two times higher with tPITC. To identify a new HIV case, 31 and 62 parents have to be counselled, and 29 and 63 children have to be tested, in the tPITC and bPITC groups, respectively. Therefore, less effort is needed with tPITC to identify a new pediatric or adolescent HIV case, and tPITC is more effective than bPITC in the context of our study.

The parents' acceptance (acceptability) of HIV testing for their children was very high using both strategies (99.7% in tPITC vs 98.8% in bPITC). The slightly higher acceptance in the tPITC group may be due to enhanced HIV awareness resulting from the contact of these parents with HIV services. Ahmed et al. reported a similar high acceptability (93.5%) in their study in Malawi [15].

The uptake of HIV testing (feasibility) among children was significantly lower in the tPITC group (56.7% vs 90.3%, $p < 0.0001$). This may be attributable to the fact that the tPITC parents living with HIV were initially seen in the hospital in the first place for their own care, and their children were less likely to be present. Similarly, low uptake of HIV testing among children in tPITC was reported in Kenya where only 14% of parents

who had initially consented to test children had followed through with the testing [16]. In our study, according to the parents' declarations, the main reasons for their inability to return to the hospital with their children for HIV testing included the lack of transport fare (38.3%), children not living with them (25.6%), and the lack of time (10.5%). These reasons should be taken with caution because the HIV testing uptake could have also been limited by parental' levels barriers, notably fear of self-disclosure, stigma and discrimination as reported by previous studies [4, 16, 20–22]. There is a need for qualitative research to provide in-depth information on parental barriers to the uptake of HIV testing for children in the context of tPITC approach implementation.

Although the HIV testing uptake was highest (90.3%) in the bPITC, nearly 10% of the children enrolled were not ultimately tested. This finding was attributable to a fraction of parents who initially consented to test their children, but they subsequently changed their decisions and did not go to the laboratory for testing. A number may have gone to the laboratory, but due to the long waiting time, they may have decided to leave without testing the child. Conducting the HIV testing on the spot or having a dedicated testing room for these children near the counseling office may have reduced the missed opportunity for testing.

In this study, pediatric HIV cases were diagnosed earlier in the tPITC group (84.8% at WHO stage 1) because this strategy tested asymptomatic children in contrast to the bPITC, in which children tested were evaluated for an illness (34.8% at WHO stage 2 and 39.1% at WHO stage 3). This finding was consistent with a previous targeted pediatric HIV testing in Malawi, where a large proportion (46.7%) of HIV infected children were diagnosed at WHO stage 1 [15]. Therefore, a pediatric HIV program could prioritize the tPITC strategy for early case identification as a means to reduce the high mortality rate associated with non-treatment of children living with HIV [23–25]. Linkage to care was significantly higher in the tPITC group (85.0% vs 52.5%, $p = 0.0018$). This finding may be explained by the fact that the large majority of parents were already in HIV care (96% of children were identified through parents on ART) and it was easier to link the children to HIV services because the parents, having seen the benefit of ART, quickly seized the treatment opportunity offered for their children who tested positive for HIV. This finding highlights the potential effect that prior enrolment of parents on ART could have on linkage of their children to care. This further demonstrates the effectiveness of the HIV care family-centered approach in enhancing pediatric HIV linkage and retention in care [26–29]. Nevertheless, in Limbe Regional Hospital, the linkage rate was statistically similar in the tPITC and bPITC groups (20.0% vs 21.4%, $p = 1$), but this rate was higher (but not statistically significant) in the tPITC group in Abong-Mbang (92.9% vs 76.2%, $p = 0.2054$) and significantly higher in Ndop (95.2% vs 40.0%, $p = 0.0144$) district hospital. In Abong-Mbang and Ndop district hospitals, we assigned staff members (linkage agents) to ensure that all children who tested positive for HIV were linked to care. Moreover, in these two new sites (through the humanitarian component of the ASPA project), nutritional kits were provided to HIV-positive children in care. Neither the linkage agent nor the nutritional support was provided at the Limbe Regional Hospital, which had the lowest linkage rate among the three sites. This finding suggests that both the linkage agent and nutritional support may have contributed meaningfully in improving linkage in the tPITC and bPITC groups. The positive effect of nutritional support in the linkage and retention of children in care has been previously demonstrated [30]. There is a need to further investigate this effect when combined with a linkage agent.

The limitations of this study were that the Limbe Regional Hospital began implementation in July 2015, while the Abong-Mbang and Ndop District Hospitals began later, in June 2016. We tweaked the implementation strategies in these 2 additional sites from lessons learned from the first site. In particular, we reinforced the follow-up of children diagnosed HIV+ to enhance linkage (introduction of a linkage agent). We also introduced the provision of nutritional kits to HIV+ children in care. These additional interventions may have contributed to increase the linkage rate in these 2 sites compared to Limbe. Thus, the results of Limbe Regional Hospital and that of Abong-Mbang and Ndop District Hospital are not comparable in all aspects. Nevertheless, because the primary objective of the study was not to compare the outcome per site, but rather, to compare the outcome of both tPITC and bPITC, the time difference in implementation per site did not affect the results of the study. In contrast, this stepwise implementation approach was found very useful because lessons learned from the first site (Limbe) informed the adjustments needed to have a more robust strategy for better linkage to care of HIV-positive children. Another potential limitation was that critically ill children were not included in our study. However, the number of these children coming to the hospital is usually marginal and their exclusion would not have affected our findings.

Conclusions

The tPITC and bPITC strategies were highly acceptable to parents to support HIV testing for their children. The tPITC had a higher yield and provided an opportunity for early detection of pediatric and adolescent HIV cases as well as linkage to care before these children become sick and present to the health facility with HIV clinical manifestations.

However, the feasibility of tPITC strategy was lower compared to bPITC, which was due to the low HIV testing uptake among children and adolescents in the former strategy. The bPITC had a higher HIV testing uptake, but a lower linkage rate. Thus, the clinical cascade for the tPITC is challenged by the HIV testing uptake gap while that of the bPITC is constrained by the ART linkage gap.

Overall, the ASPA study demonstrated the superiority of tPITC over bPITC in terms of case detection, case detection earliness, and linkage to care and treatment. However, when the required resources are available, both strategies may be promoted to fast track the achievement of the ambitious 90–90-90 targets of the UNAIDS among children and adolescents by 2020. Meeting this objective would require the implementation of strategies that are suitable to optimize the outcome of both tPITC and bPITC approaches by improving the HIV testing uptake and linkage to care and treatment, respectively.

Abbreviations

ANC: Antenatal Consultations; ART: Antiretroviral therapy; ARV: Antiretroviral Drugs; ASPA: Active Search for Pediatric HIV/AIDS; bPITC: Blanket provider-initiated testing and counseling; CD4: Cluster of differentiation 4; CI: Confidence Interval; DBS: Dot blot spot; DNA: Deoxyribonucleic acid; EID: Early Infant Diagnosis; HIV/AIDS: Human Immunodeficiency Virus/Acquired Immune Deficiency Syndrome; LRH: Limbe Regional Hospital; MTCT: Mother to Child Transmission of HIV; NDH: Ndop District Hospital; OPD: Outpatient Department; PCR: Polymerase chain reaction; PITC: Provider-initiated testing and counseling; PLHIV: People Living with HIV/AIDS; PMTCT: Prevention of Mother to Child Transmission of HIV; R4D : Research for Development International; RT1 : Rapid test 1; RT2: Rapid test 2; tPITC: Targeted provider- initiated testing and counseling; UNAIDS: The Joint United Nations Programme on HIV and AIDS; UNICEF: The United Nations Children's Fund; WHO: The World Health Organization

Acknowledgments

This study constitutes a part of the PhD Medical Research-International Health dissertation of Dr. Habakkuk Azinyui Yumo (Corresponding Author) at the Center for International Health (CIH)- Ludwig Maximilian Universität in Muenchen (Germany). He is thankful to Prof. Michael Loescher, CIH chair and all the lecturers of the PhD Medical Research-International Health for guidance and support. He is also very appreciative of the following experts who provided comments on the manuscript: Dr. Mamadou Otto Diallo, Medical Officer, CDC Atlanta, GA, USA; Prof. Dr. Jan Hendrik Richardus, Department of Public Health, Erasmus MC, University Medical Center Rotterdam, The Netherlands; Dr. Michael R. Jordan, Assistant Professor of Medicine, Tufts University School of Medicine, Boston, MA; and Dr. Isidore Sieleunou, Global Health Research Fellow, University of Montreal and R4D International, Yaounde, Cameroon.
The authors are very thankful to all of the parents and children who participated in this study. We thank all of the health personnel of the Limbe Regional Hospital, Abong-Mbang and Ndop District Hospitals for their collaboration. In particular, the Directors of the respective hospitals: Dr. Bijingni Kuwoh Pius (Limbe), Dr. Nsame Denis (Abong-Mbang) and Dr. Kwa Kedze (Ndop). The authors also appreciate the role of Dr. Titus Sabi (Camformedics e.V.), that of the ASPA Study Central Coordination Team at R4D International Foundation (Yaoundé) and all of the coordinators and research officers/data clerks of the respective sites listed as follows: Dr. Marie Balimba Njabon, Rachel Tita and Ernestine Kendowo (Limbe Regional

Hospital); Ndenkeh N. Jackson Jr., Gibero Tieseh Tandar, Moabance epse Kiringa Florence Gladys (Abong-Mbang District Hospital); Prisca Mbah-Fongkimeh Ngetemalah, Violet Mezepahyui Yumo, Wilson Nyifunda Kenyenyen, Salioh Mbinyui Mbuh (Ndop District Hospital); Hilton Nchotou Ndimuangu, Mark Benwi, Leonard Ndongo (R4D International Foundation).

Funding
The ASPA study was co-funded by: i) the Central Africa IeDEA (U01 AI096299) funded by the US National Institute of Health (NIH) through Albert Einstein College of Medicine, Bronx, New York; ii) the Else Kroener-Fresenius-Stiftung (Bad Homburg, Germany) and iii) R4D International Foundation (Yaounde, Cameroon). Camformedics e.V. (Essen, Germany) coordinated the management of the study funds between the Else Kroener-Fresenius-Stiftung and R4D International Foundation.

Authors' contributions
HAY: conceived, conceptualized and designed the study, drafted the study protocol, fundraised for the study, recruited and trained study staff, supervised data acquisition, analyzed data, interpreted the results and drafted the manuscript. CK: reviewed the study protocol, interpreted the results and reviewed the manuscript. RAA: co-supervised data acquisition, interpreted the results and reviewed the manuscript. AMN: supported data analysis, interpreted the results and reviewed the manuscript. MB: reviewed the study protocol, interpreted the results and reviewed the manuscript. DN: interpreted the results and reviewed the manuscript. KA: interpreted the results and reviewed the manuscript. TL: reviewed the study protocol, interpreted the results and reviewed the manuscript. All authors read and approved the final manuscript.

Consent for publication
This is not applicable because our manuscript does not contain any individual person's data in any form (including individual details, images or videos).

Competing interests
The authors declare that they have no competing interests.

Author details
[1]R4D International Foundation, Yaounde, Cameroon. [2]Center for International Health (CIH), Ludwig-Maximilians-Universität, München, Germany. [3]Faculty of Health Sciences, University of Bamenda, Bamenda, Cameroon. [4]University of Yaounde I, Yaounde, Cameroon. [5]CUNY Graduate School of Public Health and Health Policy, New York, USA. [6]Department of Epidemiology & Population Health, Albert Einstein College of Medicine, New York, USA. [7]Montefiore Medical Center, New York, USA.

References
1. Davies M-A, Kalk E. Provider-initiated HIV testing and counselling for children. PLoS Med. 2014;11(5):e1001650. https://doi.org/10.1371/journal.pmed.1001650.
2. UNICEF. For Every Child, End AIDS. Seventh Stocktaking Report. New York: UNICEF; 2016. https://data.unicef.org/wp-content/uploads/2016/12/HIV-and-AIDS-2016-Seventh-Stocktaking-Report.pdf. Accessed 07 Sept 2018.
3. UNICEF. Towards an AIDS-free generation Children and AIDS. Sixth Stocktaking Report. New York: UNICEF; 2013. https://www.unicef.org/publications/files/Children_and_AIDS_Sixth_Stocktaking_Report_EN.pdf. Accessed 07 Sept 2018.
4. Ahmed S, Kim MH, Sugandhi N, Phelps BR, Sabelli R, Diallo MO, et al. Beyond early infant diagnosis: case finding strategies for identification of HIV-infected infants and children. AIDS Lond Engl. 2013;27(0 2):S235–45. https://doi.org/10.1097/QAD.0000000000000099.
5. Leon N, Lewin S, Mathews C. Implementing a provider-initiated testing and counselling (PITC) intervention in Cape town, South Africa: a process evaluation using the normalisation process model. Implementation Science. 2013;8:97.
6. UNAIDS. Fact sheet 2016. Geneva: UNAIDS; 2016. www.unaids.org/sites/default/files/media_asset/20150901_FactSheet_2015_en.pdf. Accessed 07 Sept 2018.
7. UNAIDS. Fact Sheet World AIDS 2017. Geneva: UNAIDS; 2017. http://www.unaids.org/sites/default/files/media_asset/UNAIDS_FactSheet_en.pdf. Accessed 13 Aug 2017
8. UNAIDS. Country Fact Sheet Cameroon 2016. AIDSinfo. http://aidsinfo.unaids.org. Accessed 22 Sept 2017.
9. UNAIDS. 2008 Report on the Global AIDS Epidemic. Geneva: UNAIDS; 2008. http://www.unaids.org/sites/default/files/media_asset/jc1510_2008globalreport_en_0.pdf. Accessed 07 Sept 2018.
10. Yumo HA, Angwafor SA, Ayuk EM, Ndang CA. Scaling up paediatric HIV care and treatment in resource limited settings: Lessons learned from the active search for pediatric AIDS in a rural health district in northwestern Cameroon. Dakar (Senegal):2nd international interest workshop; 2008.
11. WHO and UNICEF. Policy Requirements for HIV testing and Counselling of Infants and Young Children in Health Facilities. Geneva: WHO and UNICEF; 2010. http://apps.who.int/iris/bitstream/10665/44276/1/9789241599092_eng.pdf. Accessed 07 Sept 2018.
12. Wang H, Chow SC. Sample size calculation for comparing proportions. Wiley Encyclopedia of Clinical Trials 2007. https://doi.org/10.1002/9781118445112.stat07091.
13. UNAIDS. 90–90–90-an ambitious treatment target to help end the AIDS epidemic. Geneva: UNAIDS; 2017. http://www.unaids.org/en/resources/documents/2017/90-90-90. Accessed 07 Sept 2018.
14. Abrams EJ, Strasser S. 90–90–90 – Charting a steady course to end the paediatric HIV epidemic. J Int AIDS Soc. 2015;18(Suppl 6):20296. https://doi.org/10.7448/IAS.18.7.2029.
15. Ahmed S, Sabelli RA, Simon K, Rosenberg NE, Kavuta E, Harawa M, et al. Index case finding facilitates identification and linkage to care of children and young persons living with HIV/AIDS in Malawi. Tropical Med Int Health. 2017;22(8):1021–9. https://doi.org/10.1111/tmi.12900.
16. Wagner AD, Mugo C, Njuguna IN, Maleche-obimbo E, Sherr K, Inwani IW, et al. Implementation and operational research: active referral of children of Hiv-positive adults reveals high prevalence of undiagnosed Hiv. J Acquir Immune Defic Syndr. 2016;73(5):e83–9. https://doi.org/10.1097/QAI.0000000000001184.
17. Republic of Cameroon. Cameroun Enquête Démographique et de Santé et à Indicateurs Multiples 2011. Maryland: INS-ICF International Calverton; 2012. https://dhsprogram.com/pubs/pdf/FR260/FR260.pdf. Accessed 07 Sept 2018.
18. Zoufaly A, Hammerl R, Sunjoh F, Jochum J, Nassimi N, Awasom C, et al. High HIV prevalence among children presenting for general consultation in rural Cameroon. Int J STD AIDS. 2014;25(10):742–4. https://doi.org/10.1177/0956462413518762.
19. Cohn J, Whitehouse K, Tuttle J, Lueck K, Tran T. Paediatric HIV testing beyond the context of prevention of mother-to-child transmission: a systematic review and meta-analysis. Lancet HIV. 2016 (10):e473–81. https://doi.org/10.1016/S2352-3018(16)30050-9.
20. Rwemisisi J, Wolff B, Coutinho A, Grosskurth H, Whitworth J. "What if they ask how I got it?" dilemmas of disclosing parental HIV status and testing children for HIV in Uganda. Health policy plan. Health Policy Plan. 2008;23(1):36–42.
21. Buzdugan R, Watadzaushe C, Dirawo J, Mundida O, Langhaug L, Willis N, et al. Positive attitudes to pediatric HIV testing: findings from a nationally representative survey from Zimbabwe. PLoS One. 2012;7(12):e53213. https://doi.org/10.1371/journal.pone.0053213.
22. John-Stewart GC, Wariua G, Beima-Sofie KM, Richardson BA, Farquhar C, Maleche-Obimbo E, et al. Prevalence, perceptions, and correlates of pediatric HIV disclosure in an HIV treatment program in Kenya. AIDS Care. 2013;25(9):1067–76. https://doi.org/10.1080/09540121.2012.749333.
23. Newell M-L, Brahmbhatt H, Ghys PD. Child mortality and HIV infection in Africa: a review. AIDS. 2004;18(Suppl 2):S27–34.
24. Lallemant C, Halembokaka G, Baty G, Ngo-Giang-Huong N, Barin F, Le Coeur S. Impact of HIV/Aids on child mortality before the highly active antiretroviral therapy era: a study in Pointe-Noire, republic of Congo. J Trop Med. 2010;2010. https://doi.org/10.1155/2010/897176.
25. Wagner A, Slyker J, Langat A, Inwani I, Adhiambo J, Benki-Nugent S, et al. High mortality in HIV-infected children diagnosed in hospital underscores need for faster diagnostic turnaround time in prevention of mother-to-child transmission of HIV (PMTCT) programs. BMC Pediatr. 2015;15:10. https://doi.org/10.1186/s12887-015-0325-8.

26. Phelps BR, Ahmed S, Amzel A, Diallo MO, Jacobs T, Kellerman SE, et al. Linkage, initiation and retention of children in the antiretroviral therapy cascade: an overview. AIDS Lond Engl. 2013;27(02):S207–13. https://doi.org/10.1097/QAD.0000000000000095.

27. Ruria EC, Masaba R, Kose J, Woelk G, Mwangi E, Matu L, et al. Optimizing linkage to care and initiation and retention on treatment of adolescents with newly diagnosed HIV infection. AIDS Lond Engl. 2017;31(Suppl 3): S253–60. https://doi.org/10.1097/QAD.0000000000001538.

28. Carmone A, Bomai K, Bongi W, Frank TD, Dalepa H, Loifa B, et al. Partner testing, linkage to care, and HIV-free survival in a program to prevent parent-to-child transmission of HIV in the highlands of Papua New Guinea. Glob Health Action. 2014;7:24995. https://doi.org/10.3402/gha.v7.24995.

29. Luyirika E, Towle MS, Achan J, Muhangi J, Senyimba C, Lule F, et al. Scaling up Paediatric HIV care with an integrated, family-Centred approach: an observational case study from Uganda. PLoS One. 8(8):e69548. https://doi.org/10.1371/journal.pone.0069548.

30. Kranzer K, Meghji J, Bandason T, Dauya E, Mungofa S, Busza J, et al. Barriers to provider-initiated testing and counselling for children in a high HIV prevalence setting: a mixed methods study. PLoS Med. 11(5):e1001649. https://doi.org/10.1371/journal.pmed.1001649.

18

Mothers' knowledge, attitude and practice towards the prevention and home-based management of diarrheal disease among under-five children in Diredawa, Eastern Ethiopia, 2016

Hailemariam Mekonnen Workie*🆔, Abdilahi Sharifnur Sharifabdilahi and Esubalew Muchie Addis

Abstract

Background: Diarrhea remains the 2nd leading cause of death among children under 5 globally. It kills more young children than AIDS. It would have been prevented by simple home management using oral rehydration therapy. Mothers play a central role in its management and prevention. So, the main objective of this study was to assess mothers' knowledge, attitude & practice in prevention & home-based management of diarrheal disease among under-five children in Dire Dawa, Eastern Ethiopia.

Methods: Institutional based cross-sectional study was conducted from March 15–April 14, 2016, in Diredawa among 295 Mothers who had under-five child with diarrhea in the last 2 weeks using simple random sampling method. Mothers were interviewed face to face by using pretested, standard and structured questionnaire. The data quality was assured by translation, retranslation and pretesting the questionnaire. Data were checked for completeness, consistency and then entered into Epi Info v3.1 and analyzed using SPSS v20. The descriptive statistical analysis was used to compute frequency, percentages, and mean of the findings of this study. The results were presented using tables, charts, and graphs.

Results: In this study, 295 participants were included with 100% response rate. From total 295 mothers, around two-thirds (65.2%) of them had good knowledge, but more than half of mothers (54.9%) had a negative attitude towards home-based management and prevention of diarrhea among under-five children. Regarding the attitude of the mothers, 58% had poor practice towards home-based management and prevention of diarrhea among under-five children.

Conclusion: The finding of this study showed that the attitude and practice of mothers were unsatisfactory about the prevention and home-based management of under-five diarrheal diseases. Therefore, Health education, dissemination of information, and community conversation should plan and implement to create a positive attitude and practice towards the better prevention and management of under 5 diarrheal diseases.

Keywords: Knowledge, Attitude, Practice, Mothers, Prevention, Home-based management, Diarrhea, Under-five children

* Correspondence: hailemariam2129@gmail.com
School of Nursing and Midwifery, College of Health and Medical Science,
Haramaya University, P.O. Box 235, Harar, Ethiopia

Introduction

According to WHO, Passage of 3 or more than 3 loose of stool or watery stools per day or considers as abnormal by the mothers or stools more frequent than normal for a child is considered as diarrhea [1, 2]. Diarrheal disease remains the second leading cause of death among under 5 children globally [3–6]. Nearly one in five deaths of a child – about 1.5 million each year – is due to the disease of diarrhea [4, 7]. It kills more young children than malaria HIV/AIDS, and measles together [1, 4].

Diarrheal disease is one of the commonest illnesses that has the greatest negative impact on the growth and development of infants and young children [8]. Worldwide, children whose age is less than 5 years' experience, on average, 3.2 episodes of diarrhea every year and consequently 1.87 million children will die from dehydration associated with diarrheal disease, particularly in the countries of Asia, Africa and Latin America [3].

According to Ethiopian demographic health survey (EDHS) of 2000, 2005, 2011 and 2016 the 2 weeks prevalence of diarrheal disease among under-five children was 24, 18, 13, 12% respectively [9–12]. Even though there was a double reduction of the prevalence of under 5 diarrheal diseases in the last 16 years in Ethiopia, but, still it is one of the most important public issue and major health problems of the country [9, 12].

Rotavirus is among the commonest diarrheal pathogen in children worldwide that causes about one-third of diarrhea-associated hospitalizations and 800,000 deaths per year [13–15]. Children in the poorest countries like Ethiopia account for 82% of rotavirus deaths of under-five children [16]. Rotavirus can cause intestinal losses of fluid, electrolyte and nutritional deficiency which relatively progresses rapidly to cause dehydration and death [17, 18].

Contaminated weaning food, inappropriate feeding practice, lack of clean water, poor hand washing, limited sanitary disposal of waste, poor housing conditions, and lack of access to adequate and affordable health care are aggravated factors of the under 5 diarrheal disease [6, 8, 19, 20].

Diarrheal diseases among under 5-year children can be tackled in at both primary and secondary prevention levels. The former about the improvement of sanitation and water quality but the latter is about early recognition of dehydration due to diarrhea and prompt oral rehydration using ORS (oral rehydration solution) or appropriate home available fluids. Oral rehydration solution has been proven to be effective in preventing diarrhea mortality in the community while varying degree of evidence favors the use of home available fluid [21].

Optimal infant & young child feeding practices could prevent more than 10% of deaths from diarrhea. On the other hand, better hygiene practices, particularly hand washing with soap & the safe disposal of excreta can reduce the incidence of diarrhea by 35% [1, 22].

Diarrhea is not lethal itself, the improper knowledge, poor practice and negative attitudes of mothers and their misdirected approach towards its management and prevention leads to high degree of severe dehydration and lastly death [23, 24]. Therefore, the main objective of this study was to assess the mothers' knowledge, attitude, and practice in the prevention and home-based management of diarrhea towards their under-five children in Diredawa, East Ethiopia.

Method

Study area and period

The study was conducted from March 15 –April 14, 2016, in Diredawa city. Diredawa city is one of the two administrative cities in Ethiopia. It situated and located in the eastern part of Ethiopia with 515 km from Addis Ababa (capital city of Ethiopia) and 313 from Djibouti. According to the 2011 Ethiopian Demographic health survey (EDHS), the total population of the administration was 341,834 of which 174,461 were men and 170,461 women [11]. About 233,224 (68.23%) of the population were urban inhabitants, while 31.77% were rural inhabitants. In Dire-Dawa administration there was 2 governmental and 4 private hospitals. From these, the 3 hospitals were selected for this study.

Study design and participants

A cross-sectional study design was conducted in selected Diredawa hospitals to assess mothers' knowledge, attitude & practice towards the prevention & home-based management of diarrheal disease among under-five children. Mothers who had a child less than 5 years of age with diarrhea in the last 2 weeks were included in an interview using each hospital monthly patient flow report as a sampling frame. Those mothers with a physical impairment (unable to hear and speak) and mentally ill were excluded from the study.

Sample size determination and technique

The sample size (n) required for this study was determined using a single population proportion formula $(n = (Z\alpha/2)^2 \, p(1\text{-}p)/d^2))$; whereas n = the required sample size for this study, $Z\alpha/2(1.96)$: significance level at $\alpha = 0.05$ with 95% confidence interval, p: proportion of prevalence of diarrhea in eastern region which was 22.5% [25], d: margin of error (5%) and 10% non-response rate. The final required sample size was 295. Lottery method was used to select the 3 hospitals and the sample was collected proportionally from each hospital using simple random sampling method. Each hospital monthly patient flow report was used as a sampling frame.

Operational definitions

Dehydration: It is a condition when the child loses too much water and salt from the body [2, 26]

Rehydration: The correction of dehydration with oral rehydration salts (ORS) or home prepared solution [2].

Oral Rehydration Therapy (ORT): The administration of fluid by mouth to prevent or correct the dehydration that is a consequence of diarrhea. It is a mixture of clean water, salt and sugar [2].

Good knowledge: Those mothers who answered above the mean of the knowledge questions [27].

Poor knowledge: Those mothers who answered below the mean of the knowledge questions [27].

Positive Attitude: Mothers who answered above the mean questions of the attitude were assigned as having "positive attitude" [28]

Negative Attitude: those who answered below the attitude questions were assigned as having a "negative attitude" [28]

Good practice: Mothers who able to answer above the mean of the practice questions were measured as good practice [29].

Poor Practice: Those mothers who answer below the mean of the practice questions were measured as poor practice [29].

Measurement and data collection procedure

Face to face interview was employed by using a standard and structured questionnaire that contained sociodemographic status, knowledge, attitude, practice, and health-seeking behavior questions of the mothers regarding under 5 children diarrheal diseases. There were four trained BSc nurse data collectors and 1 M.Sc. nurse as a supervisor.

Data quality control

The data quality was assured by using different methods. The standard and structured questionnaire was used (Additional file 1). The questionnaire was prepared in English and translated into the local language (Amharic, oromic, and somalic) for data collection and then re translated back into English for analysis. Two days of training was given to the data collectors and supervisors on the data collection tool and procedures. Then the questionnaire was pretested on 5% of the sample size to ensure its validity. Findings from the pretesting were utilized for modifying and adjustment of the instrument and interviewing technique. Data collectors were supervised closely by the supervisors and the principal investigators. Completeness of each questionnaire was checked by the principal investigator and the supervisors on daylily basis. Double data entry was done by two data clerks and the consistency of the entered data was cross-checked by comparing the two separately entered data.

Data processing and analysis

Immediately after the data collection was completed, each questionnaire was thoroughly reviewed for completeness and consistency by the data collectors, supervisor and investigators. Then the data were entered into Epi Info version 3.1 and analyzed using SPSS for window version 20. The descriptive statistical analysis was used to compute frequency, percentages, and mean of the findings of this study. The results were presented using tables, graphs, and result statements.

Results

A total of 295 mothers have participated in the study with a response rate of 100%. So, 295 respondents' data were included in the analysis process.

Socio-demographic characteristics of the mothers

In this study, more than half of the mothers (51.5%) were in the age of 25–34 years with the mean age of 27. Based on religion, Muslims (67.5%) and Orthodox (22%) were dominant. Regarding ethnicity, 137 (46.4%) mothers were Oromo, 121 (41.0%) Somali, 31 (10.5%) Amhara and 6 (2.1%) were from other ethnicities.

From the total participants, 275 (93.2%) were married, 113 (38.3%) were housewives and 132 (44.8%) were unable to read and write. The mean monthly family income of the respondents was 1551 Ethiopian Birr. About half of the children [146 (49.5%)] were in the age group of 6–24 months (Table 1).

Mothers knowledge about diarrhea prevention and management among under 5 children

Most of the mothers (92.5%), defined diarrhea as the passing of loose stool 3 or more times per day, while, only 8 (2.7%) mothers identified blood in the stool. Two hundred fifty-two (85.5%) respondents thought that diarrhea is caused by drinking contaminated water. Around half (51.2%) of the participants identified that weakness or lethargy is the danger sign of under-five diarrheal disease. To the contrary, only 2 (0.7%) of them knew that marked thirst for water is the danger sign of diarrheal disease (Table 2).

Regarding homemade solution, only less than half of the participants [125 (42.4%)] were used homemade solution during diarrheal disease of their child. From them, [117 (93.6%)] prepared the solution using 1/2 teaspoon of salt, and 6 teaspoons of sugar in 1 liter of water.

Around two-thirds [184 (62.4%)] of the mothers knew about the recommended volume of water for mixing a sachet of ORS (i.e., 1000 ml. of water to 1 sachet of ORS). One hundred three (34.9%) of the respondents believed that ORS should be given after the passing of every loose stool of the child, while 90 (30.4%) said that should be administered whatever child needs to drink (Table 3).

Table 1 Sociodemographic characteristics of respondents, Diredawa, East Ethiopia, 2016

Characteristic	Category	Frequency	Percentages
Age of the mother	15–24	109	36.9%
	25–34	152	51.5%
	35–44	32	10.9%
	>45	2	0.7%
Age of the child	0–5 months	60	20.3%
	6–24 months	146	49.5%
	24–59 months	89	30.2%
Marital status of the mother	Married	275	93.2%
	Single	2	0.7%
	Widowed	6	2.0%
	Divorced/separated	12	4.1%
Occupation of the mother	Housewife	235	79.7%
	Gov't/NGO employed	52	17.6%
	Self-employed	8	2.7%
Monthly income of the mother (Binned)	<=1000	106	35.9%
	1001–3000	148	50.2%
	3001 & above	41	13.9%
Mother's educational status	Unable to read and write	132	44.8%
	Primary	113	38.3%
	Secondary	29	9.8%
	Diploma and above	21	7.1%
The religion of the mother	Islam	199	67.5%
	Orthodox	65	22.0%
	Protestant	29	9.8%
	Others	2	0.7%
The ethnicity of the mother	Oromo	137	46.4%
	Somali	121	41.0%
	Amhara	31	10.5%
	Others	6	2.1%

Table 2 Maternal knowledge about under 5 diarrheal diseases in Dire Dawa, Eastern Ethiopia, 2016

Characteristic	Frequency	%
Definition of diarrhea		
Frequent passing of watery stool (3 or more times)	273	92.5%
Frequent passing of normal stool	12	4.1%
Blood in stools	8	2.7%
Greenish stools	2	0.7%
Diarrheal causes		
Teething	15	5.1%
Evil eye	24	8.1%
Contaminated water	252	85.5%
No idea	4	1.3%
Diarrheal danger signs		
Becoming weak or lethargic	151	51.2%
Repeated vomiting/vomiting everything	103	34.9%
Fever and blood in the stool	37	12.5%
Marked thirst for water	2	0.7%
Others	2	0.7%

Mother's attitudes toward prevention and home-based management of under-five diarrhea

From the total respondents, the majority of them [162 (55%)] disagreed towards the provision of oral rehydration solution at home for the treatment of under-five diarrheal diseases. Similarly, most of the participants [181 (61.4%)] disagreed with the statement "mothers can treat their children's diarrheal disease at home". Around half of the mothers, 152 (51.5%) believed that their child dislikes the taste of oral rehydration solution (Figs. 1, 2, and 3).

Practices of mothers towards the prevention and home management of diarrhea among under-five children

Only one-quarter of the mothers [77 (26.1%)] breastfed their child more than usual while majority 178 (60.3%) breastfed less than usual during the diarrheal episodes. Likewise, only 83 (28.1%) offered a drink more than usual during diarrheal episodes but most of the mothers 181 (61.4%) offered a drink for their child less than usual during the diarrheal episodes. Concerning feeding, 99 (33.6%) of mothers offered food more than usual to eat during the diarrheal episodes and 185 (62.7%) of the mother offered less than usual. Most of the mothers (67.8, 84.7% & 100%) responded that they usually wash their hands before preparing food, after preparing food, and after defecation respectively (Table 4).

Mothers care-seeking behavior and places during their children diarrheal episode

Almost all of the mothers [289 (98.0%)] sought medical treatment for their children during the time of diarrheal diseases. From those who sought care for their child's diarrhea, the majority [179 (60.7%)] visited hospitals for the treatment of diarrhea, and 9 (3.1%) went to the traditional practitioner (Table 5).

The overall level of knowledge, attitude, and practice of mothers in prevention and home-based management of diarrhea among under-five children

Knowledge was assessed by asking, whether the mothers know about ORS and what the benefits of ORS, and so on. Mothers who respond above the mean of the questions correctly were assigned as having "good knowledge" while mothers who answered below the mean were regarded as having "poor knowledge":

Table 3 Respondents' knowledge about the correct use of ORS, Diredawa, East Ethiopia, 2016

Variable	Categories	Freq.	%
How is ORS prepared?	1 sachet of ORS- 300 ml (1 coke bottle) of water	25	8.5%
	1 sachet of ORS- 500 ml (1 small size of mineral bottle) of water	56	18.9%
	1 sachet of ORS- 600 ml (1 beer bottle) of water	25	8.5%
	1 sachet of ORS- 1000 ml (1 l) of water	184	62.4%
	1 sachet of ORS- 1500 ml (1.5 l or large size of mineral bottle) of water	5	1.7%
How often should ORS be given?	Once a day	50	17.0%
	2–3 times a day	52	17.6%
	Whatever child wants to drink	90	30.5%
	After the passing of very loose stool	103	34.9%
How long should the mixed ORS last?	24 h. (1 day)	255	86.4%
	48 h. (2 days)	33	11.2%
	72 h. (3 days)	4	1.4%
	96 h. (4 days)	3	1.0%

Also, the attitude was assessed whether they agree or disagree towards the taste of ORS to their child, or whether they agree or disagree that ORS is the first choice in the management of diarrhea and so on. Mothers who answered above the mean questions were assigned as having "positive attitude" and those who answer below the mean were assigned as having "negative attitude".

Like others, the overall practice of mothers was measured by asking how is ORS prepared, how often is it given and how long should a mixed ORS last and so on. Mothers who answered above the mean questions were assigned as having "good practices" whereas those who did not be assigned as having "poor practice".

Based on these criteria, 192 (65.2%) of the mothers had good knowledge and 103 (34.9%) had poor knowledge about the prevention and home-based management of under 5 diarrheal diseases. Regarding the attitude, more than half of the mothers (54.9%) had a negative attitude and only 133 (45.1%) had a positive attitude towards the prevention and home-based management of under 5 diarrheas. From the total of mothers participated in this study, only 124 (42%) of them had a good practice and the remaining 171 (58%) had poor practice towards prevention and home-based management of under 5 diarrheas.

Discussion

This study has assessed mothers' knowledge, attitude, and practices towards the prevention and home-based management of under 5 diarrheal diseases in Diredawa city, Eastern Ethiopia. Based on the findings, the majority of

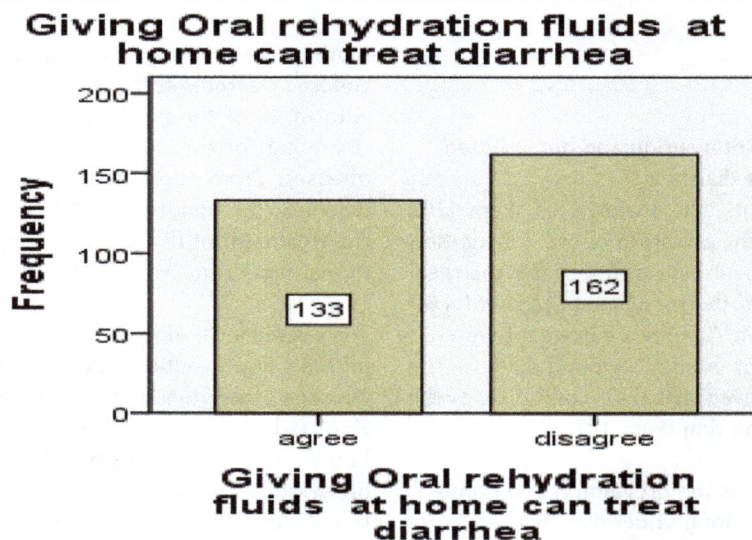

Fig. 1 Mothers attitude toward giving oral rehydration therapy at home in Diredawa, Eastern Ethiopia, 2016

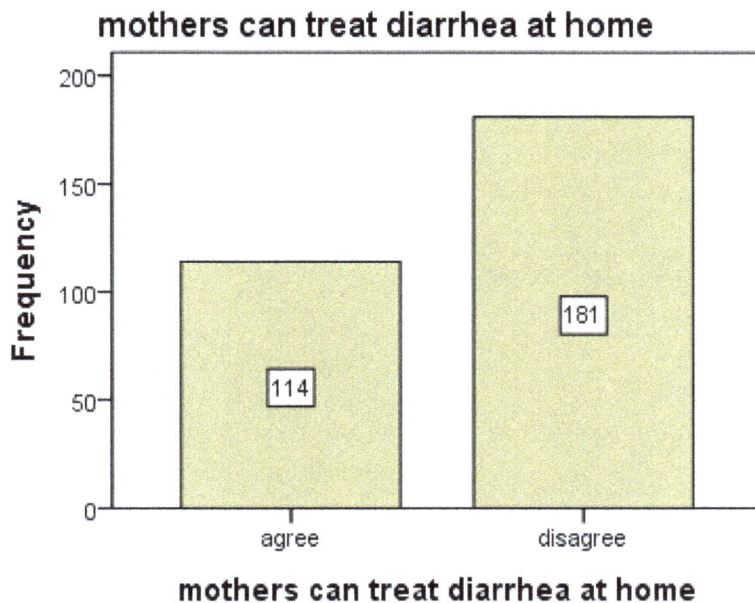

Fig. 2 Mothers attitude towards the statement of "Mothers can treat diarrhea at home" in Dire Dawa, Eastern Ethiopia, 2016

the respondents (65.2, 54.9, and 58%) had good knowledge, negative attitude and poor practice about the prevention and home-based management of under 5 diarrheal diseases respectively.

The finding of this study showed that 65.2% of mothers had a good knowledge about prevention and home-based management of diarrhea among under-five children. A similar finding was observed in Fenoteselam,

Ethiopia (65.9%) [29]. On the contrary, this finding is higher than studies done in Kashan, Iran (28.8%), Fagita Lekoma, Ethiopia (56.2%), and Assosa, Ethiopia (37.5%) [27, 28, 30]. This is mainly due to the fact that Dire Dawa city is a bigger and more urbanized city with many mass media.

Most of the mothers (92.2%) defined diarrhea correctly (as the passing of loose stool 3 or more times per day);

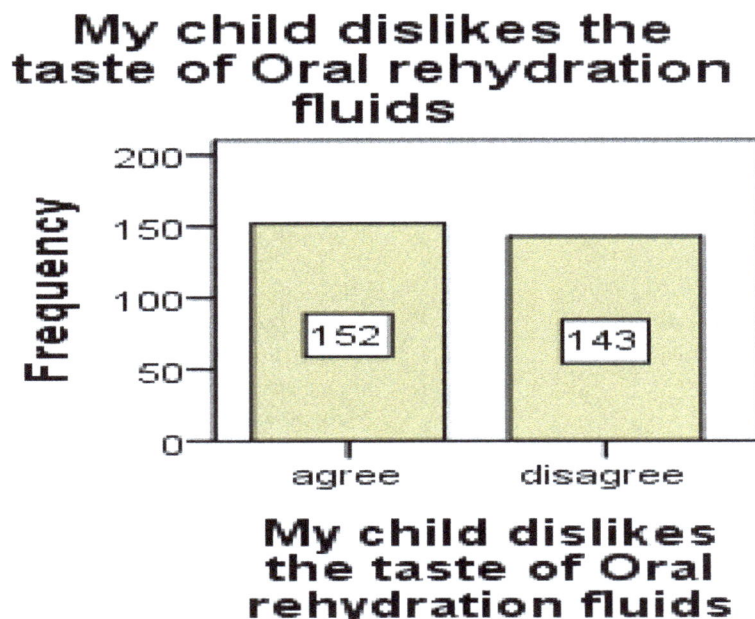

Fig. 3 Mothers attitude about the taste of oral rehydration fluid by their children, Diredawa, Eastern Ethiopia, 2016

Table 4 Maternal feeding practices during child's diarrheal episode and hand washing behaviors in Dire Dawa, 2016

Characteristic	Category	n	%
When (Name) had diarrhea, did you breastfeed him/her less than usual, about the same amount, or more than usual?	Less	178	60.3%
	Same	35	11.9%
	More	77	26.1%
	Child not breastfed	4	1.4%
	Don't know	1	0.3%
When (Name) had diarrhea, was he/she offered less than usual to drink, about the same amount, or more than usual to drink?	Less	181	61.4%
	Same	31	10.5%
	More	83	28.1%
	Nothing to drink	0	0.0%
	Don't know	0	0.0%
Was (name) offered less than usual to eat, about the same amount, or more than usual to eat?	Less	185	62.7%
	Same	11	3.7%
	More	99	33.6%
	Nothing to eat	0	0.0%
	Don't know	0	0.0%
When do you wash hands with soap	Before food preparation	200	67.8%
	Before feeding children	250	84.7%
	After defecation	295	100.0%
	Never	0	0.0%
	Other	0	0.0%

which is much higher than other studies done in Fagita Lekoma, Ethiopia (65.4%), Karachi, Pakistan (52.5%) [24, 27]. Similarly, in this study, two hundred fifty-two (85.5%) respondents thought that diarrhea is caused by drinking contaminated water; that is significantly higher than studies conducted in Pakistan, India, Mali, and Western Ethiopia [24, 28, 31, 32]. The probable explanation of the discrepancy might be due to the presence of many mass media and health facilities in the city, which may disseminate information to the population and create good knowledge towards under-five diarrheal diseases.

Table 5 Mothers' care-seeking behavior and place sought for care in Dire Dawa, Eastern Ethiopia, 2016

Characteristic	Category	n	%
Did you seek advice or treatment from someone outside of the home for (Name's) diarrhea?	Yes	289	98.0%
	No	6	2.0%
Where did you first go for advice or treatment?	Hospital	179	60.7%
	Health center	91	30.8%
	Health post	0	0.0%
	PVO center	0	0.0%
	Clinic	16	5.4%
	Traditional practitioner	9	3.1%

Less than half of the participants (42.4%) were used homemade solution during diarrheal disease of their child. The result different from the Heidedal community (90%), Taung district (83.6%), Swaziland community (97%) of South Africa [33]. This might be due to the fact that most of the mothers in the city sought medical treatment for their children during the time of diarrheal diseases.

Around two-thirds [184 (62.4%)] of the mothers knew about the recommended volume of water for mixing a sachet of ORS. This is much less than other studies done in Ethiopia (85.4%), Pakistan (75.5%), Nepal (70%), and India (76.7%) [24, 27, 31, 34]. This could be justified by the fact that these mothers might not be familiar with ORS mixing due to lack of education.

Also, the majority of the mothers agreed that ORT can replace lost fluid but they disagreed ORT is the first-choice management of diarrhea. Similarly, a study done in Mali showed that majority of mothers knew ORT can replace lost fluid but its inability to stop diarrhea caused them to seek additional treatments such as antibiotics and traditional medicines to treat diarrhea [32].

This study indicated that 42% of mothers had good practice in prevention and home-based management of diarrhea. This is compiled with the finding of Northwest, Ethiopia (44.9%), but the opposite was observed in studies conducted in Assossa District (62.9%) and Awi zone

(37.6%), [27–29]. The difference may be due to the difference of the study area, period and sample size.

In this study, 61.4 and 62.7% of the mother offered fluid and feeding less than usual to their child during the diarrheal episodes respectively. In the same way, more than 70% of mothers in Kenya and 19.6% of mothers in India decrease fluid intake and feeding during the diarrheal episodes [31, 35]. To the contrary, other studies in Bangladesh and Pakistan showed that more than 50 and 71% of mothers were in favor of giving food and fluids during the diarrheal illness of the child [24, 36]. Majority of the mothers in this study area were uneducated and this might be the major reason for the discrepancy as uneducated mothers could not have the opportunity to get information from books, newspaper, and other reading sources. The other possible reason for the decrement of fluid intake and feeding during diarrheal illness by the mothers might be due to the fear of more vomiting and lose of watery stool.

Most of the mothers (67.8% & 100%) usually wash their hands before preparing food, and after defecation respectively. But in Assossa, Ethiopia only 11.7, and 16%, of the mothers was wash their hands before preparing food, and after defecation respectively [28]. To contrary, in Bangladesh, 60.0 and 3.1% don't wash their hands before food preparation and after defecation respectively [36]. This variation might be due to differences in culture, sociodemographic and information access.

Almost all of the mothers [289 (98.0%)] in the present study sought medical treatment for their children during the time of diarrhea diseases which much different from Fagita Lekoma, Ethiopia (71.6%), Karachi, Pakistan (52.5%) and Assossa, Ethiopia (62.4%) [24, 27, 28]. As Diredawa is a highly urbanized city, mothers have more opportunity to access health facilities within the near distance.

Conclusions

The finding of this study showed that the attitude and practice of mothers were unsatisfactory about the prevention and home-based management of under-five diarrheal diseases. Therefore, Health education, dissemination of information, and community conversation should plan and implement to create a positive attitude and practice towards the better prevention and management of under 5 diarrheal diseases.

Strength and limitation of the study

As there was no the same study in the study area, it can use as a baseline for other studies. Similarly, it can also be a blueprint to conduct an interventional study in the particular area.

The limitation of this study is that it was not possible to establish a temporal relationship between the

exposure and outcome variable as this study design was a cross-sectional study. Additionally, determinant factors for the negative attitude and poor practice of the mothers were not included due to the limitation of time and resource. So, another study is needed to determine these associated factors.

Abbreviations
EDHS: Ethiopian Demographic and Health Survey; EPI: Expanded Program on Immunization; FMOH: Federal Ministry of Health; HIV: Human Immunodeficiency Virus; IMNCI: Integrated Management of Neonatal and Childhood Illnesses; IV: Intra-venous; Kg: Kilograms; MDG: Millennium Development Goal; Ml: Milliliters; ORS: Oral rehydration salt; ORT: Oral Rehydration Therapy; RHFs: Recommended Home Fluids; SPSS: Statistical Package for Social Science; SSS: Sugar Salt Solution; SSW: Sugar-Salt- Water; UNICEF: United Nations International Children Emergency Fund; WHO: World Health Organization

Acknowledgments
We would like to thank Dilchora, Yemariam Work and Bilal hospital for giving us the permission to conduct this research in their hospital. Our sincere gratitude and appreciation forward data collectors and participants without whom it would not be realized.

Funding
This research didn't receive grants from any funding agency in the public, commercial or not-for-profit sectors.

Authors' contributions
All the authors had a substantial contribution from conception to the acquisition of data. HM & AS had a great contribution to study design, analysis, and interpretation of the findings. HM drafted the manuscript. All authors revised the paper carefully for important intellectual contents. All authors read and approved the final manuscript.

Competing interests
The authors declare that they have no competing interests.

References
1. WHO, UNICEF. WHO-UNICEF joint statement on the clinical management of acute diarrhea. Geneva: World Health Assembly; 2004.
2. World Health Organization. Diarrhoeal disease Fact sheet N°330. 2013 [Available from: https://web.archive.org/web/20140717205014/http://www.who.int/mediacentre/factsheets/fs330/en/]. Accessed 15 May 2016.
3. World Health Organization. The treatment of diarrhoea: a manual for physicians and other senior health workers. Geneva: WHO; 2005. WHO/CDD/SER/80.2; 2013
4. Wardlaw T, Salama P, Brocklehurst C, Chopra M, Mason E. Diarrhoea: why children are still dying and what can be done. Lancet. 2010;375(9718):870–2.
5. Kosek M, Bern C, Guerrant RL. The global burden of diarrhoeal disease, as estimated from studies published between 1992 and 2000. Bull World Health Organ. 2003;81(3):197–204.
6. Black RE, Morris SS, Bryce J. Where and why are 10 million children dying every year? Lancet. 2003;361(9376):2226–34.
7. Walker CLF, Aryee MJ, Boschi-Pinto C, Black RE. Estimating diarrhea mortality among young children in low and middle income countries. PLoS One. 2012;7(1):e29151.
8. Motarjemi Y, Kaferstein F, Moy G, Quevedo F. Contaminated weaning food: a major risk factor for diarrhoea and associated malnutrition. Bull World Health Organ. 1993;71(1):79–92.
9. Central Statistical Agency. Ethiopian demographic health survey (EDHS), 2000. Addis Ababa and Calverton: Central Statistical Agency and ICF International; 2001.
10. Demographic E. Health survey 2005. Central statistical agency. Addis Ababa, Ethiopia, RC Macro, Calverton, Maryland, USA. 2006.
11. CSA, International I. Ethiopia demographic and health survey 2011. Addis Ababa and Calverton: Central Statistical Agency and ICF International; 2012. p. 430.

12. Central Statistical Agency (CSA) [Ethiopia], ICF. Ethiopia Demographic and Health Survey 2016. Addis Ababa, Ethiopia, and Rockville, Maryland, USA: CSA and ICF; 2016.

13. Parashar UD, Bresee JS, Gentsch JR, Glass RI. Rotavirus. Emerg Infect Dis. 1998;4(4):561.

14. Parashar UD, Gibson CJ, Bresee JS, Glass RI. Rotavirus and severe childhood diarrhea. Emerg Infect Dis. 2006;12(2):304–6.

15. Walker CLF, Rudan I, Liu L, Nair H, Theodoratou E, Bhutta ZA, et al. Global burden of childhood pneumonia and diarrhoea. Lancet. 2013;381(9875): 1405–16.

16. Parashar UD, Hummelman EG, Bresee JS, Miller MA, Glass RI. Global illness and deaths caused by rotavirus disease in children. Emerg Infect Dis. 2003; 9(5):565–72.

17. King CK, Glass R, Bresee JS, Duggan C, Control CfD, Prevention. Managing acute gastroenteritis among children. MMWR Recomm Rep. 2003;52(1):16.

18. O'Ryan M, Lucero Y, O'Ryan-Soriano MA, Ashkenazi S. An update on management of severe acute infectious gastroenteritis in children. Expert Rev Anti-Infect Ther. 2010;8(6):671–82.

19. Prüss A, Kay D, Fewtrell L, Bartram J. Estimating the burden of disease from water, sanitation, and hygiene at a global level. Environ Health Perspect. 2002;110(5):537.

20. Keusch GT, Fontaine O, Bhargava A, Boschi-Pinto C, Bhutta ZA, Gotuzzo E, et al. Diarrheal diseases. In: Disease control priorities in developing countries, vol. 2; 2006. p. 371–88.

21. Munos MK, Walker CL, Black RE. The effect of oral rehydration solution and recommended home fluids on diarrhoea mortality. Int J Epidemiol. 2010; 39(Suppl 1):i75–87.

22. Benenson AS, Chin J, Heymann DL. Control of communicable diseases manual. Washington, DC: American Public Health Association; 1995.

23. Hackett KM, Mukta US, Jalal CS, Sellen DW. Knowledge, attitudes and perceptions on infant and young child nutrition and feeding among adolescent girls and young mothers in rural Bangladesh. Matern Child Nutr. 2015;11(2):173–89.

24. Mumtaz Y, Zafar M, Mumtaz Z. Knowledge attitude and practices of mothers about diarrhea in children under 5 years. J Dow Uni Health Sci. 2014;8(1):3-6.

25. Mengistie B, Berhane Y, Worku A. Prevalence of diarrhea and associated risk factors among children under-five years of age in eastern Ethiopia: a cross-sectional study. Open J Prev Med. 2013;3(07):446.

26. Gosling P. Dorland's illustrated medical dictionary: 30th Edition. Australasian Chiropractic & Osteopathy. 2003;11(2):65.

27. Desta BK, Assimamaw NT, Ashenafi TD. Knowledge, practice, and associated factors of home-based Management of Diarrhea among caregivers of children attending under-five Clinic in Fagita Lekoma District, Awi zone, Amhara regional state, Northwest Ethiopia, 2016. Nurs Res Pract. 2017;2017: 8084548.

28. Merga N, Alemayehu T. Knowledge, perception, and management skills of mothers with under-five children about diarrhoeal disease in indigenous and resettlement communities in Assosa District, Western Ethiopia. J Health Popul Nutr. 2015;33(1):20–30.

29. Amare D, Dereje B, Kassie B, Tessema M, Mullu G, et al. Maternal Knowledge and Practice Towards Diarrhoea Management in Under Five Children in Fenote Selam Town, West Gojjam Zone, Amhara Regional State, Northwest Ethiopia, 2014. J Infect Dis Ther. 2014;2:182. https://doi.org/10.4172/2332-0877.1000182.

30. Ghasemi AA, Talebian A, Masoudi Alavi N, Moosavi G. Knowledge of mothers in management of diarrhea in under-five children, in Kashan, Iran. Nurs Midwifery Stud. 2013;1(3):158–62.

31. Saurabh S, Shidam UG, Sinnakirouchenan M, Subair M, Hou LG, Roy G. Knowledge and practice regarding oral rehydration therapy for acute diarrhoea among mothers of under-five children in an urban area of Puducherry India. Natl J Community Med. 2014;5(1):100–4.

32. Ellis AA, Winch P, Daou Z, Gilroy KE, Swedberg E. Home management of childhood diarrhoea in southern Mali--implications for the introduction of zinc treatment. Soc Sci Med. 2007;64(3):701–12.

33. Dippenaar H, Joubert G, Nel R, Bantobetse M, Opawole A, Roshen K. Homemade sugar-salt solution for oral rehydration: knowledge of mothers and caregivers. S Afr Fam Pract. 2005;47(2):51–3.

34. Ansari M, Ibrahim MI, Hassali MA, Shankar PR, Koirala A, Thapa NJ. Mothers' beliefs and barriers about childhood diarrhea and its management in Morang district, Nepal. BMC Res Notes. 2012;5:576.

35. Othero DM, Orago AS, Groenewegen T, Kaseje DO, Otengah PA. Home management of diarrhea among underfives in a rural community in Kenya: household perceptions and practices. East Afr J Public Health. 2008;5(3): 142–6.

36. Rabbi SE, Dey NC. Exploring the gap between hand washing knowledge and practices in Bangladesh: a cross-sectional comparative study. BMC Public Health. 2013;13:89.

19

Adherence to the neonatal resuscitation algorithm for preterm infants in a tertiary hospital in Spain

Silvia Maya-Enero[1]* ⓘ, Francesc Botet-Mussons[1], Josep Figueras-Aloy[1], Montserrat Izquierdo-Renau[2], Marta Thió[2] and Martin Iriondo-Sanz[2]

Abstract

Background: There is evidence that delivery room resuscitation of very preterm infants often deviates from internationally recommended guidelines. There were no published data in Spain regarding the quality of neonatal resuscitation. Therefore, we decided to evaluate resuscitation team adherence to neonatal resuscitation guidelines after birth in very preterm infants.

Methods: We conducted an observational study. We video recorded resuscitations of preterm infants < 32 weeks' gestational age and evaluated every step during resuscitation according to a score-sheet specifically designed for this purpose, following Carbine's method, where higher scores indicated that more intense resuscitation maneuvers were required. We divided the score achieved by the total possible points per patient to obtain the percentage of adherence to the algorithm. We also compared resuscitations performed by staff neonatologists to those performed by pediatricians on-call. We compared percentages of adherence to the algorithm with the Chi-square test for large groups and Fisher's exact test for smaller groups. We compared assigned Apgar scores with those given after analyzing the recordings and described them by their median and interquartile range. We measured the interrater agreement between Apgar scores with Cohen's kappa coefficient. Linear and logarithmic regressions were drawn to characterize the pattern of algorithm adherence. Statistical analysis was performed using SPSS V.20. A p-value < 0.05 was considered significant. Our Hospital Ethics Committee approved this project, and we obtained parental written consent beforehand.

Results: Sixteen percent of our resuscitations followed the algorithm. The number of mistakes per resuscitation was low. Global adherence to the algorithm was 80.9%. Ventilation and surfactant administration were performed best, whereas preparation and initial steps were done with worse adherence to the algorithm. Intubation required, on average, 2.2 attempts; success on the first attempt happened in 33.3% of cases. Only 12.5% of intubations were achieved within the allotted 30 s. Many errors were attributable to timing. Resuscitations led by pediatricians on-call were performed as correctly as those by staff neonatologists.

Conclusions: Resuscitation often deviates from the internationally recognized algorithm. Perfectly performed resuscitations are infrequent, although global adherence to the algorithm is high. Neonatologists and pediatricians need intubation training.

Keywords: Neonatal resuscitation, Video recording, Very preterm infant, Delivery room

* Correspondence: smaya1@clinic.cat
[1]Neonatology Service, Hospital Clínic, seu Maternitat, ICGON (Institut Clínic de Ginecologia, Obstetrícia i Neonatologia), Barcelona University, Sabino de Arana, 1, 08028 Barcelona, Spain
Full list of author information is available at the end of the article

Background

Neonatal resuscitation (NR) is the most frequently performed resuscitation in hospitals [1–3]. Infants that are more immature are more likely to require support. Approximately 85% of very preterm neonates need intervention during transition after birth and their viability and prognosis greatly depend on the care they receive in the delivery room (DR) [4–6]. Most preterm infants initiate breathing after birth, but they often have a weak, insufficient respiratory drive. Guidelines recommend tactile stimulation (warming, drying and rubbing the back or soles of the feet) to stimulate breathing. Guidelines exist to standardize and optimize resuscitation. However, there is evidence that the sequence and quality of interventions during NR often deviate from guidelines [3, 7–11]. Video recording has been widely used for educational and clinical quality assessment purposes, with good acceptance by caregivers [12, 13]. It is inexpensive, it does not interfere with resuscitation, and it offers data to assess performance accurately. Video reviewing reinforces teamwork and permits identification and amendment of errors that otherwise could be neglected. Combining the recording of physiological parameters (ECG, pulse oximetry (PO), capnography and respiratory function monitoring) with video images helps audit performance [12–15]. There is a lack of information about adherence to NR guidelines in Spain. Consequently, we sought to evaluate adherence to NR guidelines in very preterm neonates at our hospital. Our main hypothesis was that resuscitation often deviates from the algorithm. A secondary hypothesis was that staff neonatologists perform better than pediatricians on-call because they work only with neonates and have more experience on average, whereas pediatricians are younger and work with children up to 18 years.

Methods

We conducted this observational study at Hospital Clínic de Barcelona, a tertiary referral center in Spain where approximately 150 babies < 32 weeks' gestational age (GA) are born every year. Our Hospital Ethics Committee approved this project. We recorded and analyzed these infants' resuscitations after obtaining written parental informed consent. We aimed to analyze as many NRs as possible. However, given the difficulties in obtaining parental consent in such moments of stress, we aimed to analyze a representative sample of at least one-third of all NRs performed. Thus, we decided to record 50 resuscitations. We had planned to obtain the data in 1 year, although it took us longer (16 months), as fewer candidates were born during the study period than expected. This study was the basis for the doctoral thesis of the main author (see link in http://www.ub.edu/medicina/doctorat/lectura.htm May 27, 2011). However, the

data were never published. The authors believe that the results and conclusions may be perfectly applicable today.

Inclusion criteria: All babies < 32 weeks GA were candidates for inclusion in this study. When the pediatrician was required in the delivery room, parents were approached for consent to record the NR. After obtaining written consent, the resuscitator began recording the NR, and that case was included in the study.

All infants were resuscitated under a radiant heater equipped with a neonatal automatic ventilator (Babylog 2, Dräger Medical, Drägerwerk AG & Co. KGaA, Lübeck, Germany) that included an oxygen blender and could provide Continuous Positive Airway Pressure (CPAP) and Positive Pressure Ventilation (PPV) and with a pulse-oximeter (Nellcor™ NPB-295, Minneapolis, MN, USA). A Sony Handycam DCR-SR 32 E (Sony, Tokyo, Japan) digital video camera attached to the upper left side of the radiant warmer recorded the newborn, the hands of the resuscitators and the PO screen. The clinical team turned the recording on before the baby was born.

We designed an evaluation sheet to score 12 domains in each resuscitation (Table 1) according to the algorithm of the Spanish Society of Neonatology, adapted from the ILCOR 2005 guidelines (see Fig. 1). We assigned a numerical score to every resuscitation, following Carbine's previously described method [16]: we awarded 2 points for every correct decision and proper procedure, 1 point for delayed interventions or inadequate technique, and 0 points for indicated procedures that were omitted or for inappropriate procedures (for details of how we scored each domain, see Table 1). The total score per resuscitation ("resuscitation score") ranged from 4 to 22 points. A higher score indicated that more intense resuscitation was required. We obtained the percentage of adherence to the algorithm by dividing the score achieved (X) by the maximum possible score per patient that is, X of a potential of (4–22) points, as a percentage. We registered admission temperature and Apgar scores at 1, 5 and 10 minutes (min) as assigned by the caregiver and after video recording review.

We compared two groups of resuscitators: staff neonatologists (group N) and pediatricians on-call (group P). Neonatologists on-call performed a few of the resuscitations after-hours.

Statistic analysis

We present the characteristics of our study population and its subgroups using the median, standard deviation (SD) and range for quantitative variables (gestational age, birth weight, temperature at admission and adherence to the algorithm and resuscitation score). We

Table 1 Data collection sheet

Patient's identification:		Gestational age:	
Birth weight:		Sex:	
Twin? 1st or 2nd of 2		Time and date of birth	
C-section?			
Apgar score: assigned: 1 min: 5 min: 10 min:			
Apgar score: camera: 1 min: 5 min: 10 min:			
Admission temperature: ºC			
Analyzed aspects	0 points	1 point (any technical error in a correctly indicated maneuver is awarded 1 point; the main errors and examples are listed in every domain)	2 points
Heat loss prevention measures[a]	Not performed	No cap; baby dried with towels and then placed in a plastic wrap; if towels were used, they had to be replaced by new, preheated ones	Well done (dried and towels replaced OR plastic wrap)
Head in a "sniffing position"[a]	Not performed	Head in hyperextension or bent or to a side	Well done
Suctioning	Not performed when indicated	Done after the first 20 s; for more than 5 s; incorrect order (nasal suction before oral); incorrect suction catheter (not 8 F); excessively introduced catheter (more than 10 cm)	Well done
Stimulation	Not performed when indicated: inactive, apneic or not spontaneously breathing, or gasping, or bradycardic	Stimulation performed on other places than the back or the soles of the feet. Too aggressive (not gentle rubbing)	Well done
Preductal PO probe	Not placed in a baby who needed CPAP, PPV or oxygen	Not preductal (left hand or wrist, foot)	Preductal (right hand or wrist)
Administration of oxygen	Not used in a baby who needed it	Given free-flow oxygen; not administered with PPC or PPV; not discontinued when color or SpO_2 improved; use of initial FiO_2 other than 0.3	Well done
Administration of CPAP	Mandatory if < 28 weeks GA or ≥ 29 with a positive initial evaluation but distress	Evident mask leak; incorrect mask/cannula size	Well done
Administration of mask PPV	Not performed when needed	Initiation after the first 20 s; use of a self-inflating bag instead of an automatic or manual ventilator; incorrect mask size; incorrect rate (not 40-60 rpm); mask leak; not re-evaluated for response (HR and color) after 30 s	Well done
Intubation	Not performed when needed	Duration of each intubation attempt (time from the introduction of the laryngoscope blade to the mouth to its removal) > 30 s); incorrect size of the endotracheal tube; position of the endotracheal tube not checked (auscultation/chest wall rise/inserted to correct depth); lack of ventilation between intubation attempts, Number of intubation attempts; Unplanned extubation	Well done
Chest compressions	Not performed when needed	Incorrect method (other than 2 thumbs or 2 fingers); incorrect area (other than lower third of the sternum); incorrect depth (not one third of the anterior-posterior diameter of the chest); incorrect rate (not 90 bpm); incorrect coordination with ventilation (not 3:1); initiation without correct ventilation; Not re-evaluated for response	Well done
Epinephrine administration	Not performed when needed	Not administered after 30 s of CC if heart rate < 60 bpm; Dose and route of administration	Well done
Surfactant administration	Not performed when indicated: intubated and < 28 or ≥ 29 weeks GA and FiO_2 ≥ 0.3	Not administered at 10 min of life; Dose	Well done
Total points			

[a]Always mandatory
If PPV, CC or drugs are necessary, breathing, heart rate and color must be reassessed every 30 s.
Min Minutes, *PO* Pulse-Oximeter, *CPAP* Continuous Positive Airway Pressure, *PPV* Positive Pressure Ventilation, *GA* Gestational Age, *CC* Chest Compressions

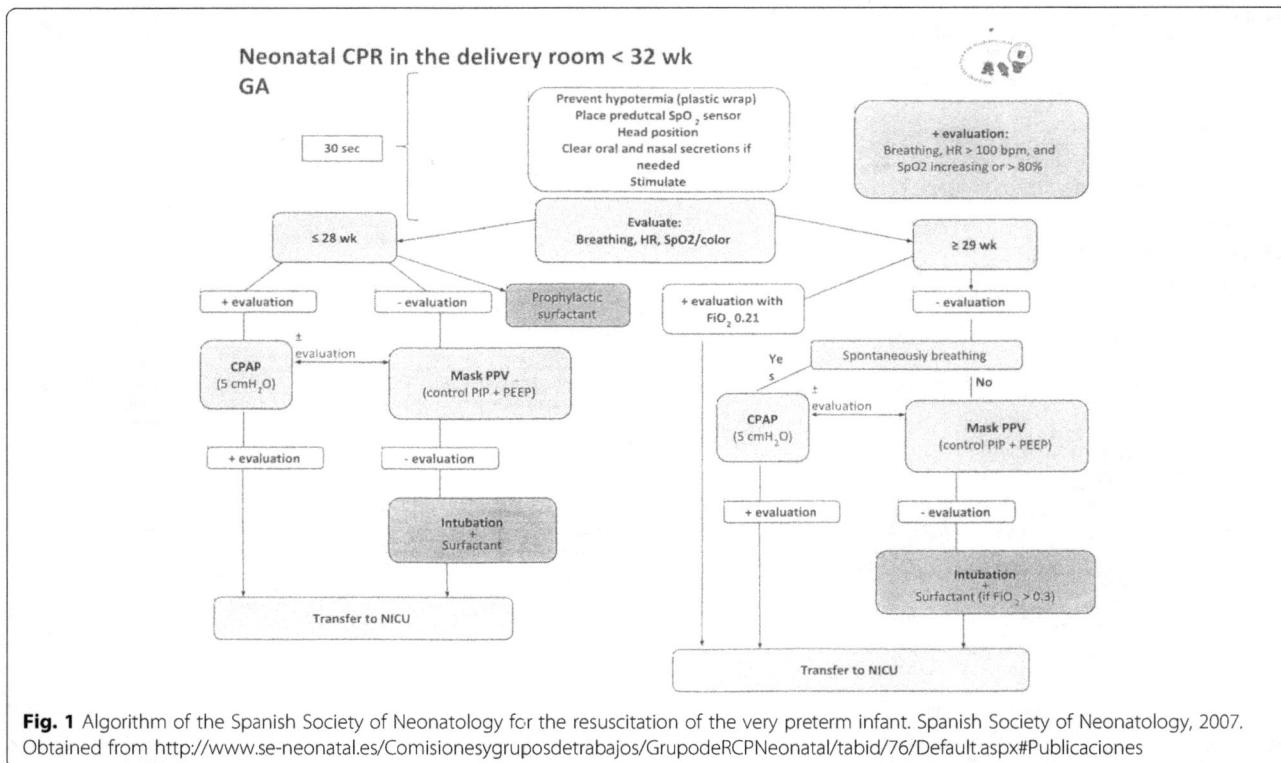

Fig. 1 Algorithm of the Spanish Society of Neonatology for the resuscitation of the very preterm infant. Spanish Society of Neonatology, 2007. Obtained from http://www.se-neonatal.es/Comisionesygruposdetrabajos/GrupodeRCPNeonatal/tabid/76/Default.aspx#Publicaciones

confirmed homogeneity of our subgroups in terms of gestational age, birth weight and resuscitation score. We used the Shapiro-Wilk test to evaluate normality in our subgroups. We compared normally distributed quantitative variables with a paired T-test between our two groups. For nonnormally distributed quantitative variables, we used the Mann-Whitney U test to compare the two groups.

We compared percentages of adherence to the algorithm for every domain with the Chi-square test for large groups and with Fisher's exact test for smaller groups (fewer than 5 cases). Linear and logarithmic regressions were drawn to characterize the pattern of adherence to the algorithm.

We compared assigned Apgar scores with those given after analyzing the recordings and described them by their median and interquartile range (IQR). We measured

interrater agreement between Apgar scores with Cohen's kappa coefficient.

Statistical analysis was performed using SPSS (SPSS for Windows, V.20, Chicago, Illinois, USA). A p-value < 0.05 was considered significant.

Results

Between April 2008 and August 2009, 162 infants < 32 weeks GA were born in our center. We analyzed 50 resuscitations (30.6%), a representative sample of the population. Groups N (staff neonatologists) and P (pediatricians on-call) were homogeneous. Tables 2 and 3 show the characteristics of our population and subgroups.

Global adherence to the algorithm was $80.9 \pm 14.2\%$, with no differences between groups N and P ($81.5 \pm 12.7\%$ in group N versus $80.7 \pm 15.0\%$ in group P, $P = 0.93$, Mann-Whitney U), and was independent of the

Table 2 Characteristics of our population and neonates < 32 weeks GA born during the study period

Characteristic	Study patients ($n = 50$)	Neonates < 32 weeks GA born during the study period ($n = 162$)	P[c]
Gestational age, SD (weeks) (range)	$29^4 \pm 2^5$ (25^5–31^6)	$29^1 \pm 2$ (24^1–31^6)	NS (0.24)[a]
Male (%)	26/50 (52%)	88/162 (54.3%)	NS (0.07)[b]
BW, SD (g) (range)	1181 ± 368 (460–2015)	1201 ± 377 (340–2475)	NS (0.75)[a]
Twins (%)	19/50 (38)	81/162 (50)	NS (0.13)[b]
BW < 1500 g (%)	42/50 (84)	131/162 (80.8)	NS (0.61)[b]
C-section (%)	33/50 (66)	94/162 (58)	NS (0.31)[b]

SD Standard Deviation, *BW* Birth Weight, *GA* Gestational Age. [a]Paired T- test, [b]Chi-square, [c]Indicates significance at the $P < 0.05$ level. NS: non-significant

Table 3 Subgroups in our study

Characteristic	Group N (staff neonatologists) (n = 18)	Group P (pediatricians oncall) (n = 32)	p[d]
GA (weeks, SD) (range)	$29^4 \pm 1^6$ (25^5–31^6)	$29^3 \pm 1^4$ (26^0–31^6)	NS (0.90)[a]
Male (%)	8/18 (44.4)	18/32 (56.2)	NS (0.61)[b]
BW (g, SD) (range)	1091 ± 418 (460–1900)	1232 ± 333 (720–2015)	NS (0.20)[a]
RS (possible points) (range)	12.66 ± 4.39 (6–20)	13.96 ± 3.71 (6–20)	NS (0.29)[c]

Group N Staff Neonatologists, *group P* Pediatricians On-call, *GA* Gestational Age, *SD* Standard Deviation, *BW* Birth Weight, *RS* Resuscitation Score. [a]Paired T-test, [b]Chi-square, [c]Mann-Whitney U test, [d]Indicates significance at the P < 0.05 level. NS: non-significant

number of interventions required. Eight resuscitations (16%) were technically correct; 15/50 (30%) failed in one domain; 12/50 (24%) in two; 5/50 (10%) in three; 6/50 (12%) in four; 2/50 (4%) in five; and 2/50 (4%) in seven. The mean (SD) resuscitation score was 13.5 (3.9) points/ resuscitation (range: 6–20). Table 4 analyzes the adherence to the algorithm by domains.

Table 5 shows results from measures to prevent heat loss and its relation to admission temperature. We found no differences between the group that received correct measures to prevent hypothermia and the group that did not. Intubation differentiated intensive (16–20 total possible points) from mild resuscitation (6–16 points). Infants who did not need intubation (*n* = 36) had a mean global adherence to the algorithm of 83%. Deviations from the algorithm in this group did not correlate with the intensity of resuscitation (R^2 = 0.0013).

Some errors we observed
Heat loss prevention
Twelve percent of patients were placed in plastic wrap after drying. When only dried, the technique was correct in 58.1% (18/31) of cases; 22.6% (7/31) did not have the towels changed, and 19.3% (6/31) had no cap. Only 22.4% of patients (11/49) were normothermic (36.5–37.5 °C); 73.5% (36/49) were hypothermic. More critically ill patients were more likely to receive worse anti-hypothermia measures because they were being subjected to other procedures: ventilation, intubation, chest compressions (CC) and surfactant administration. Sixty-eight percent of patients (13/19) in whom heat loss prevention was incorrect had a resuscitation score ≥ 14 points, which means that they received at least ventilatory support.

Clearing the airway with a suction catheter
The following errors were observed: oral without nasal suctioning, 16.7%; undue suction (over 5 s, range 31–50 s), 8.3%; use of a larger catheter than recommended, 8.3%; delayed suctioning after 20 s, 6.2%, or after ventilation, 4.2%; incorrect suctioning order (first nasal), 2.1%; and excessive introduction of the catheter, 2.1%. We observed no episodes of severe bradycardia during suctioning.

Table 4 Adherence to the algorithm

Domain	Indicated (%)	Performed (%)	Adherence to the algorithm (%) (PO/TTPx100)			
			Global	Group N	Group P	p[3]
Heat loss prevention	100 (50/50)	100 (50/50)	62 (31/50)	66.7 (12/18)	59.4 (19/32)	NS (0.84)[2]
Head in a "sniffing" position	100 (50/50)	94 (47/50)	94 (47/50)	94.4 (17/18)	93.7 (30/32)	NS (0.71)[1]
Clearing the airway	96 (48/50)	96 (48/50)	62.5 (30/48)	55.6 (10/18)	66.7 (20/30)	NS (0.59)[2]
Stimulation	64 (32/50)	30 (15/50)	93.3[4] (14/15)	80 (4/5)	100 (10/10)	NS (0.33)[1]
Placing a preductal pulse-oximeter probe	82 (41/50)	90.2 (37/41)	63.4 (26/41)	76.9 (10/13)	57.1 (16/28)	NS (1.49)[1]
Administration of oxygen	68 (34/50)	68 (34/50)	94.1 (32/34)	100 (10/10)	91.3 (21/23)	NS (0.48)[1]
CPAP	60	60	100	100	100	–
Administration of PPV	60 (30/50)	96.7 (29/30)	79.3 (23/29)	60 (6/10)	85 (17/20)	NS (0.14)[1]
Intubation	32 (16/50)	87.5 (14/16)	0 (0/16)	0 (0/5)	0 (0/11)	–
CC	4 (2/50)	2 (1/50)	0	0	0	–
Epinephrine administration	?	4 (2/50)	0	0	0	–
Surfactant administration	24 (12/50)	20 (10/50)	100[4] (10/10) 83.3 (10/12)[5]	75 (3/4)	87.5 (7/8)	NS (0.58)[1]

PO Points Obtained, *TPP* Total Possible Points, *Group N* Staff Neonatologists, *Group P* Pediatricians On-call, *CPAP* Continuous Positive Airway Pressure, *PPV* Positive Pressure Ventilation, *CC* Chest Compressions. [1]Fisher's exact test, [2]Chi-square, [3]Indicates significance at the P < 0.05 level, [4]when done, [5]when indicated. NS: non-significant

Table 5 Heat loss prevention

Group	Heat loss prevention adherence to algorithm (%) (PO/TPP)	P[c]	Admission temperature (C) (range)	P[c]
Total	62 (31/50)		36.0 ± 0.6 (34.6–37.8)	
Group N	66.7 (12/18)	NS (0.84)[a]	35.8 ± 0.7 (34.6–37.6)	NS (0.09)[b]
Group P	59.4 (19/32)		36.1 ± 0.6 (35.0–37.8)	
Correct heat loss prevention measures (n = 31)			36.1 ± 0.7 (35.0–37.8)	NS (0.60)[b]
Incorrect heat loss prevention measures (n = 19)			36.0 ± 0.6 (34.6–36.9)	

[a]Chi-square
[b]Paired T-test
[c]Indicates significance at the $P < 0.05$ level. NS non-significant, PO Points Obtained, TPP Total Possible Points, Group N Staff Neonatologists, Group P Pediatricians On-call

Stimulating breathing

One baby was stimulated when unnecessary, and 32% (16/50) who needed stimulation did not receive it, particularly those in worse condition. One baby had his face rubbed.

Administration of PPV

One patient was intubated without previous PPV. We observed the following errors: undue delay in starting PPV (at 56, 60 and 69 s) in 10.3% of cases (3/29), use of a self-inflating bag instead of a ventilator in 6.9% of patients (2/29), ventilation without previous suctioning when airway was obstructed in 6.9% (2/29), lack of ventilation between intubation attempts in 3.4% (1/29), and face mask leak in 3.4% (1/29). We did not use a respiratory function monitor, so we could not objectively document leaks; however, in one patient, the lack of a mask seal was obvious. In some patients, more than one mistake occurred.

Intubation

All intubations deviated from the algorithm. Two of 16 (12.5%) patients could not be intubated after several attempts; their indication for intubation was respiratory distress. They were transferred to the Neonatal Intensive Care Unit (NICU) with CPAP and intubated under sedation. The mean number of intubation attempts was 2.2 (range 1–6); success on the first attempt happened in 33.3% of cases; on second attempt, 38.9%; on third attempt, 16.7%; and 11.1% needed more than three attempts (5 and 6). We analyzed 40 intubation attempts. Two unplanned extubations after surfactant administration (due to incorrect securing of the tube) required reintubation. In all intubation cases, at least one attempt took longer than recommended (30 s). Mean duration to perform intubation was 58.8 ± 23.4 s (range 17–128 s). Only 5 of 40 intubations (12.5%) were achieved within 30 s.

Chest compressions and epinephrine administration

CC technique was correct, but it was initiated late. Despite correct intubation and ventilation, one newborn was bradycardic at 3:59 min, and CCs were started at 7:22 min. One patient received epinephrine without previous CCs, and another received epinephrine when CCs were started.

The median (IQR) assigned Apgar scores at 1, 5 and 10 min were 7 (5.7–9), 9 (8–10) and 10 (8–10). The median (IQR) Apgar scores after reviewing NRs were 7 (5–9), 9 (6.7–10) and 9 (7.7–10). Agreement at the three time points was acceptable (Kappa coefficient 0.35). Interrater reliability in evaluating Apgar scores was moderate at 1, 5 and 10 min (Cohen's kappa coefficients: 0.57, 0.60 and 0.44, respectively).

Our resuscitation team obtained a median of 10 points per resuscitation (red line), regardless of the resuscitation score (blue line), which means that resuscitations with a resuscitation score above 10 were poorly done (Fig. 2). Figure 3 shows that the relationship between the resuscitation score and the points obtained was nearly logarithmic ($R^2 = 0.7053$), which means that resuscitators scored very few additional points as the resuscitation intensity increased.

Discussion

All our patients were resuscitated in our dedicated room for resuscitation, which provides a setting similar to that in the NICU. Vento [4, 6] suggested that incorporating an intensive care environment into the DR could enhance survival and reduce the morbidity of extremely low birth weight (BW) infants. Among our study population, we found a high percentage of hypothermia (73.5%), which led us to make some changes in our resuscitation room to reduce hypothermia: we increased the temperature to 26 °C by keeping the doors locked and installed a heater next to the resuscitation cot. We use heated, humidified gases for ventilation.

Several authors have proven that performance often deviates from guidelines. Our study is the first report on adherence to the neonatal resuscitation algorithm for very preterm infants in a tertiary care center in Spain.

Carbine was the first to use video recording to evaluate NR [16]. We based our study on his publication and adopted his scoring system. Carbine found deviations in 54% of NRs. We evaluated more aspects and may have detected more errors (84%). We believe

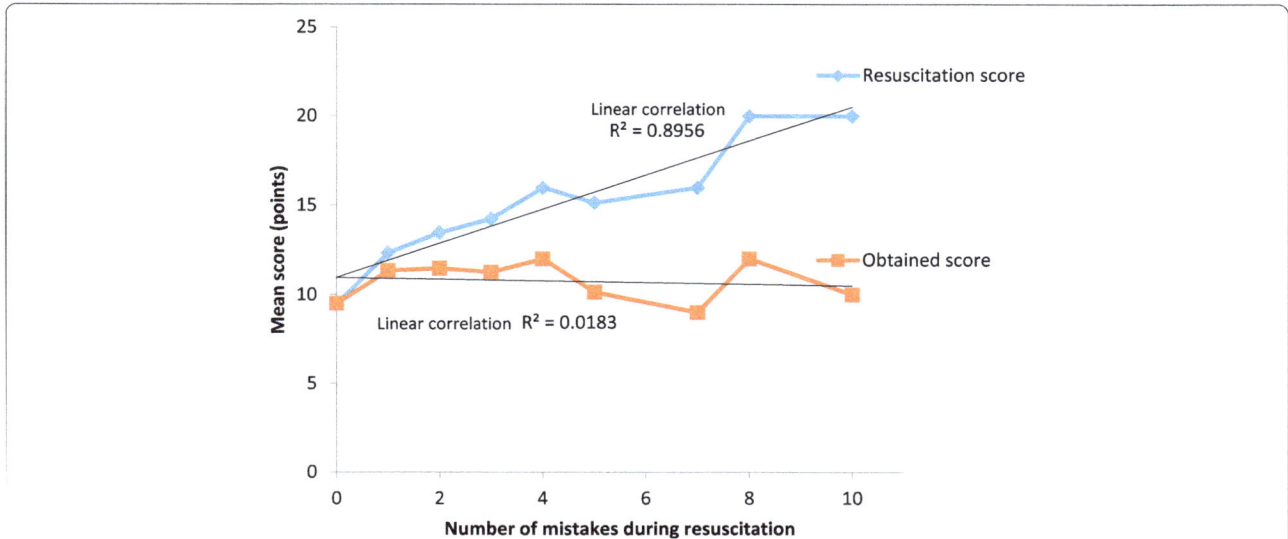

Fig. 2 Correlation between the number of errors during resuscitation and the mean obtained resuscitation score (red line) and the maximum resuscitation score (blue line). The difference between the blue and red lines was the average of virtually lost points

that our resuscitation score was higher: 22% of Carbine's patients only required stimulation (whereas 64% of ours needed stimulation); 80% required stimulation and oxygen, and only 7% needed PPV (vs our 80% respiratory support and 32% intubation). Carbine reported errors in the mask ventilation rate. We considered the use of a self-inflating bag an error, as we used an automatic ventilator. Consequently, we did not find this error. Only 28.6% of Carbine's cases involving PPV had no deviations, which is worse than our 72.7% rate of proper ventilation. Among Carbine's infants, 58.3% were intubated on the first attempt (vs our 33.3%), and only 33.3% (vs our 87.5%) were intubated within the established time limit. Like Carbine,

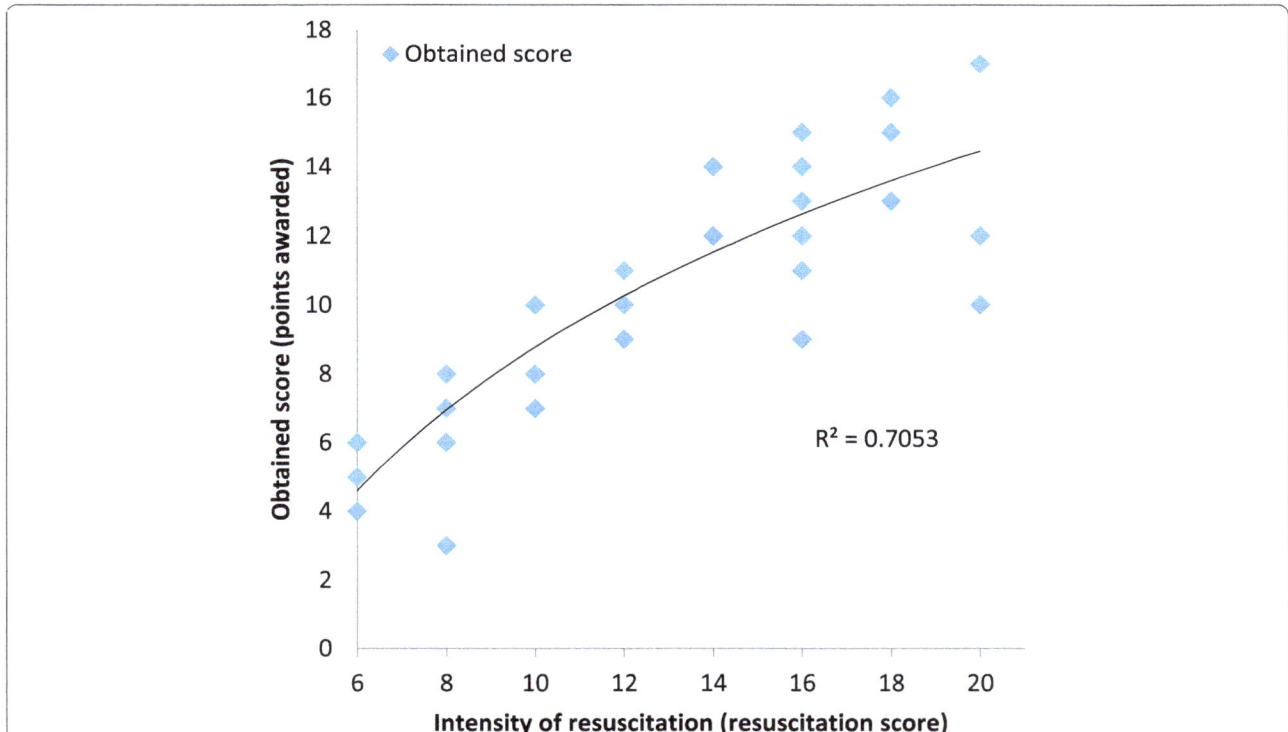

Fig. 3 Relationship between intensity of resuscitation and obtained score

we observed that perfect resuscitations were more likely for less intense interventions. None of our patients who required intubation received a perfect resuscitation.

Similar to Dekker [17], we observed that stimulation was often indicated but not performed, and when it was applied, it was most often indicated. Dekker's infants who received no stimulation required intubation more often (18 vs 7%); in our case, 62.5% of intubated infants had not been stimulated and 25% of stimulated infants did not require intubation. However, 18.7% of infants (6/32) who were stimulated were also intubated afterward.

By using video recording at a Nepalese tertiary hospital, Lindbäck [10] identified deviation from guidelines in over 50% of resuscitations. Most errors concerned the use of bag-and-mask ventilation (which we did not evaluate, as ventilating with a bag and mask was an error in our study), suction and excessive use of oxygen. Their results seem more favorable than ours. However, Lindbäck did not focus on preterm infants.

Gelbart [8] reported that the demanding technical skills scored higher than the more basic steps of resuscitation because technique is taught, whereas clinical assessment, communication skills and teamwork need practice. He found that invasive ventilation and surfactant administration were best performed, with median scores of 100%, whereas the performance of preparation and initial steps (69%) and assessment and communication of heart rate (75%) was worse. In our patients, most errors took place during the initial steps as well, whereas administration of CPAP, PPV and surfactant were performed better. Surfactant was administered in 83.3% of our cases when indicated. Technique was always correct, although two patients who required it did not receive it; the PO was not functioning, and the pediatrician preferred to administer it in the NICU with proper monitoring.

Schilleman [9] used video recording to evaluate compliance with NR guidelines in a population similar to ours, although our patients were in better conditions according to the Apgar scores. Schilleman found that deviations mainly occurred within the first 30 s because caregivers needed more time to perform the initial steps and mainly involved the way ventilation was given. As such, Schilleman suggested that 1 min be allowed for the initial evaluation, which is what the current ILCOR guidelines allow.

No intubations were perfectly performed. We analyzed 40 intubation attempts. Success occurred on the first attempt in 33.3% of cases and on the second attempt in 38.9%; more than three attempts (5 and 6) were required in only 11.1% of cases. In all intubation cases, at least one attempt took longer than recommended. Only 12.5% of intubations took place within the allotted 30 s. Other authors have reported similar deficiencies. Lane [18] reported a mean duration for successful attempts of 27.3 s; 30% infants were intubated on the first attempt, 30% on the second, 20% on the third, and 20% required more than three. Success was higher for 30 s, and no infants decompensated between 20 and 30 s; 20% of successful attempts took longer than 40 s. Finer and Rich's [3, 15] overall success rate for intubation was 33% within the allotted 20 s and 56% within 30 s. They reported an average of at least three attempts to successfully intubate infants < 1000 g. Our intubation success rate was higher than that reported by Finer and Rich. We needed, on average, 2.2 attempts to intubate infants < 1000 g (range 1–5), but unfortunately, it took longer (median (SD) 58.1 s (23.4), range 17–128 s). O'Donnell [19] analyzed intubation attempts in 31 infants (mean GA 28 weeks and BW 1227 g). Intubation attempts were often unsuccessful and successful attempts often took more than 30 s (17% were successful within 20 s, 20% between 20 and 29 s, and 25% > 30 s). Konstantelos [7] needed a median of 2 attempts, and 47 (25–60) s for intubation, and only 11% were successful within the allotted time. Wozniak [20] analyzed intubation attempts in preterm infants (795 g median BW, 25 weeks' GA) and reported a mean duration of 35 s and 2 attempts. Like Konstantelos [21], we believe that the lack of medication for intubation and surfactant administration are the reasons for the longer time needed for intubation. Because health care providers often underestimate the passage of time during NR, it is difficult to realize when the allotted time has passed. The American Academy of Pediatrics NRP used to allow 20 s for intubation, but since several studies reported that it often took longer [3, 16, 18, 19, 21] and that infants did not decompensate between 20 and 30 s, the current limit is 30 s [20].

As Fig. 2 shows, resuscitators obtained, on average, 10 points per patient regardless of the intensity of resuscitation, which means that caregivers did not score more points in more complex resuscitations. There are two reasons for the constant red line: a) some initial, common mistakes in heat loss prevention, suctioning and a postductal PO probe placement prevented most mild NRs (mean resuscitation score of 13 points) from scoring higher, and b) the points corresponding to almost all complex domains (intubation, chest compressions or epinephrine administration) were lost. The consequence is the flat line in the relationship between mistakes and the obtained score. However, the more mistakes that occur in a NR, the higher the resuscitation score (blue line, $R^2 = 0.895$), meaning that complex domains (the area above the red line) are lost in terms of obtained points. Not surprisingly, the relationship between the resuscitation score and the obtained score (Fig. 3) followed a strong logarithmic pattern ($R^2 = 0.705$). This finding means that although more points are possible, the resuscitator team would gain little benefit from those complex domains. More emphasis must be placed on the initial steps, which are common to most NRs, and especially on training for complex skills such as intubation.

This study has some limitations. Its purpose was to evaluate adherence to NR guidelines. For this reason, all mistakes counted equally, although it is obvious that not all the deviations are equally serious: some are mild and nontranscendental (for example, duration of oral suctioning) whereas others are potentially harmful (like timing and route of epinephrine administration). The same mistake could have consequences or not, depending on the patient. For example, placing a postductal PO probe in a patient who does not receive oxygen or ventilatory support has no impact on the maneuvers performed but may lead to hyperoxia in an intubated neonate. Only 16% of our resuscitations perfectly followed the algorithm, but the number of mistakes per resuscitation was low, and global adherence to the algorithm was 80.9%. We acknowledge that the value of global adherence in itself has little meaning without the proper analysis of the main and more critical errors. Another limitation of our study is the lack of feedback of our findings to the resuscitation team. We designed the study to assess adherence to the algorithm and find the most common errors. In the pilot study, we did not consider an active intervention with the resuscitation team. Sharing our findings with them would probably improve performance. In most cases, the resuscitation team consisted of two neonatologists or two pediatricians on-call. All of them are trained in neonatal resuscitation, although their expertise varies from more than 30 years to only a few months after completing a residency. However, 38% of our patients were twins, which may worsen performance, as in some cases, there was only one caregiver per patient [22]. All our medical staff was aware of this study when it started, and we periodically reminded them about it. All the neonatologists and pediatricians who work at our hospital participated in this study. The medical staff turned the video camera on, automatically consenting to be recorded, when they were called to the DR. Recording usually began minutes before the neonate was born but sometimes began when the newborn arrived at the resuscitation room.

Similar to many other previous studies, our study demonstrated that deviations from the algorithm exist. Many of the errors have to do with timing: some maneuvers take longer than allotted, and personnel are not aware of this [23].

We compared performance of staff neonatologists with pediatricians on-call. We thought that the neonatologists would perform better since they work with only newborns and are subspecialized in neonatology, whereas after-hour on-call pediatricians who cover this shift often do not work with only newborns. We observed no differences between these two groups, which means that we have a good team of pediatricians who perform as well as neonatologists. This is a positive aspect to consider. Although global adherence to the algorithm was high, mistakes were common despite our staff's training.

In line with other authors [8, 22–25], we found a discrepancy in Apgar scores, particularly when the Apgar was not 9/10/10, and the staff attending the delivery commonly overestimated the score. It is easy to score 9/10/10 if no resuscitation is necessary, whereas it is difficult to remember the patient's situation at 5 and 10 min when resuscitation is required. Video recording scores tended to be lower than scores given by neonatologists (47.1% at 1 min, 73.3% at 5, 88.9% at 10). Gelbart [8] also found overestimation of Apgar scores by a median value of 2 points at 1 and 5 min. As other authors suggest, we believe that memories of a stressful past event can be inaccurate, and Apgar scores are usually calculated afterward [24].

Finally, we are aware that our study sample was small. We aimed to analyze 50 resuscitations due to the difficulty in obtaining written consent before resuscitation started. Nonetheless, we managed to record one-third of our potential cases, which is a significant sample. The ILCOR guidelines have changed twice since we conducted this study, and some actions that we considered mistakes would now be correct, for example, supporting transition rather than keeping timing strict or not suctioning routinely. While it is true that our data are old, and a few aspects are outdated, our aim was to assess our performance in terms of adherence to the algorithm, that is, if our physicians performed according to the written rules, not the appropriateness of the algorithm. Our results would probably be similar today. Even though only one person reviewed the recordings, the camera was in a good position, and the scoring system was clear, so this bias is likely minimal. There was no feedback given to the resuscitation team during the study period, but our findings could serve as both a starting point for further studies and a teaching tool. As far as we know, there are no similar studies published in Spain to date.

Conclusions

Resuscitation of very preterm newborns often deviates from guidelines. Perfectly performed resuscitations are infrequent, although global adherence to the algorithm is high. Resuscitations led by pediatricians on-call and neonatologists are performed equally correct. Intubation training may improve complex resuscitations the most.

Abbreviations

bpm: Beats Per Minute; BW: Birth Weight; C: Celsius; CC: Chest Compressions; CPAP: Continuous Positive Airway Pressure; DR: Delivery Room; GA: Gestational Age; ILCOR: International Liaison Committee on Resuscitation; min: Minute; NICU: Neonatal Intensive Care Unit; NR: Neonatal Resuscitation; NRP: Neonatal Resuscitation Program; PO: Pulse-Oximeter; PPV: Positive Pressure Ventilation; s: Second; SD: Standard Deviation; Temp: Temperature

Acknowledgements

We would like to thank the medical and nursing NICU staff for participating and taking ownership during the realization of this project. We thank all the neonatologists and pediatricians on-call for supporting this study.

Authors' contributions

SM conceptualized and designed the study, carried out the initial analyses, drafted the initial manuscript and approved the final manuscript as submitted. FB helped to conceptualize and design the study, reviewed and revised the manuscript, and approved the final manuscript as submitted. JF helped to design the study, helped to carry out the statistical analyses, reviewed and revised the manuscript, and approved the final manuscript as submitted. MI-R helped to carry out the initial analyses, reviewed and revised the manuscript, and approved the final manuscript as submitted. MT helped to conceptualize and design the study, helped to develop the neonatal resuscitation algorithm for very preterm infants (2007), reviewed and revised the manuscript, and approved the final manuscript as submitted. MI-S helped to conceptualize and design the study, helped to develop the neonatal resuscitation algorithm for very preterm infants (2007), reviewed and revised the manuscript, and approved the final manuscript as submitted.

Competing interests

The authors have no financial relationships relevant to this article to disclose.' I declare that I have no competing interests.

Author details

[1]Neonatology Service, Hospital Clínic, seu Maternitat, ICGON (Institut Clínic de Ginecologia, Obstetrícia i Neonatologia), Barcelona University, Sabino de Arana, 1, 08028 Barcelona, Spain. [2]Neonatology Service, Hospital Sant Joan de Déu, BCNatal (Centre de Medicina Maternofetal i Neonatal de Barcelona, Hospital Sant Joan de Déu, Hospital Clínic), Barcelona University, Passeig de Sant Joan de Déu, 2, 08950 Esplugues de Llobregat, Barcelona, Spain.

References

1. Perlman JM, Wyllie J, Kattwinkel J, Wyckoff MH, Aziz K, Guinsburg R, et al. Part 7: Neonatal Resuscitation: 2015 International Consensus on Cardiopulmonary Resuscitation and Emergency Cardiovascular Care Science With Treatment Recommendations. Pediatrics. 2015. https://doi.org/10.1542/peds.2015-3373D.
2. https://data.unicef.org/topic/child-survival/neonatal-mortality/ (accessed 2017 July 25).
3. Finer N, Rich W. Neonatal resuscitation for the preterm infant: evidence versus practice. J Perinatol. 2010. https://doi.org/10.1038/jp.2010.115.
4. Vento M, Cheung PY, Aguar M. The first golden minutes of the extremely-low-gestational-age neonate: a gentle approach. Neonatology. 2009. https://doi.org/10.1159/000178770.
5. Izquierdo-Renau M, Gómez-Robles C, Pino-Vázquez A. Lección 12. El recién nacido muy prematuro (<32 semanas). In: Sociedad Española de Neonatología. Manual de Reanimación Neonatal. 4th edition. Editorial Ergon. Madrid 2017. Pages 167-180. ISBN: 9788416732494. Spanish.
6. Vento M, Aguar M, Leone TA, Finer NN, Gimeno A, Rich W, et al. Using intensive care technology in the delivery room: a new concept for the resuscitation of extremely preterm neonates. Pediatrics. 2008. https://doi.org/10.1542/peds.2008-1422.
7. Konstantelos D, Ifflaender S, Dinger J, Rüdiger M. Suctioning habits in the delivery room and the influence on postnatal adaptation - a video analysis. J Perinat Med. 2015. https://doi.org/10.1515/jpm-2014-0188.
8. Gelbart B, Hiscock R, Barfield C. Assessment of neonatal resuscitation performance using video recording in a perinatal centre. J Paediatr Child Health. 2010. https://doi.org/10.1111/j.1440-1754.2010.01747.x.
9. Schilleman K, Siew ML, Lopriore E, Morley CJ, Walther FJ, Te Pas AB. Auditing resuscitation of preterm infants at birth by recording video and physiological parameters. Resuscitation. 2012. https://doi.org/10.1016/j.resuscitation.2012.01.036.
10. Lindbäck C, KC A, Wrammert J, Vitrakoti R, Ewald U, Målqvist M. Poor adherence to neonatal resuscitation guidelines exposed; an observational study using camera surveillance at a tertiary hospital in Nepal. BMC Pediatr. 2014. https://doi.org/10.1186/1471-2431-14-233.
11. Finer NN, Rich W. Neonatal resuscitation: toward improved performance. Resuscitation. 2002;53(1):47–51.
12. Murphy MC, O'Donnell CPF, McCarthy LK. Attittudes of staff members towards video recording in the delivery room. Arch Dis Child Fetal Neonatal Ed. 2018. https://doi.org/10.1136/archdischild-2017-313789.
13. den Boer MC, Houtlosser M, van Zanten HA, Foglia EE, Engberts DP, Te Pas AB. Ethical dilemmas of recording and reviewing neonatal resuscitation. Arch Dis Child Fetal Neonatal Ed. 2018. https://doi.org/10.1136/archdischild-2017-314191.
14. Van Vonderen JJ, van Zanten HA, Schilleman K, Hooper SB, Kitchen MJ, Witlox RS, et al. Cardiorespiratory Monitoring during Neonatal Resuscitation for Direct Feedback and Audit. Front Pediatr. 2016. https://doi.org/10.3389/fped.2016.00038.
15. Rich WD, Leone T, Finer NN. Delivery room intervention: improving the outcome. Clin Perinatol. 2010. https://doi.org/10.1016/j.clp.2010.01.011.
16. Carbine DN, Finer NN, Knodel E, Rich W. Video recording as a means of evaluating neonatal resuscitation performance. Pediatrics. 2000;106:654–8.
17. Dekker J, Martherus T, Cramer SJE, van Zanten HA, Hooper SB, Te Pas AB. Tactile stimulation to stimulate spontaneous breathing during stabilization of preterm infants at birth: a retrospective analysis. Front Pediatr. 2017;5:61. https://doi.org/10.3389/fped.2017.00061.
18. Lane B, Finer N, Rich W. Duration of intubation attempts during neonatal resuscitation. J Pediatr. 2004. https://doi.org/10.1016/j.jpeds.2004.03.003.
19. O'Donnell CP, Kamlin CO, Davis PG, Morley CJ. Endotracheal intubation attempts during neonatal resuscitation: success rates, duration, and adverse effects. Pediatrics. 2006. https://doi.org/10.1542/peds.2005-0901.
20. Wozniak M, Arnell K, Brown M, Gonzales S, Lazarus D, Rich W, et al. The 30 second rule: the effects of prolonged intubation attempts on oxygen saturation and heart rate in preterm infants in the delivery room. Minerva Pediatr. 2018. https://doi.org/10.23736/S0026-4946.16.04469-8.
21. Konstantelos D, Dinger J, Ifflaender S, Rüdiger M. Analyzing video recorded support of postnatal transition in preterm infants following a c-section. BMC Pregnancy Childbirth. 2016. https://doi.org/10.1186/s12884-016-1045-2.
22. Layouni I, Danan C, Durrmeyer X, Dassieu G, Azcona B, Decobert F. Video recording of newborn resuscitation in the delivery room: technique and advantages. Arch Pediatr 2011; doi: https://doi.org/10.1016/S0929-693X(11)71094-6. French.
23. Trevisanuto D, De Bernardo G, Res G, Sordino D, Doglioni N, Winer G, et al. Time Perception during Neonatal Resuscitation. J Pediatr. 2016. https://doi.org/10.1016/j.jpeds.2016.07.003.
24. McCarthy LK, Morley CJ, Davis PG, Kamlin CO, O'Donnell CP. Timing of interventions in the delivery room: does reality compare with neonatal resuscitation guidelines? J Pediatr. 2013. https://doi.org/10.1016/j.jpeds.2013.06.007.
25. Schilleman K, Witlox RS, van Vonderen JJ, Roegholt E, Walther FJ, te Pas AB. Auditing documentation on delivery room management using video and physiological recordings. Arch Dis Child Fetal Neonatal Ed. 2014. https://doi.org/10.1136/archdischild-2014-306261.

20

Medication administration error and contributing factors among pediatric inpatient in public hospitals of Tigray, northern Ethiopia

Zeray Baraki[1], Mebrahtu Abay[2]*[iD], Lidiya Tsegay[1], Hadgu Gerensea[1], Awoke Kebede[1] and Hafte Teklay[3]

Abstract

Background: Medication administration error is a medication error that occurs while administering a medication to a patient. A variety of factors make pediatrics more susceptible to medication errors and its consequences. In low-income countries, like Ethiopia, there is no sufficient evidence regarding medication administration error among pediatrics. The aim of this study is, therefore, to determine the magnitude and factors associated with medication administration error among pediatric population.

Methods: A prospective observational based cross sectional study design was conducted from January to April 2017. Data collection was done using pre-tested structured questionnaire and blind observation checklist to health professionals in charge of administering selected medications. A total of 1282 medication administrations were obtained using single population proportion formula from patients in the selected public hospitals and the samples were selected using multistage sampling technique. Multivariable logistic regression using odds ratio and 95% confidence interval was used to determine the relationship between the independent and dependent variables. Variables with p-value < 0.05 were considered as independent factors for medication administration error.

Result: A total of 1251 medication administrations were observed from 1251 patients. The occurrence of medication administration error was 62.7% with 95% CI (59.6%, 65.0%), wrong dose being the most common type of medication administration error with an occurrence rate of 53.7%. Medications administered for pediatric patients less than 1 month age, administered by bachelor degree holder health professionals, prepared in facilities without medication preparation room, prepared in facilities without medication administration guide and administer for patients who have two or more prescribed medications were more likely to have medication administration error than their counterparts with AOR (95% CI) of 7.54(2.20–25.86), 1.52 (1.07–2.17), 13.45 (8.59–21.06), 4.11 (2.89–5.85), and 2.42 (1.62–3.61), respectively.

Conclusion: This study has revealed that there is high occurrence of medication administration error among pediatric inpatients in public hospitals of Tigray, Northern Ethiopia.. Age of patients, educational level of medication administrators, availability of the medication preparation room and guide, and the number of medications given per single patient were statistically significant factors associated with occurrence of medication administration error.

Keywords: Medication administration error, Pediatrics, Inpatient, Tigray, Ethiopia

* Correspondence: gmebrahtuabay@gmail.com
[2]Department of Epidemiology and Biostatistics, School of Public Health, College of Health Sciences, Aksum University, P. O. Box: 298, Aksum, Ethiopia
Full list of author information is available at the end of the article

Background

Medication administration has been defined by the Nursing Interventions Classification (NIC) as "preparing, giving and evaluating effectiveness of prescribed and non-prescribed medications; whereas a medication administration error is a medication error that occurs while administering a medication to a patient" [1]. The National Coordinating Council for Medication Error Reporting and Prevention (NCC MERP) states that "A medication error is any preventable event that may cause or lead to inappropriate medication use or patient harm while the medication is in the control of the health care professional, patient, or consumer" [2]. Despite the existence of increased levels of awareness and developments in technology designed to reduce such errors, high rate of medication error continue over the past decade [3].

The major consequences of medication administration errors (MAE) are patient morbidity and mortality. It can, indirectly, also affect patients, families and health care providers by cost implications, prolonged hospital stays and psychological impact since errors erode public confidence to health care services. Medication administration errors are potentially more harmful and have a higher incidence rate in the pediatric population than in the adult population. The rate of MAE with potential for injury within pediatric health care was 1.1%, which is three times higher than in a separate corresponding hospital study on adults, which revealed only 0.35% [4]. One of the factors that make the pediatric population more susceptible to medication errors include availability of different dosage forms of the same medication, which can lead to dosing errors. Unlike adults, most medication dosing of pediatric patients are based upon body weight, which requires a dosage calculation and hence can expose to an error [5]. Furthermore, children, in comparison to adults, are often unable to adequately communicate when they are experiencing an adverse effect and have a limited internal physiological capacity to buffer medication errors [5].

The prevalence of MAE is still high even in developed countries like United States of America (USA). Its prevalence among hospitalized pediatric patients in USA was 67% in 2004; 42,000 pediatric inpatients experience a preventable administration error, 21% of which are caused by MAE [6, 7]. In the UK, in 2012, among acutely admitted patients to hospital 178 of 6821 children had an adverse drug reaction because of MAE [8]. Similarly, in the Latin American country Argentina, for a total of 1174 observed medication administrations in neonatal and pediatric intensive care units wards, 99 had MAE [9]. In India, 313(68.5%) out of 457 medications administered had MAE [10]. In Nigeria, between July 2006 and December 2007, there have been 40 suspected adverse drug reactions (ADRs) out of 53 administered medications [11]. In Ethiopia, in 1020, from a total of 52 patients who had a total of 218 medication administrations, 196(89.9%) MAEs were occurred [12].

Although MAEs of all sorts are investigated throughout the developed world, the issue has only lightly been explored in the low-income countries like Ethiopia. There is dearth of in-depth information regarding a problem and contributing factors of MAE, particularly in a hospitalized pediatric population of Ethiopian health institutions. Hence, this study was intended to assess occurrence of MAE and associated factors among pediatric patients who admitted in selected public hospitals of Tigray, Ethiopia.

Methods

Study design and setting

In Central, Northwest and West zones of Tigray region, Ethiopia, there are 19 hospitals, six of which are public general hospitals. A prospective observation-based cross sectional study was carried out in these six public general hospitals of from September 2016 to August 2017.. Each of the public general hospitals serves for about 1–1.5 million population [13].

Study population and sampling

The source populations are all hospitalized pediatric patients who were admitted in the pediatric ward, pediatric ICU and neonatal ICU of public general hospitals found in the selected Zones of Tigray region, northern Ethiopia. The study populations are all sampled hospitalized pediatric patients who were admitted in the pediatric ward, pediatric ICU and neonatal ICU of the public general hospitals.

The sample size was determined based on a single population proportion (p) formula n = [(z∞/2)2 p(1-p)]/ d^2, with the assumptions of 95% of confidence level, 5%α, 2% margin of error and 89.9% occurrence of MAE, from a study conducted in Jima University specialized hospital, Jima, Ethiopia [12]. By using a design effect of 1.4 and 5% non-response rate, a total sample size of 1282 medication administrations was obtained. Using the multistage sampling technique, out of the seven zones in the region, three zones were selected by the simple random sampling method and then six hospitals were proportionally selected from the three zones. Allocation of the sample among the six hospitals was done proportional to the number of expected admissions of pediatric patients in each hospital. Finally, sampling frames of medication administration were then prepared from the pediatric and neonatal units of each hospitals and simple random sampling method was used to draw one sample administered medication for each patient.

Data collection tool and quality assurance mechanisms

Data were collected through an observational checklist from the health professionals in charge of administering medications to observe the procedure of administration and interviewee- administered-structured-questionnaire was used to assess the socio-demographic and experience related factors of health professionals as well as socio-demographic factors of patients. The tool contains four components, part I (socio-demographic variables), part II (medication related variables), part III (facility and equipment related variables) and part IV (medication administration related variables). The questionnaire contains open and closed ended questions, which was adopted contextually from the WHO standard (right) of medication administration and NCC MERP recommendation for safe medication administration [14–16]. The data was collected by six midwives and twelve nurses, who were following their MSc during the data collection period, under supervision of six MSc holder nurses,. The data collection period ranged from January 10, 2017 to April 10, 2017 (Additional file 1).

To assure data quality, training was given for the data collectors by the principal investigator for three consecutive days. The data collection tool was pre-tested on 100 medication administrations and all corrections and amendment were considered 2 weeks prior to the actual data collection period in three primary hospitals.. Health professionals who were going to be observed while administering medications to each patient were informed about the work prior to the commencement of data collection, but the entire purpose of the study was not disclosed in order to ensure that the findings are unbiased. Six supervisors, on a daily bases, reviewed and checked the collected data for completeness, clearness and consistency and if there were any incorrectly filled and missed data. In cases of such findings they were sending back for immediate correction.

Variables in the study

The outcome variable, medication administration status, is a binary outcome categorized as with MAE and without MAE. The independent variables include: patient related factors (age, sex, weight, reason for admission and type of medication received by the patient), administrator related factors (educational level, work experience, patient-administrator ratio, whether proper administration and documentation was done or not, mediation related factors (type, dose and route of administration), and facility and infrastructure related factors (access of equipment, proper environment, institutional guide, drug information and patient information for medication administration).

Operational definitions

Omitted drug error: when there is failure to administer a prescribed medication

Unauthorized drug error: when the prescriber did not authorize the medication administered

Dose error: when the medication dose, strength or quantity given is different from that of prescribed

Patient error: when a medication of one patient is wrongly given to another patient

Route error: when a medication is given on a wrong route of administration

Time error: when there is greater than one-hour difference between the ordered time and the time the medication is administered

Medication administration error (MAE): when there is an occurrence of a single or combination of the above listed errors while administering a medication to a patient [17, 18].

Data management and analysis procedures

After checking the data for its completeness, missing values, and coding of questionnaires, data were entered in to computer and data processing and analysis were done using SPSS version 21 software. Multiple administration errors in a single medication administration were counted as one MAE. Medication administration status was determined for each observed administrations. Data were summarized and described using frequency with percentage for categorical variables and mean with standard deviation for continuous variables. Bivariable and multi-variable logistic regression models with 95% confidence intervals were used to determine the relationship between the independent variables and the dependent variable. Independent variables with p-value < 0.3 in the bivariable logistic regression were included into the multi-variable logistic regression model and variables with P-value < 0.05 in the final model were considered as independent determinants of MAE. Model fitness was checked by Hosmer Lemeshow test statistics. Data were also presented using tables and graphs.

Results

Distribution of medication administration across socio-demographic characteristics

A total of 1251 medication administration was observed from 1251 pediatrics patients with a 97.58% response rate. Observations were made among the patients range between the age of 1 day and 14 years with a mean age of 25.32 months and a standard deviation of 45.36 months. The mean weight of the patients was 8.02 Kilograms with a standard deviation of 8.75 Kilograms. The mean experience level of health professionals in charges of medication administrations was 13.89 months with a standard deviation of 10.84 months. The health professionals in charge of medication administration were taking care of up to 25 patients per day with a mean of 8.73 patients and standard deviation of 7.69 patients per day. About three-fourth (75.6%) of the medications were administered by health professionals who have a Bachelor degree (Table 1).

Distribution of medication administrations across different factors

All administered medications were running with availability of medication card index and without an amount

Table 1 Medication administration distribution across socio-demographic characteristic of pediatric inpatients (n = 1251)

Characteristic		Number	Percent
Age of patient in completed months	≤ 1	664	53.1
(mean = 2.32 months, SD = 45.36 months)	2–12	199	15.9
	13–60	195	15.6
	> 60	193	15.4
Weight of the patient in complete kilograms	≤ 10	992	79.3
(mean = 8.02 kg and SD = 8.75 kg)	11–20	102	8.2
	> 20	157	12.5
Work experience of health professionals	≤ 12 months	850	67.9
(mean = 13.90 months and SD = 10.84 months)	13–24 months	207	16.6
	> 24 months	194	15.5
Educational level of medication administrator	Student	9	0.7
	Diploma	296	23.7
	Bachelor degree	946	75.6
Patient to medication administrator ratio	≤ 4	295	23.6
	5–10	744	59.5
	> 10	212	16.9

perfuse fixer set. About one third (34.8%) of medication administrations were done in a place where medication preparation room is available. Nearly two-third (64%) of medications was prepared in a place where a computer or medication calculator is available to determine its dose. Six hundred forty seven (51.7%) medications were prepared in a ward, which had no medication administration guide, and 160 (12%) medications were prepared in a ward, which had no documentation system or medication sheet. Almost all (98%) and (93.7%) of the medications observed were administered through intravenous (IV) route and had prepared in the medication room with available standard weight measurement, respectively. Seven hundred eighty-seven (62.9%) medications were observed for patients who had taken two different medications and 769 (61.5%) medications were administered two times (BID) per day (Table 2).

Occurrence and types of medication administration errors

The occurrence of MAE from the total 1251 observed medications administration was 62.7% with a 95% CI (59.6%, 65.0%). The types of MAEs in decreasing their prevalence are administering of wrong dose, administering in the wrong time, medication omission, administering a wrong patient, administering via a wrong route,

administering un-prescribed medication and administering a wrong drug, which accounts for 665(85.4%), 429 (55.1%), 18(2.3%), 5(0.6%), 4 (0.5%), 2 (0.3%) and 1(0.1%), respectively (Table 3).

The five commonest drugs, which contributed for the MAEs, are ampicillin, ceftriaxone, gentamicin, cloxacilline and metronidazole, with a magnitude of 263(33.76%), 190 (24.39%), 166 (21.31%), 73 (9.37%) and 34 (4.36%), respectively (see Fig. 1).

Factors associated with medication administration error

From the socio-demographic variables, age of the patients and educational level of health professionals in charge of administering medications were found as significant independent factors associated with MAE.

Medications administered to neonatal patients aged < 1 month, 1–12 months and 13–60 months were about 7.5, 10.8 and 5.7 times more likely to have MAE than patients aged more than 60 months, with AOR(95% CI) of *7.54 (2.20–25.86), 10.84(3.15–37.31)* and *5.69(1.83–17.70), respectively.* Bachelor degree holder medication administrator health professionals were about 1.5 times higher risk of conducting MAE than diploma holder health professionals with AOR (95% CI) of *1.52(1.07–2.17).*

Regarding the health facility and drug related variables, availability of medication preparation room, the number of drug prescriptions per patient and availability of medication administration guide were found to be significant independent factors associated with MAE. Medications prepared without the availability of the medication preparation room were about 13.5 times at higher risk of MAE as compared to medications prepared in rooms available for medication preparation with AOR(95% CI) of 13.45 (8.59–21.06). Medications prepared in a place where there is no availability of medication administration guide were about 4 times more likely to have MAE than their counterparts, with AOR(95% CI) of *4.11* (2.89–5.85). Medications which administered among patients who had two prescribed medication types and those who had three or more prescribed medication types were about 2.5 and 1.9 times more likely to have MAE than patients who had single prescribed drug with AOR(95% CI) of 2.46(1.62–3.61) and 1.86(1.14–3.03), respectively. The less experience of health professionals was a factor found to be prevented for MAE. Health professionals in charge of medication administration who have been working in the pediatrics unit for less than 12 months were 63% less likely to commit medication administration error than those experienced above 24 months with AOR (95% CI) of 0.37(0.21–0.65) (Table 4).

Table 2 Medication administration distribution across different factors among pediatric inpatients ($n = 1251$)

Characteristic		Number	Percent
Availability of medication preparation room	Yes	435	34.8
	No	816	65.2
Availability of leveled medication shelf	Yes	856	68.4
	No	395	31.6
Availability of computer or calculator	Yes	801	64
	No	450	36
Availability of medication administration guide	Yes	604	48.3
	No	647	51.7
Availability of standard weight measurement	Yes	1172	93.7
	No	79	6.3
Availability of documentation system	Yes	1091	87.2
	No	160	12.8
Number of medication per a single patient	1	248	19.8
	2	787	62.9
	3 and above	207	16.6
	4 medication	9	0.7
Medication frequency to be administer	When needed (PRN)	6	0.5
	Daily (QD)	226	18.0
	Twice a day (BID)	769	61.5
	Three times a day (TID)	71	5.7
	Four times a day (QID)	163	13
	Every 4 h	16	1.3
Medication administration route	Intravenous (IV)	1226	98.0
	Intramuscular (IM)	8	0.6
	Oral (PO)	17	1.4

Discussion

The study determined the occurrence of medication administration error occurred in all public general hospitals of Tigray, Ethiopia. From the total of 1251 medication administrations, 779 (62.7%, 95% CI: (59.6–65.0%) MAEs was observed. The occurrence of MAE in this study is *consistent* with another study conducted in Nigeria teaching hospital [19], with an incidence or prevalence of 59%. However, the occurrence of MAE in this study is *higher than* that of a study done in France [10, 20], which showed an occurrence rate of *27%*. Similarly, the most common type of medication administration error of both studies was wrong dose. The occurrence of MAE in study is *lower than* the occurrence of MAE found from a study conducted at the Jimma University specialized hospital, Ethiopia, 2010 [12] and another study done in a teaching hospital of India [10, 20] with a rate of 89.9% and 68.5%, respectively. This discrepancy may be because of the difference in

educational level, experience level and training of the health professionals and the more developed and equipped facilities and guidelines in the teaching hospital than the general hospitals.

The commonest type of medication responsible for MAE was ampicillin with an error prevalence of 33.8%. This finding is supported by other studies conducted in Jimma University specialized hospital, Ethiopia [12, 21] and in teaching hospital of UK [12, 21] with an occurrence rate of 24.7% and 44%, respectively. This might be related to the frequent administration of ampicillin drug for many diseases than the other drugs. This means that a drug with the highest probability of administration has at the same time high chance of occurrence of MAE.

Adjusting for all other factors, medications administered among pediatric patients less than one-month age, between 1 month and 1 year of age and between 1 year and 5 years of age had higher-risk occurrence of MAE than above 5 years of age. This finding is concordant with the study done in

Table 3 Occurrence and types of MAE among pediatric inpatients ($n = 1251$)

Characteristic		Number	Percent
Medication administration status	Right medication administration	472	37.3; 95% CI (35.0, 40.0)
	Medication administration error	779	62.7; 95% CI (59.6, 65.0)
Omission of medication ordered	No	1233	98.6
	Yes	18	1.4
Patient drug mismatch	Drug gave to the right patient	1246	99.6
	Drug gave to the wrong patient	5	0.4
Medication type	Right drug	1238	99.9
	Wrong drug	1	0.1
Dose appropriateness	Right does	574	46.3
	Wrong dose	665	53.7
Route of administration	Right route	1235	99.7
	Wrong route	4	0.3
Time appropriateness	Right time	810	65.4
	Wrong time	429	34.6
Prescription status	Prescribed drug	1249	99.8
	Un-prescribed drug	2	0.2

Argentina which showed that infants less than 1 year were 2.61 times more likely to have MAE than above 1 year children [9]. This may point towards the availability of a variety of dosage forms of medications for younger children (infants and neonates) than older children. This might make professionals to be prone to make an error in calculation of dose.

Medications administered by professionals with an educational level of BSc. degree, were 1.52 times more likely to have a risk of MAE than medication administered by diploma holder professionals. This finding is congruent with another study done in a referral hospital of the University of Gondar, Ethiopia, 2016 which shows that medications administered by nurses with the educational level of BSc. degree were 2.51 times more likely to commit MAEs than diploma holders [22]. This important finding of both studies in the country may indicate that the education policy for diploma level is more focused on skill as compared to the degree level, which could more emphasize on theoretical part. The same reason could contribute to the factor in this finding which found that professionals who have longer duration of experience have had committed more MAEs; this could be because freshly employed professionals may have little negligence in preparing and administering medications than senior professionals. A study from Nigerian hospital also concluded that workload was one of the factors that affect the occurrence of MAE [19].

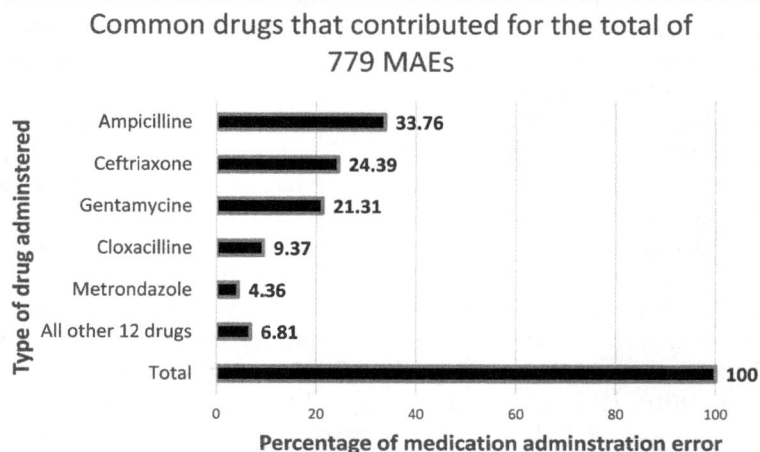

Fig. 1 Percentage of types of drugs contributed for the different types of MAEs

Table 4 Factors associated with MAE among pediatric inpatients

Variable		MAE		COR (95% CI)	AOR (95% CI)
		Yes	No		
Age of patient in months	> 60	65	128	1	1
	13–60	107	88	2.394 (1.588–3.610)	5.69 (1.83–17.70)*
	1–12	155	44	6.937 (4.430–10.864)	10.84 (3.15–37.31)**
	< 1	452	212	4.199 (2.988–5.900)	7.54 (2.20–25.86)**
Educational level of medication administrators	Diploma	155	155	1	1
	Degree	624	322	1.875 (1.444–2.436)	1.52 (1.07–2.17)*
Experience of medication administrators	> 24 months	177	17	1	1
	13–24 months	117	90	0.125 (0.71–0.220)	0.78 (0.41–1.51)
	≤ 12 months	485	365	0.128 (0.76–0.214)	0.37 (0.21–0.65)**
Availability of medication preparation room	Yes	146	289	1	1
	No	633	183	6.847 (5.289–8.864)	13.45 (8.59–21.06)**
Availability of leveled medication shelf	Yes	502	354	1	1
	No	277	118	1.655 (1.283–2.136)	0.89 (0.11–1.31)
Availability of medication administration guide	Yes	286	318	1	1
	No	493	154	3.559 (2.796–4.531)	4.11 (2.88–5.85)**
Number of medication per a single patient	One	126	122	1	1
	Two	523	264	1.918 (1.436–2.562)	2.46 (1.62–3.61)**
	Three and above	130	86	1.464 (1.012–2.117)	1.86 (1.14–3.03)*

COR crude odds ratio, *AOR* adjusted odds ratio, *CI* confidence interval*significant at *p*-value 0.05, **significant at *p*-value 0.01

In this study, the higher number of medications given for a single patient had the higher MAE. Patients received two and more than two medications at the same time, are about 2.5 and 2 times more likely to have MAE than patients who receive single medication, respectively. This could be because patients received more than one drug at a time might be prone to confuse professionals in administering the appropriate dosage and time of medication as per the prescription.

Regarding the health facility related factors, lack of availability of medication preparation room and lack of availability of medication administration guide line were found to be significant predictors of MAE. Lack of availability of the medication preparation room/s and lack of availability of medication administration guide/s were about 13 and 4 times more likely to have MAE than their counterparts, respectively. It is obvious that professionals lacked these services would definitely make more MAE.

Conclusion

The occurrence of medication administration error was found to be high in this study. Age of patients, educational level of medication administrators, availability of medication preparation room and guide and a number of medications given per single patient were statistically significant factors associated with occurrence of medication administration error. Tigray regional health office, medical directors and other responsible bodies of the

hospitals should work in providing updated medication administration guidelines, enough space or room for medication preparation, continuous training for health professionals. The health professional should devote their time in updating themselves on how to administer medications to their patients safely and appropriately.

Abbreviations
AOR: Adjusted Odds Ratio; CI: Confidence Interval; COR: Crude Odds Ratio; ICU: Intensive Care Unit; MAE: Medication Administration Error; NCC MERP: National Coordinating Council for Medication Error Reporting and Prevention; NIC: Nursing Interventions Classification; WHO: World Health Organization

Acknowledgments
Our deep gratitude goes to study participants, the health professionals and pediatric patients from whom data sources are taken. We feel thankful to the data collectors and supervisors in that this study would have been not possible without their significant contribution. In addition, we want to acknowledge the Aksum University for funding this valuable work.

Funding
Aksum University research and publication office funded the project.

Authors' contribution
ZB, HT, AK and LT develop the proposal. ZB, MA, AK, LT, HG and HT enter, clean and analyze the data. MA and ZB wrote the first draft of the manuscript. All authors wrote and read the final draft of the manuscript.

Competing interests
All authors declared that they have no competing interest.

Author details
[1]Department of Neonatal Nursing, School of Nursing, College of Health Sciences, Aksum University, Aksum, Ethiopia. [2]Department of Epidemiology and Biostatistics, School of Public Health, College of Health Sciences, Aksum University, P. O. Box: 298, Aksum, Ethiopia. [3]Department of Biomedical Sciences, School of Medicine, College of Health Sciences, Aksum University, Aksum, Ethiopia.

References
1. Bulecheck G, Butcher, H et al. Nursing intervention classification. 2008. Available at: https://www.elsevier.com/books/nursing-interventions-classification-nic/bulechek/978-0-323-10011-3
2. NCCMERP. What is medication error. 2013.Available at:www.nccmerp.org/recommendations-statements.
3. Cafazzo JA, Trbovich P, Cassano-Piche A, Chagpar A, Rossos PG, Vicente KJ, et al. Human factors perspectives on a systemic approach to ensuring a safer medication delivery process. Healthcare Quarterly. 2009;12(Sp).
4. Kaushal R, Bates DW, Landrigan C, McKenna KJ, Clapp MD, Federico F, et al. Medication errors and adverse drug events in pediatric inpatients. JAMA. 2001;285(16):2114–20.
5. Payne CH, Smith CR, Newkirk LE, Hicks RW. 2.2 pediatric medication errors in the Postanesthesia care unit: analysis of MEDMARX data. AORN J. 2007;85(4):731–40.
6. Hicks R, Becker S, Cousins D. MEDMARX data report: a chartbook of medication error findings from the perioperative settings from 1998-2005. Rockville: MD: USP center for the advancement of patient safety; 2006.
7. Woods D, Thomas E, Holl J, Altman S, Brennan T. Adverse events and preventable adverse events in children. Pediatrics. 2005;115(1):155–60.
8. Gallagher RM, Mason JR, Bird KA, Kirkham JJ, Peak M, Williamson PR, et al. Adverse drug reactions causing admission to a paediatric hospital. PLoS One. 2012;7(12):e50127.
9. Otero P, Leyton A, Mariani G, Cernadas JMC. Medication errors in pediatric inpatients: prevalence and results of a prevention program. Pediatrics. 2008;122(3):e737–e43.
10. Parihar M, Passi GR. Medical errors in pediatric practice. Indian Pediatr. 2008;45(7):586.
11. Oshikoya KA, Chukwura H, Njokanma OF, Senbanjo IO, Ojo I. Incidence and cost estimate of treating pediatric adverse drug reactions in Lagos. Nigeria Sao Paulo Medical Journal. 2011;129(3):153–64.
12. Feleke Y, Girma B. Medication administration errors involving paediatric in-patients in a hospital in Ethiopia. Tropical Journal of Pharmaceutical Research. 2010;9(4).
13. FDRE MOH. Guideline for implementation of a patient referral system. May: Addis Ababa, Ethiopia; 2010. Available at: https://www.medbox.org/et-guidelines-others/ethiopia-guideline-for-implementation-of-a-patient-referral-system/preview
14. Elliott M, Liu Y. The nine rights of medication administration: an overview. Br J Nurs. 2010;19(5):300.
15. NCCMERP. Recommendations to enhance accuracy of administration of medications. 2015. Available at: http://www.nccmerp.org/recommendations-enhance-accuracy-administration-medications
16. WHO. Report on the Web-Based Modified Delphi Survey of the International Classification for Patient Safety Overview, 2007. Available at: www.who.int/patientsafety/taxonomy/ps_modified_delphi_survey.pdf
17. Medication Errors, International Council of Nurses. ICN; c1899–2010 [cited 2 Feb 2010]. Available at: http://www.icn.ch/matters_errors.htm
18. Kenneth NB, Flynn EA, Pepper GA, Bates DW, Mikeal RL. Medication error observed in 36 health care facility. ARCH INTEN MED. 2002;162(16):162–72.
19. Demehin A, Babalola O, Erhun W. Pharmacists and nurses perception of medication errors in a Nigerian University teaching hospital. International Journal of Health Research. 2008;1(2):51–61.
20. Prot S, Fontan JE, Alberti C, Bourdon O, Farnoux C, Macher MA, et al. Drug administration errors and their determinants in pediatric in-patients. Int J Qual Health Care. 2005;17(5):381–9.
21. Ross L, Wallace J, Paton J. Medication errors in a paediatric teaching hospital in the UK: five years operational experience. Arch Dis Child. 2000;83(6):492–7.
22. Bifftu BB, Dachew BA, Tiruneh BT, Beshah DT. Medication administration error reporting and associated factors among nurses working at the University of Gondar referral hospital, Northwest Ethiopia, 2015. BMC Nurs. 2016;15(1):43.

21

Clinical and genetic Rett syndrome variants are defined by stable electrophysiological profiles

Conor Keogh[1], Giorgio Pini[2], Adam H. Dyer[1], Stefania Bigoni[3], Pietro DiMarco[2], Ilaria Gemo[2], Richard Reilly[4] and Daniela Tropea[5,6*]

Abstract

Background: Rett Syndrome (RTT) is a complex neurodevelopmental disorder, frequently associated with epilepsy. Despite increasing recognition of the clinical heterogeneity of RTT and its variants (e.g Classical, Hanefeld and PSV(Preserved Speech Variant)), the link between causative mutations and observed clinical phenotypes remains unclear. Quantitative analysis of electroencephalogram (EEG) recordings may further elucidate important differences between the different clinical and genetic forms of RTT.

Methods: Using a large cohort ($n = 42$) of RTT patients, we analysed the electrophysiological profiles of RTT variants (genetic and clinical) in addition to epilepsy status (no epilepsy/treatment-responsive epilepsy/treatment-resistant epilepsy). The distribution of spectral power and inter-electrode coherence measures were derived from continuous resting-state EEG recordings.

Results: RTT genetic variants (MeCP2/CDLK5) were characterised by significant differences in network architecture on comparing first principal components of inter-electrode coherence across all frequency bands ($p < 0.0001$). Greater coherence in occipital and temporal pairs were seen in MeCP2 vs CDLK5 variants, the main drivers in between group differences. Similarly, clinical phenotypes (Classical RTT/Hanefeld/PSV) demonstrated significant differences in network architecture ($p < 0.0001$). Right tempero-parietal connectivity was found to differ between groups ($p = 0.04$), with greatest coherence in the Classical RTT phenotype. PSV demonstrated a significant difference in left-sided parieto-occipital coherence ($p = 0.026$). Whilst overall power decreased over time, there were no difference in asymmetry and inter-electrode coherence profiles over time. There was a significant difference in asymmetry in the overall power spectra between epilepsy groups ($p = 0.04$) in addition to occipital asymmetry across all frequency bands. Significant differences in network architecture were also seen across epilepsy groups ($p = 0.044$).

Conclusions: Genetic and clinical variants of RTT are characterised by discrete patterns of inter-electrode coherence and network architecture which remain stable over time. Further, hemispheric distribution of spectral power and measures of network dysfunction are associated with epilepsy status and treatment responsiveness. These findings support the role of discrete EEG profiles as non-invasive biomarkers in RTT and its genetic/clinical variants.

Keywords: Rett syndrome, MeCP2, CDKL5, EEG, Network

* Correspondence: tropead@tcd.ie
[5]Neuropsychiatric Genetics, Trinity Centre for Health Sciences, St. James's Hospital, D8 Dublin, Ireland
[6]Trinity College Institute of Neuroscience (TCIN), Lloyd Building, Trinity College Dublin, Dublin 2, Ireland
Full list of author information is available at the end of the article

Background

Rett Syndrome (RTT) is a rare neurodevelopmental disorder affecting 1 in 10,000–20,000 live female births [1–3]. Patients with RTT typically undergo normal development for the first 18 months of life, followed by a period of stagnation and subsequent regression in cognitive and psychomotor abilities. The disorder is characterised by several well-defined stages consisting of: (I) early onset stagnation, (II) developmental regression, (III) pseudostationary period and (IV) late motor deterioration [4]. Further, the clinical picture in RTT is complicated by associated clinical problems, most notably a high incidence of epilepsy which is frequently resistant to treatment, as well as gastro-intestinal problems, gait disturbance, scoliosis, osteopenia and cardiorespiratory dysfunction [4].

Increasing attention has been drawn to this rare disorder as a consequence of the discovery of causative mutations in *MeCP2* (Methyl CpG Binding Protein 2), a gene involved in brain development, neuronal structure and synaptic function [5, 6], in the majority (80–85%) of cases [7]. Further, a rarer variant of Rett Syndrome characterised by mutations in the *CDKL5* (Cyclin-Dependent Kinase-Like 5) gene, a regulator of *MeCP2* which also has important roles in brain development and neuronal maturation [8], suggests a common underlying mechanism related to abnormalities in synapse formation in Rett Syndrome.

Whilst the molecular underpinnings of RTT suggest a single common pathway of abnormal synaptic regulation during development, RTT is increasingly recognised as a clinically heterogenous disorder with widely varying clinical phenotypes [4]. Among the best characterised are the Hanefeld variant, closely linked to mutations in *CDKL5*; these patients may not show the same development and regression pattern with which is characteristic of the classical RTT phenotype, but have a pathognomonic early onset of seizures [9, 10]. The Preserved Speech Variant (PSV), or "Zappella" variant, which is characterised by relatively preserved speech in addition to a less severe clinical picture [11, 12], associated with mutations in the same gene as the Classic variant (*MeCP2*), further highlights the clinical heterogeneity observed, even in the context of mutations in the same causative gene.

Our increasing knowledge of the genetic underpinnings of RTT variants is therefore paired with a relatively poor understanding of the specific neuropathological changes brought about by these genetic abnormalities, and how these reflect the variability observed at the clinical level. Greater elucidation of the nature of these changes may offer insights into the pathological mechanisms underlying RTT variants, as well as offering potential biomarkers for diagnosis, classification and prognostication. Given the lack of correspondence between the genetics and the clinical presentation, it is predicted that specific patterns of abnormality in central nervous system structure and function may be responsible for the differences observed in the separate phenotypes. A suitable "endophenotype", which may act as an intermediary between the underlying molecular pathology and clinical presentation, may therefore be a characterisation of nervous system functioning using the analysis of quantitative electrophysiological data.

While initial EEG analysis have supported the presence of electrophysiological abnormalities in RTT, a quantitative analysis of how continuous resting-state electrophysiological features relate to specific genetic and phenotypic variants of RTT has been absent [13–17]. A thorough analysis of the differences between these subtypes may therefore offer novel insight into the mediation of clinical phenotypes and how these relate to the underlying genetics.

Notably, EEG metrics have proven to be a valuable tool to understand the pathophysiology of brain dysfunction in related disorders. This is the case for Autism Spectrum Disorder (ASD), which has been the subject of many electrophysiological studies as reviewed elsewhere [18–20]. In studies examining cortical connectivity in ASD, robust patterns of network-level dysfunction have been demonstrated by several authors [21, 22]. Despite evidence that many genes related to ASD have pervasive roles in neurodevelopment, synaptic formation and maintenance in a similar manner to those underlying RTT and related subtypes [23], whether abnormalities at the network level are seen in RTT and its subtypes has never been explored. Such approaches offer the potential to investigate whether genetic and clinical subtypes of RTT are associated with specific abnormalities in network-level architecture, which may offer greater insight into the nature and classification of these groups.

The importance of electrophysiological abnormalities is further underlined by high rates of co-morbid epilepsy in RTT. The associated epilepsy is frequently resistant to treatment and represents a significant clinical problem in this patient cohort. In a large study of RTT patients, epilepsy was present in two-thirds (64.2%) of patients with all-type RTT, with treatment-resistant epilepsy in under one fifth (17.2%) [4]. Epilepsy is present in all of those with the Hanefeld variant of RTT [4]. It follows from the clinical differences in seizure presence and response to treatment that there may be underlying electrophysiological differences within the different RTT phenotypes. The relationship between epilepsy status and electrophysiological characteristics in RTT has, however, never been investigated.

In the present study we therefore characterised the electrophysiological features of the major genetic and clinical subtypes of RTT. In addition, we examined whether differences in these features were associated with epilepsy status and treatment responsiveness in this patient group. Our analysis demonstrates that RTT variants are characterised by specific abnormalities in EEG parameters which are stable across time, further parsing the neurobiological and clinical heterogeneity in these increasingly characterised subgroups, and that EEG measures have the potential to act as endophenotypes in these disorders, with a potential role in diagnosis, classification and prognostication.

Methods

Subject recruitment

Patients were recruited from the Tuscany Rett Centre, Italy. All experiments were undertaken in accordance with the Declaration of Helsinki and approved by the Ethical Committee: approval ID: 12720. Patients' families gave consent and for collection and use of the data for scientific purposes. 42 patients were recruited, with a mean age of 7.69 +/− 5.22 years. Further details on patient demographics are available anonymously in Additional file 1: Appendix 1 and Table S1.

Data collection

Clinical, genetic and electrophysiological data was recorded for each participant. In any case where the relevant clinical or genetic information was not available for a specific patient, that patient was excluded from electrophysiological analysis. Clinical data was available for 35, genetic data for 40 and epilepsy status for 42 patients.

Clinical characterisation

Clinical phenotype was recorded for each patient based on their presentation. This was divided into the common Classic phenotype, the rarer, more severe, Hanefeld variant, and the rare but milder Preserved Speech Variant (PSV) [9]. Epilepsy status was also measured for each patient, recorded as No Epilepsy, Epilepsy or Treatment Resistant Epilepsy based on (1) whether there was clinical evidence of epilepsy and (2) whether epilepsy responded to medical management.

Genetic characterisation

Causative mutations were identified for each patient. These were recorded based on the gene affected: *MeCP2*, the gene most commonly implicated in Rett Syndrome [7], and *CDKL5*, a more rarely affected gene associated with more severe clinical presentations [8].

Electrophysiological characterisation

Electroencephalographic (EEG) data was recorded using an eight-electrode montage, with electrodes in frontal, temporal, parietal and occipital locations bilaterally (see Additional file 1: Figure S1, for a schematic of electrode montage). Reference electrodes were placed on the mastoid processes. The ground electrode was placed in position FpZ (midline sagittal plane). Recordings were made from awake subjects seated for a minimum of 20 min continuously at rest (range: 20 min to 204 to minutes, mean 59 min). Recordings were sampled at a rate of 128 Hz. All recordings were carried out under the same testing conditions.

Preprocessing

The first and last five minutes of each recording were discarded to reduce contamination with movement artefacts. Data were then visually inspected to verify recording quality. Data were split into ten-minute epochs and an automated artefact rejection algorithm run. All remaining epochs were manually examined. The first sufficiently artefact-free epoch was extracted from each recording for analysis in order to ensure inclusion of stationary signals without wide epileptic abnormalities. In order to ensure that these results were not impacted by undetected artefacts, all analyses were repeated using a series of combinations of shorted epochs which were then averaged (see Additional file 1: Appendix 2: Epoch Length). Results were consistent across each iteration, and so the results of the ten-minute epochs are presented here.

All recordings were transformed to a common eight-electrode montage (see Fig. 1, Additional file 1), with any additional channels present in individual subjects discarded.

Data were baseline corrected by subtraction of the mean of all channels, re-referenced to the average of all scalp channels and digitally filtered offline at 1 Hz - 50 Hz.

Feature extraction

In order to characterise differences in electrophysiology within Rett Syndrome subtypes, a profile of electrophysiological features was derived using custom MatLab scripts.

Spectral power

Overall power spectra were calculated over the full ten minute epochs by Fourier Transform, allowing gross assessment of differences in the 1 - 50 Hz range and evaluation of the spatial distribution of the overall power.

Individual frequency bands were assessed by isolating theta (4 Hz − 8 Hz), alpha (8 Hz − 12 Hz), beta (12 Hz − 30 Hz), delta (0.5 Hz − 4 Hz) and gamma (> 30 Hz) bands [24]. This allowed characterisation of the distribution of activity at specific oscillatory frequencies across the scalp.

Overall power was assessed using the mean of the individual channel spectra. This was measured in absolute power (dB). Power in individual bands was normalised

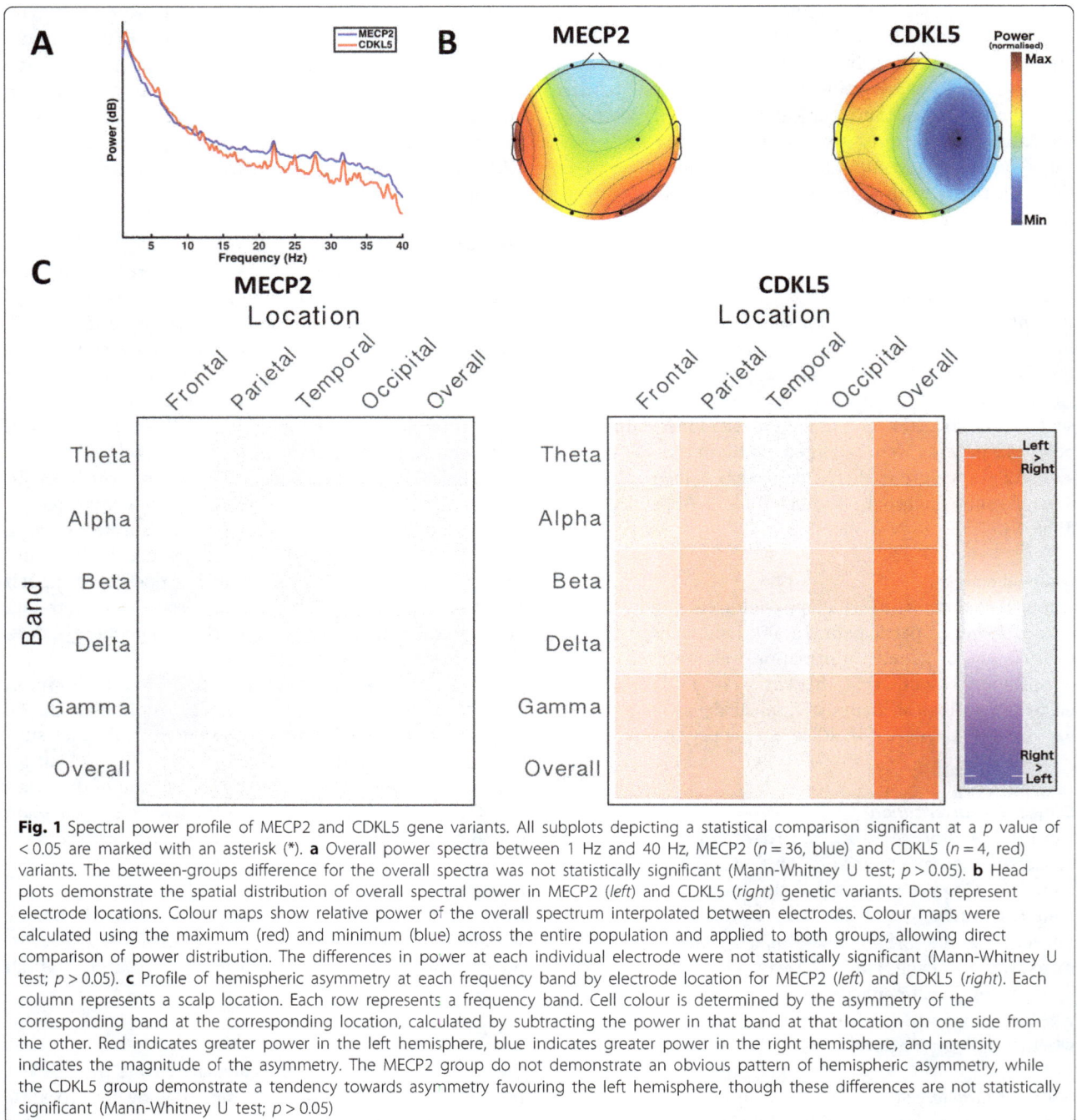

Fig. 1 Spectral power profile of MECP2 and CDKL5 gene variants. All subplots depicting a statistical comparison significant at a p value of < 0.05 are marked with an asterisk (*). **a** Overall power spectra between 1 Hz and 40 Hz, MECP2 ($n = 36$, blue) and CDKL5 ($n = 4$, red) variants. The between-groups difference for the overall spectra was not statistically significant (Mann-Whitney U test; $p > 0.05$). **b** Head plots demonstrate the spatial distribution of overall spectral power in MECP2 (*left*) and CDKL5 (*right*) genetic variants. Dots represent electrode locations. Colour maps show relative power of the overall spectrum interpolated between electrodes. Colour maps were calculated using the maximum (red) and minimum (blue) across the entire population and applied to both groups, allowing direct comparison of power distribution. The differences in power at each individual electrode were not statistically significant (Mann-Whitney U test; $p > 0.05$). **c** Profile of hemispheric asymmetry at each frequency band by electrode location for MECP2 (*left*) and CDKL5 (*right*). Each column represents a scalp location. Each row represents a frequency band. Cell colour is determined by the asymmetry of the corresponding band at the corresponding location, calculated by subtracting the power in that band at that location on one side from the other. Red indicates greater power in the left hemisphere, blue indicates greater power in the right hemisphere, and intensity indicates the magnitude of the asymmetry. The MECP2 group do not demonstrate an obvious pattern of hemispheric asymmetry, while the CDKL5 group demonstrate a tendency towards asymmetry favouring the left hemisphere, though these differences are not statistically significant (Mann-Whitney U test; $p > 0.05$)

with respect to overall power to give a measure of relative power. Each of these results represents the mean of the power measures within that band.

Asymmetry

Relative activity of each hemisphere was assessed in order to evaluate whether there was a marked dominance of one hemisphere, suggestive of abnormalities in distribution of activity. This was calculated by subtracting the overall power in the right hemisphere from power in the left hemisphere.

Profiles of hemispheric symmetry were further characterised by examining the asymmetry in overall power between corresponding electrode pairs, allowing evaluation of the distribution of power in frontal, temporal, parietal and occipital regions specifically. Asymmetry profiles were then derived for each frequency band, allowing investigation of hemispheric dominance within individual bands.

Network measures

Interactions between electrodes were evaluated in order to provide an assessment of network function [25]. Measures of inter-electrode coherence were derived for each electrode pair through calculation of the cross-spectrum of two channels normalised by the power spectra of both channels, repeated for each unique pair:

$$C(\omega) = \frac{S_{xy}(\omega)^2}{S_{xx}(\omega)\,S_{yy}(\omega)}$$

This provides a measure of the phase stability between the signals at each electrode, with high degrees of inter-electrode coherence indicating functional connectivity between the two electrodes. Coherence is measured on a scale of 0 (no coherence) to 1 (full coherence).

In order to evaluate overall differences in network architecture between groups while avoiding large numbers of statistical comparisons, dimensionality reduction was carried out using a principal component analysis performed on the inter-electrode coherence measures for each subject. The first principal components, accounting for the highest degree of variance within the coherence measures, were then compared between groups to evaluate differences in overall networks.

Higher-order network architecture was visualised by deriving covariance matrices of inter-electrode coherence measures.

Longitudinal analysis

We followed up nine subjects (mean age 6.33 +/- 4.33 years) at an interval of 10–14 months and re-assessed their electrophysiological profiles to evaluate whether the observed patterns were stable features of RTT subtypes.

This group consisted of 7 patients with *MeCP2* mutations (all Classic phenotype) and 2 with *CDKL5* mutations; analysis of the *MeCP2* subgroup demonstrated similar results to the overall group, while the small number of *CDKL5* subjects prevented a subgroup analysis of this group. As the results of the *MeCP2* group and the pooled group followed the same pattern, the results for the overall group are presented.

Statistical comparisons

As a consequence of the relatively small numbers of the rare variants of Rett Syndrome, nonparametric statistical tests were used throughout to avoid assumptions of normality within the small subgroups. Kruskal-Wallis H testing was used for multi-group comparisons, and

Mann-Whitney U tests were used for pairwise comparisons. Wilcoxon signed-rank tests were used for comparison of paired data in longitudinal analyses. All tests were two-tailed.

In order to avoid large numbers of statistical comparisons, analysis was initially restricted to overall data, or to measures derived from dimensionality reduction methods (principal component analysis of inter-electrode coherence measures), with further exploration of subgroups based on initial evaluation of overall measures.

All results are reported as mean +/- standard deviation. All data processing was performed blinded to patient characteristics.

Subsampling

As the patient population is dominated by the more common variants of Rett Syndrome, a subsampling method was employed to re-analyse the features between groups in order to verify that results were not skewed by the uneven distribution of Rett subtypes. Samples of four subjects were drawn from the large *MeCP2* group and compared to the *CDKL5* group across all main features compared. This was repeated with 15 randomly drawn subsamples and the results analysed to ensure consistency.

These results demonstrated consistency across multiple subsamples, and were consistent with the results obtained using the full population, indicating that the results were not biased by the uneven distribution of Rett subtypes. As a result, the results of comparisons using the larger overall population are presented here. The full results of the subsampled analysis can be found in Additional file 1: Appendix 3: Subsampling Results.

Experimental design

Patient recruitments and clinical analyses were performed by personnel who were not involved in EEG analysis. Processing and feature extraction algorithms were applied to all recordings without consideration of presentation, genetics or other clinical parameters.

Results
Electrophysiological profiles of genetic variants

In order to assess whether the effects of different pathogenic mutations were mediated through distinct patterns of electrophysiological dysfunction, we compared the electrophysiological profiles of groups with confirmed mutations in *MeCP2* (*n* = 36) and *CDKL5* (*n* = 4).

Spectral power profile

The power spectra of the *MeCP2* and *CDKL5* groups between 1 Hz and 40 Hz were compared (Fig. 1).

We found no significant difference in the overall power spectra of the genetic variants (*MeCP2*: 2.5 +/- 8.57,

CDKL5: 1.75 +/− 8.63; $p = 1$, Mann-Whitney U test), indicating no gross difference in the overall electrical activity of the cortex between groups (Fig. 1a).

We then analysed the distribution of the overall power across the eight electrodes (Fig. 1b). The *MeCP2* variant demonstrated a pattern of high relative power in temporal and occipital regions bilaterally with relatively low power in frontal regions. The *CDKL5* variant show a pattern of diffuse high power in the left hemisphere, with low power throughout the right hemisphere. Quantitative assessment of these differences in distribution were not statistically significant ($p > 0.05$, Mann-Whitney U test; see Additional file 1: Table S2, for results of comparisons of overall spectrum at each electrode location).

The distribution of power within individual EEG bands was investigated (Additional file 1: Figure S2). We found that the patterns suggested by the overall power spectrum were evident within individual frequency bands (see Additional file 1: Table S3, for results of comparisons of each frequency band).

We then measured hemispheric asymmetry to evaluate differences in the balance of cortical functioning between groups (Fig. 1c). The *MeCP2* group does not exhibit a major pattern of hemispheric dominance, while the *CDKL5* group trends toward left hemispheric dominance in all areas and across all bands. This trend, however, was not statistically significant (*MeCP2*: 0.11 +/− 16.00 vs. 11.92 +/− 26.69; $p = 0.60$, Mann-Whitney U test). (see Additional file 1: Table S4, for comparisons of asymmetry at each electrode location).

Network measures

In order to assess whether different pathogenic mutations resulted in distinct patterns of network dysfunction, we analysed patterns of inter-electrode coherence.

We compared the first principal components of inter-electrode coherence measures across all frequency bands, and we found a statistically significant difference in network architecture between genetic variants ($p < 0.0001$, Mann-Whitney U test), suggesting that genetic variants of Rett Syndrome are associated with discrete patterns of network dysfunction. A comparison restricted solely to measures within the overall spectrum was also statistically significant ($p = 0.026$, Mann-Whitney U test). A breakdown of the percentage of the total variance explained by each of the first five principal components for each group can be found in Additional file 1: Table S5.

We then evaluated the overall network architecture for each group by deriving a covariance matrix of inter-electrode coherence measures (Fig. 2a). This representation demonstrates the overall patterns of network activity between and across frequency bands.

We explored the nature of network-level differences between groups. The spatial distribution of electrode pairs found to have a statistically significant difference in coherence in the overall power spectrum between groups (using a threshold of $p < 0.05$, Mann-Whitney U test) and a profile of the direction and magnitude of these differences is illustrated in Fig. 2.

We identified occipital (O1 & O2 pairs) and temporal (T3 & T4 pairs) as the primary drivers of differences between groups (Fig. 2a), suggesting that differences in occipito-temporal network function may result from differences in the underlying causative mutation (see Additional file 1: Table S6, for coherence measures between each electrode pair). The *MeCP2* variant showed greater coherence in each of these connections (Fig. 2b), suggesting that this mutation is associated with greater network function in these areas, while the *CDKL5* variant has less activity in these networks.

Electrophysiological profiles of phenotypic variants

In order to assess whether differences in network function evident between genetic variants were conserved at the phenotypic level, acting as a bridge between genetic abnormalities and the observed clinical phenotype, we evaluated differences in electrophysiological profile between Classic ($n = 26$), Hanefeld ($n = 4$) and PSV ($n = 5$) phenotypic groups.

Spectral power profile

We characterized the power spectra of the Classic, Hanefeld and PSV phenotypic groups between 1 Hz and 50 Hz (Fig. 3).

The overall power spectra of the phenotypic variants (Fig. 3a) demonstrates a trend towards higher power in the Classic group at higher frequencies, though we found that this difference was not statistically significant (Classic: 4.27 +/− 8.80, Hanefeld: 1.75 +/− 8.63, PSV: 0.71 +/− 4.42; $p = 0.73$, Kruskal-Wallis H test).

The distribution of the overall power across the scalp suggested gross differences in the activity of specific brain regions between phenotypes (Fig. 3b). However, quantitative assessment of these difference in distribution by comparisons of overall power between corresponding electrode sites was not statistically significant ($p > 0.05$, Kruskal-Wallis H test; see Additional file 1: Table S7, for results of comparisons of overall spectrum at each electrode location).

A similar analysis within individual bands demonstrated similar patterns to that observed for the overall spectrum (Additional file 1: Figure S5). (see Additional file 1: Table S8, for results of comparisons of each frequency band).

We then measured hemispheric asymmetry between groups (Fig. 3c). The Classic group does not exhibit a major pattern of hemispheric dominance, while the Hanefeld group trends toward left hemispheric dominance. The PSV group also demonstrates a less marked

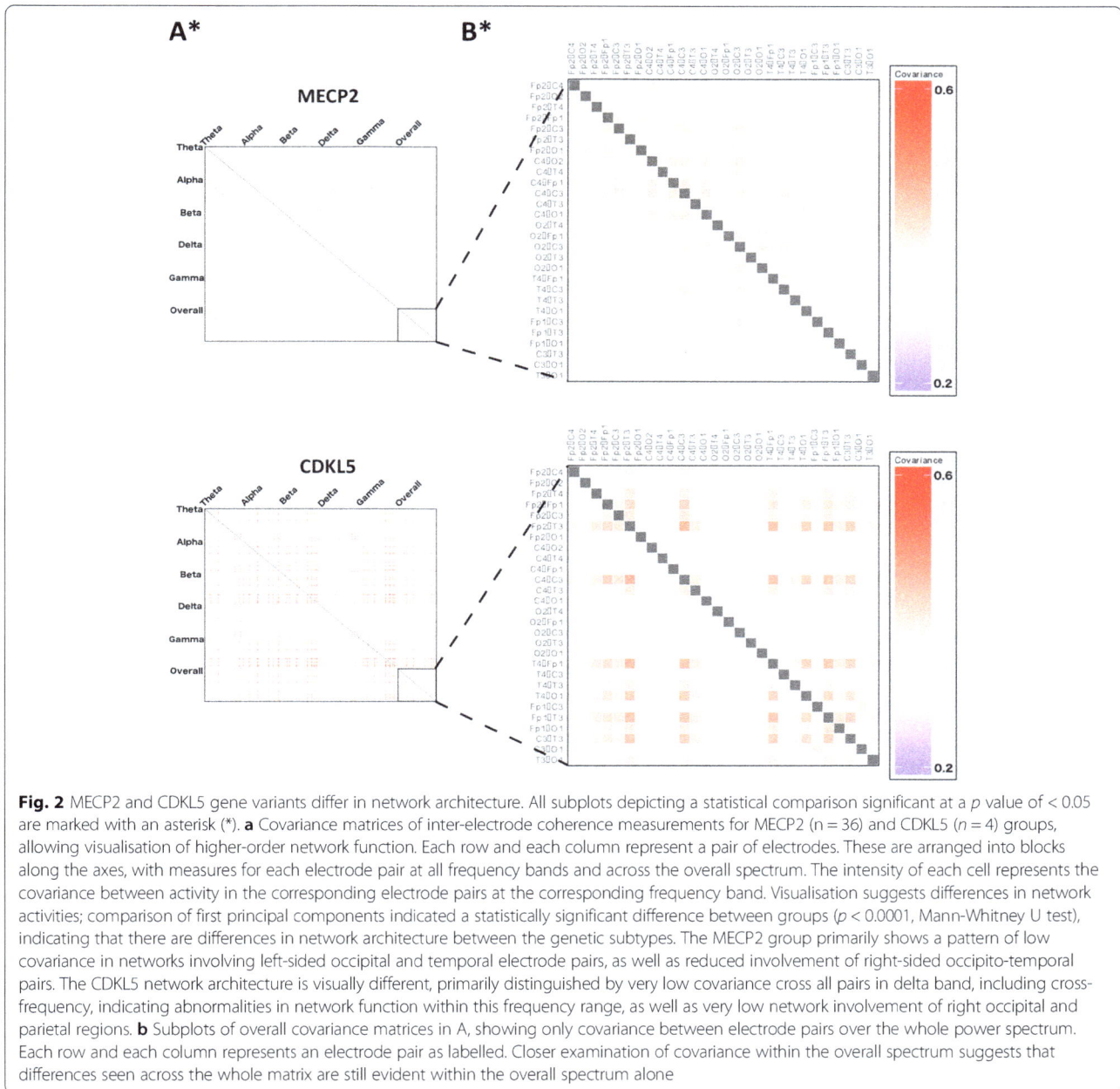

Fig. 2 MECP2 and CDKL5 gene variants differ in network architecture. All subplots depicting a statistical comparison significant at a *p* value of < 0.05 are marked with an asterisk (*). **a** Covariance matrices of inter-electrode coherence measurements for MECP2 (n = 36) and CDKL5 (*n* = 4) groups, allowing visualisation of higher-order network function. Each row and each column represent a pair of electrodes. These are arranged into blocks along the axes, with measures for each electrode pair at all frequency bands and across the overall spectrum. The intensity of each cell represents the covariance between activity in the corresponding electrode pairs at the corresponding frequency band. Visualisation suggests differences in network activities; comparison of first principal components indicated a statistically significant difference between groups (*p* < 0.0001, Mann-Whitney U test), indicating that there are differences in network architecture between the genetic subtypes. The MECP2 group primarily shows a pattern of low covariance in networks involving left-sided occipital and temporal electrode pairs, as well as reduced involvement of right-sided occipito-temporal pairs. The CDKL5 network architecture is visually different, primarily distinguished by very low covariance cross all pairs in delta band, including cross-frequency, indicating abnormalities in network function within this frequency range, as well as very low network involvement of right occipital and parietal regions. **b** Subplots of overall covariance matrices in A, showing only covariance between electrode pairs over the whole power spectrum. Each row and each column represents an electrode pair as labelled. Closer examination of covariance within the overall spectrum suggests that differences seen across the whole matrix are still evident within the overall spectrum alone

trend towards left hemispheric dominance. Comparison of differences in overall asymmetry between groups was not statistically significant, however (Classic: − 0.48 +/− 17.38, Hanefeld: 11.92 +/− 26.69, PSV: 2.38 +/− 17.39; *p* = 0.87, Kruskal-Wallis H test). (see Additional file 1: Table S9, for comparisons of asymmetry at at each electrode location).

Network measures
We compared profiles of network-level activity between phenotypes. Comparison of first principal components of inter-electrode coherence measures across all frequency bands demonstrated a statistically significant difference in network architecture between phenotypes (*p* < 0.0001, Kruskal-Wallis H test), suggesting a role for network dysfunction in the mediation of observed clinical subtypes. A breakdown of the percentage of the total variance explained by each of the first five principal components for each group can be found in Additional file 1: Table S10.

We evaluated higher-order network function for each group using covariance matrices of inter-electrode coherence measures (Fig. 4a).

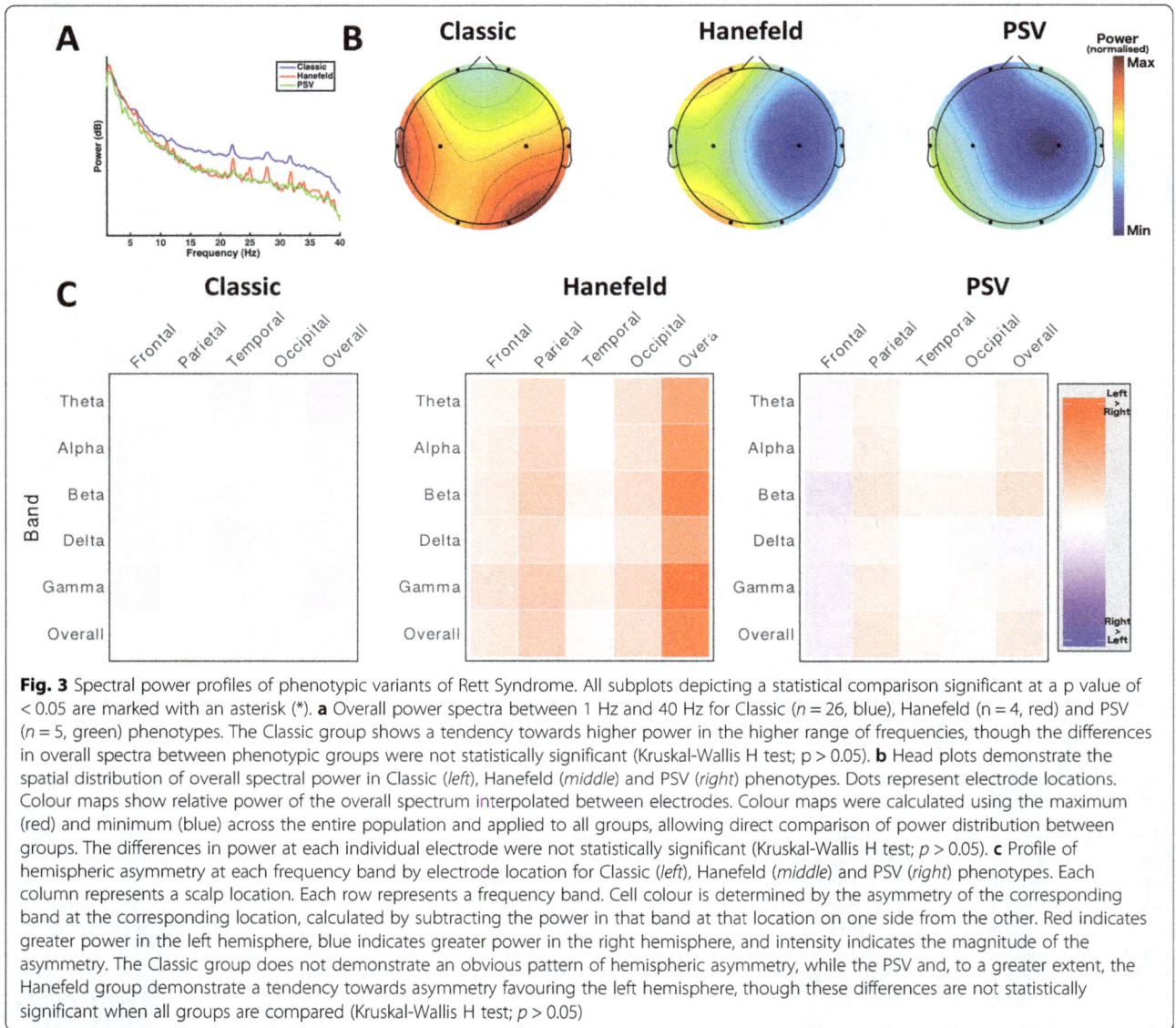

Fig. 3 Spectral power profiles of phenotypic variants of Rett Syndrome. All subplots depicting a statistical comparison significant at a p value of < 0.05 are marked with an asterisk (*). **a** Overall power spectra between 1 Hz and 40 Hz for Classic (n = 26, blue), Hanefeld (n = 4, red) and PSV (n = 5, green) phenotypes. The Classic group shows a tendency towards higher power in the higher range of frequencies, though the differences in overall spectra between phenotypic groups were not statistically significant (Kruskal-Wallis H test; p > 0.05). **b** Head plots demonstrate the spatial distribution of overall spectral power in Classic (*left*), Hanefeld (*middle*) and PSV (*right*) phenotypes. Dots represent electrode locations. Colour maps show relative power of the overall spectrum interpolated between electrodes. Colour maps were calculated using the maximum (red) and minimum (blue) across the entire population and applied to all groups, allowing direct comparison of power distribution between groups. The differences in power at each individual electrode were not statistically significant (Kruskal-Wallis H test; p > 0.05). **c** Profile of hemispheric asymmetry at each frequency band by electrode location for Classic (*left*), Hanefeld (*middle*) and PSV (*right*) phenotypes. Each column represents a scalp location. Each row represents a frequency band. Cell colour is determined by the asymmetry of the corresponding band at the corresponding location, calculated by subtracting the power in that band at that location on one side from the other. Red indicates greater power in the left hemisphere, blue indicates greater power in the right hemisphere, and intensity indicates the magnitude of the asymmetry. The Classic group does not demonstrate an obvious pattern of hemispheric asymmetry, while the PSV and, to a greater extent, the Hanefeld group demonstrate a tendency towards asymmetry favouring the left hemisphere, though these differences are not statistically significant when all groups are compared (Kruskal-Wallis H test; p > 0.05)

We explored the patterns of network activity differentiating the groups and found statistically significant differences in coherence of electrode pairs in the overall power spectrum between phenotypes (using a threshold of *p* < 0.05, Kruskal-Wallis H test). The results of this are shown in Fig. 4.

Right temporo-parietal connectivity (T4-C4) was found to differ between clinical phenotypes (*p* = 0.04), consistent with the patterns observed in the covariance matrices, with the Classic phenotype (0.42 +/- 0.22) demonstrating the greatest coherence, followed by PSV (0.34 +/- 0.19) and then Hanefeld (0.21 +/- 0.05), suggesting that specific network-level dysfunctions may play a role in determining the Rett phenotype expressed (see Additional file 1: Table S11, for coherence measures between each electrode pair).

Characterising the PSV variant

Having determined that network level dysfunctions may differ across clinical phenotypes and hence play a role in mediating the clinical presentation of a given mutation, we compared the PSV variant (*n* = 5) directly to a group of Classic phenotype (*n* = 26) with mutations in same gene (MeCP2).

Notably, comparison of the inter-electrode coherence profiles of PSV and Classic groups demonstrated a statistically significant difference in left-sided parieto-occipital coherence (PSV: 0.55 +/- 0.07, Classic: 0.39 +/- 0.17; *p* = 0.026, Mann-Whitney U test), shown in Additional file 1: Figure S8. This suggests a role for parieto-occipital network function in mediating the phenotype of PSV variant Rett syndrome, with increased left-sided parieto-occipital connectivity potentially associated with a preservation of speech function.

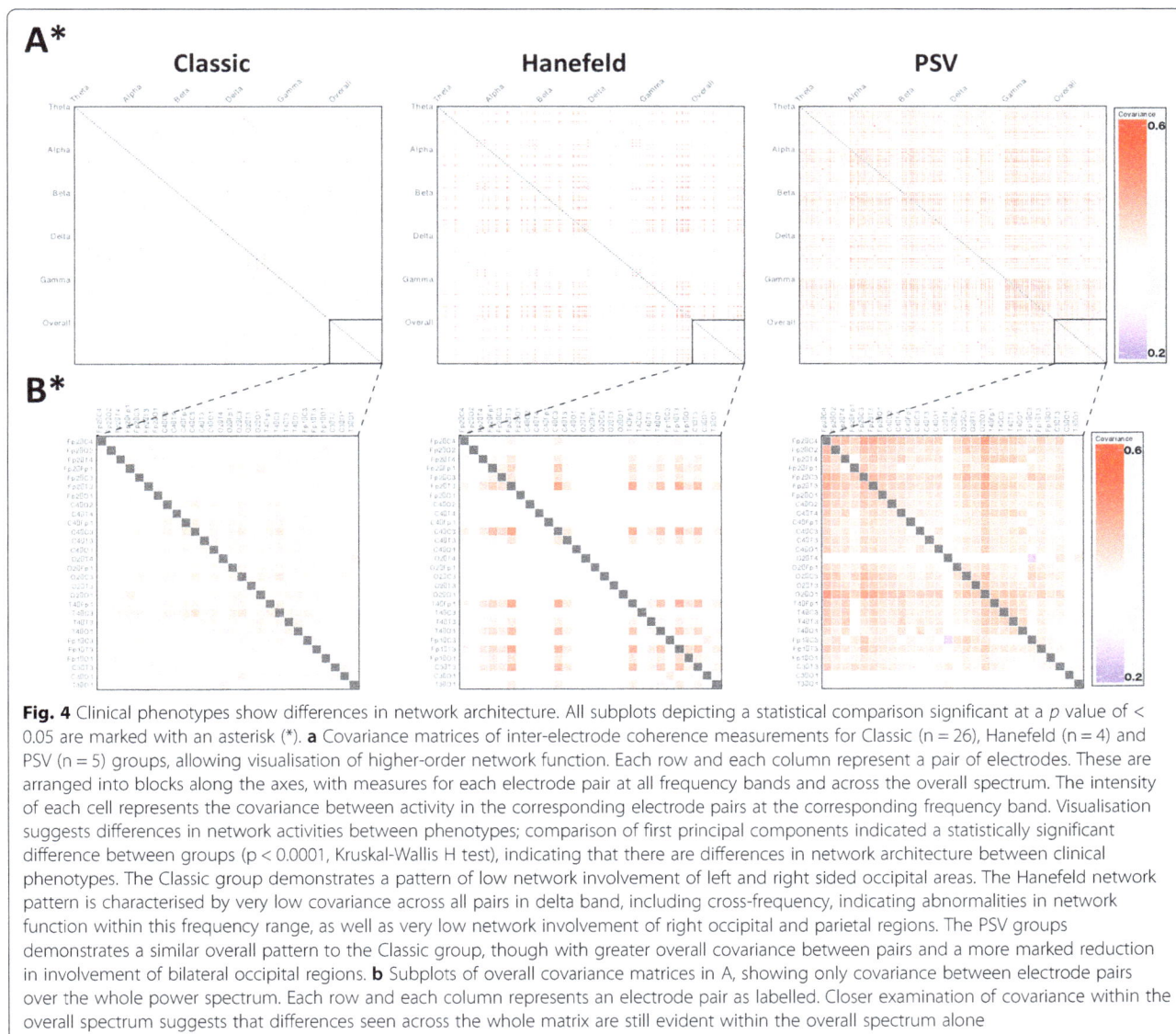

Fig. 4 Clinical phenotypes show differences in network architecture. All subplots depicting a statistical comparison significant at a p value of < 0.05 are marked with an asterisk (*). **a** Covariance matrices of inter-electrode coherence measurements for Classic (n = 26), Hanefeld (n = 4) and PSV (n = 5) groups, allowing visualisation of higher-order network function. Each row and each column represent a pair of electrodes. These are arranged into blocks along the axes, with measures for each electrode pair at all frequency bands and across the overall spectrum. The intensity of each cell represents the covariance between activity in the corresponding electrode pairs at the corresponding frequency band. Visualisation suggests differences in network activities between phenotypes; comparison of first principal components indicated a statistically significant difference between groups (p < 0.0001, Kruskal-Wallis H test), indicating that there are differences in network architecture between clinical phenotypes. The Classic group demonstrates a pattern of low network involvement of left and right sided occipital areas. The Hanefeld network pattern is characterised by very low covariance across all pairs in delta band, including cross-frequency, indicating abnormalities in network function within this frequency range, as well as very low network involvement of right occipital and parietal regions. The PSV groups demonstrates a similar overall pattern to the Classic group, though with greater overall covariance between pairs and a more marked reduction in involvement of bilateral occipital regions. **b** Subplots of overall covariance matrices in A, showing only covariance between electrode pairs over the whole power spectrum. Each row and each column represents an electrode pair as labelled. Closer examination of covariance within the overall spectrum suggests that differences seen across the whole matrix are still evident within the overall spectrum alone

Longitudinal analysis

Comparison of spectral power profiles at baseline and at follow-up revealed changes in the power and distribution of frequency bands over time (Fig. 5). We found a generalised decrease in overall power across the scalp, and also in individual bands ($p < 0.05$, Wilcoxon signed rank test; see Additional file 1: Table S12, for comparisons of power at each electrode location at baseline and at follow-up). This pattern of decreasing power with age is particularly evident in left frontal (Fp1) and parietal (C3) regions. This suggests that spectral power profiles, repeated over ten-minute epochs at each sample point, are not entirely stable with time.

Notably, we found no statistically significant differences in comparisons of asymmetry (see Additional file 1: Table S13)

or inter-electrode coherence profiles (see Additional file 1: Table S14) at follow up ($p > 0.05$, Wilcoxon signed rank test). This indicates that patterns of network activity are stable across time, and as a result network features that characterise specific subgroups of Rett Syndrome may have a role as valuable markers, as well as providing insights into the link between genetic mutation and clinical syndrome.

Notably, the absolute change in overall power measures was not significantly correlated with severity of disease as assessed by the International Severity Score ($r = 0.62$, $p = 0.072$), nor was the change in overall asymmetry ($r = -0.03$, $p = 0.94$). These relationships remained true when the differences were normalised with respect to the follow-up interval to give a rate of change (power: $r = 0.59$, $p = 0.09$; asymmetry: r = -0.03, $p = 0.93$).

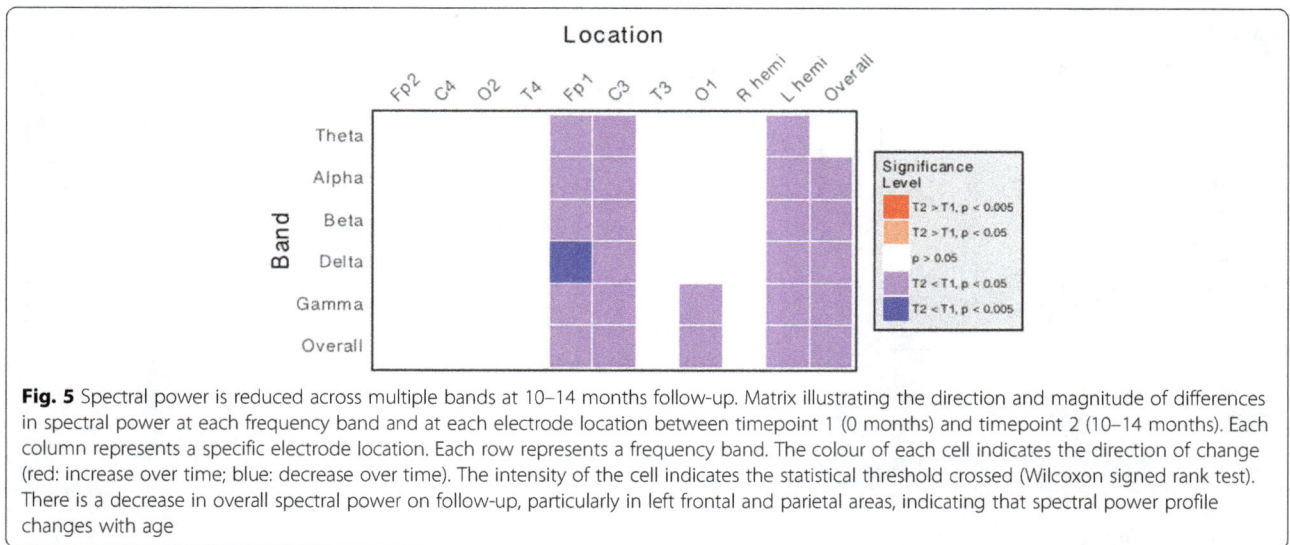

Fig. 5 Spectral power is reduced across multiple bands at 10–14 months follow-up. Matrix illustrating the direction and magnitude of differences in spectral power at each frequency band and at each electrode location between timepoint 1 (0 months) and timepoint 2 (10–14 months). Each column represents a specific electrode location. Each row represents a frequency band. The colour of each cell indicates the direction of change (red: increase over time; blue: decrease over time). The intensity of the cell indicates the statistical threshold crossed (Wilcoxon signed rank test). There is a decrease in overall spectral power on follow-up, particularly in left frontal and parietal areas, indicating that spectral power profile changes with age

Electrophysiological characterisation of epilepsy status

Patients were divided into No Epilepsy ($n = 18$), Epilepsy ($n = 16$) or Resistant Epilepsy ($n = 8$) groups in order to investigate whether these subtypes are characterised by specific functional patterns which may act as electrophysiological biomarkers of epilepsy status.

Spectral power profile

The power spectra of the No Epilepsy, Epilepsy and Resistant epilepsy status groups between 1 Hz and 50 Hz were characterised (Fig. 6).

Although the Epilepsy group trends towards lower power across the spectrum, there was no statistically significant difference in overall power between the epilepsy status groups (No Epilepsy: 4.12 +/− 8.93 Epilepsy: − 0.24 +/− 9.22 Resistant: 5.69 +/− 8.78; $p = 0.16$, Kruskal-Wallis H test), indicating no gross difference in overall cortical electrical activity between groups (Fig. 6a).

The distribution of the overall power across the scalp was investigated (Fig. 6b). Although visualization suggests differences in distribution of power, quantitative assessments of these differences were not statistically significant ($P > 0.05$, Kruskal-Wallis H test; see Additional file 1: Table S15, for results of comparisons of overall spectrum at each electrode location).

The distribution of power within individual bands was investigated (Additional file 1: Figure S9). The distribution of all frequency bands is broadly similar within groups, with a similar pattern to that seen in the overall spectrum (see Additional file 1: Table S16, for results of comparisons of each frequency band).

Hemispheric asymmetry

Measures of hemispheric asymmetry were compared between epilepsy groups to evaluate whether there are differences in the balance of cortical functioning between groups (Fig. 6c).

Comparison of asymmetry in the overall power spectra demonstrated a statistically significant difference between groups in occipital regions (No Epilepsy: − 2.50 +/− 5.81 Epilepsy: 0.78 +/− 4.60 Resistant: 3.41 +/− 6.01; $p = 0.04$, Kruskal-Wallis H test), suggesting that differences in asymmetry across the full spectrum may differentiate between epilepsy status groups.

Further exploration of the hemispheric asymmetry profiles showed a pattern of statistically significant differences in asymmetry between groups ($p < 0.05$, Kruskal-Wallis H test; (see Additional file 1: Table S17, for comparisons of asymmetry at each electrode location)). The differences in occipital asymmetry seen in the overall spectrum were evident across all frequency bands (Additional file 1: Figure S10), indicating that patterns in the balance of activity in occipital areas is associated with epilepsy status.

The direction of differences in pairwise comparisons indicates that the Resistant group has the highest level of hemispheric asymmetry in occipital regions, while the Epilepsy group still has greater asymmetry than those in the No Epilepsy group. This suggests a pattern of increasing severity with increasing left-hemispheric predominance.

Network measures

Profiles of network-level activity were compared between phenotypes in order to assess whether epilepsy status was associated with differences in patterns of network dysfunction (Fig. 7).

Comparison of first principal components of inter-electrode coherence measures across all frequency bands demonstrated a statistically significant difference in network architecture between groups (p = 0.04), Kruskal-Wallis H

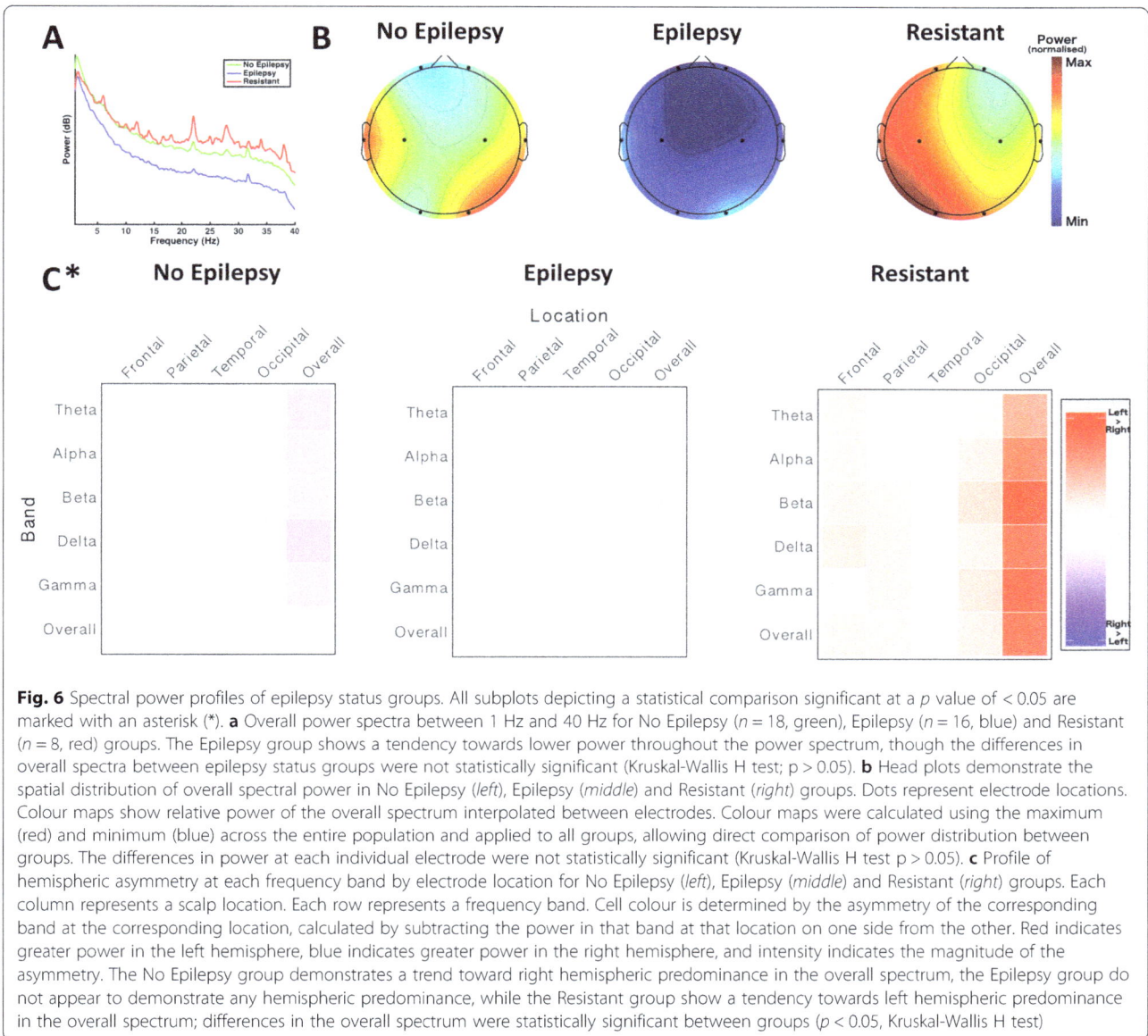

Fig. 6 Spectral power profiles of epilepsy status groups. All subplots depicting a statistical comparison significant at a *p* value of < 0.05 are marked with an asterisk (*). **a** Overall power spectra between 1 Hz and 40 Hz for No Epilepsy (*n* = 18, green), Epilepsy (*n* = 16, blue) and Resistant (*n* = 8, red) groups. The Epilepsy group shows a tendency towards lower power throughout the power spectrum, though the differences in overall spectra between epilepsy status groups were not statistically significant (Kruskal-Wallis H test; p > 0.05). **b** Head plots demonstrate the spatial distribution of overall spectral power in No Epilepsy (*left*), Epilepsy (*middle*) and Resistant (*right*) groups. Dots represent electrode locations. Colour maps show relative power of the overall spectrum interpolated between electrodes. Colour maps were calculated using the maximum (red) and minimum (blue) across the entire population and applied to all groups, allowing direct comparison of power distribution between groups. The differences in power at each individual electrode were not statistically significant (Kruskal-Wallis H test p > 0.05). **c** Profile of hemispheric asymmetry at each frequency band by electrode location for No Epilepsy (*left*), Epilepsy (*middle*) and Resistant (*right*) groups. Each column represents a scalp location. Each row represents a frequency band. Cell colour is determined by the asymmetry of the corresponding band at the corresponding location, calculated by subtracting the power in that band at that location on one side from the other. Red indicates greater power in the left hemisphere, blue indicates greater power in the right hemisphere, and intensity indicates the magnitude of the asymmetry. The No Epilepsy group demonstrates a trend toward right hemispheric predominance in the overall spectrum, the Epilepsy group do not appear to demonstrate any hemispheric predominance, while the Resistant group show a tendency towards left hemispheric predominance in the overall spectrum; differences in the overall spectrum were statistically significant between groups (*p* < 0.05, Kruskal-Wallis H test)

test), suggesting aberrations of network architecture with epilepsy status. A breakdown of the percentage of the total variance explained by each of the first five principal components for each group can be found in Additional file 1: Table S18.

Higher-order network function was visualised using covariance matrices of inter-electrode coherence measures (Fig. 7a).

The patterns of network activity differentiating the groups were explored. No individual electrode pairs were found to differ significantly between epilepsy status groups in the overall spectrum (*p* > 0.05, Kruskal-Wallis H test), indicating that despite the overall differences in network architecture, differences in the strength of individual electrode pairs between epilepsy status groups are not sufficiently large to reach statistical significance (see Additional file 1: Table S19, for coherence measures between each electrode pair).

These results indicate that there are differences in overall electrophysiological profile based on epilepsy status, and that these groups are primarily differentiated electrophysiologically by asymmetry of electrical activity in the occipital region in Rett Syndrome, with increasing severity associated with the presence of epilepsy and with treatment-resistance, as well as differences in overall network architecture.

Characterising epilepsy & treatment resistance
Having established that electrophysiological differences exist between epilepsy status groups, the Epilepsy and

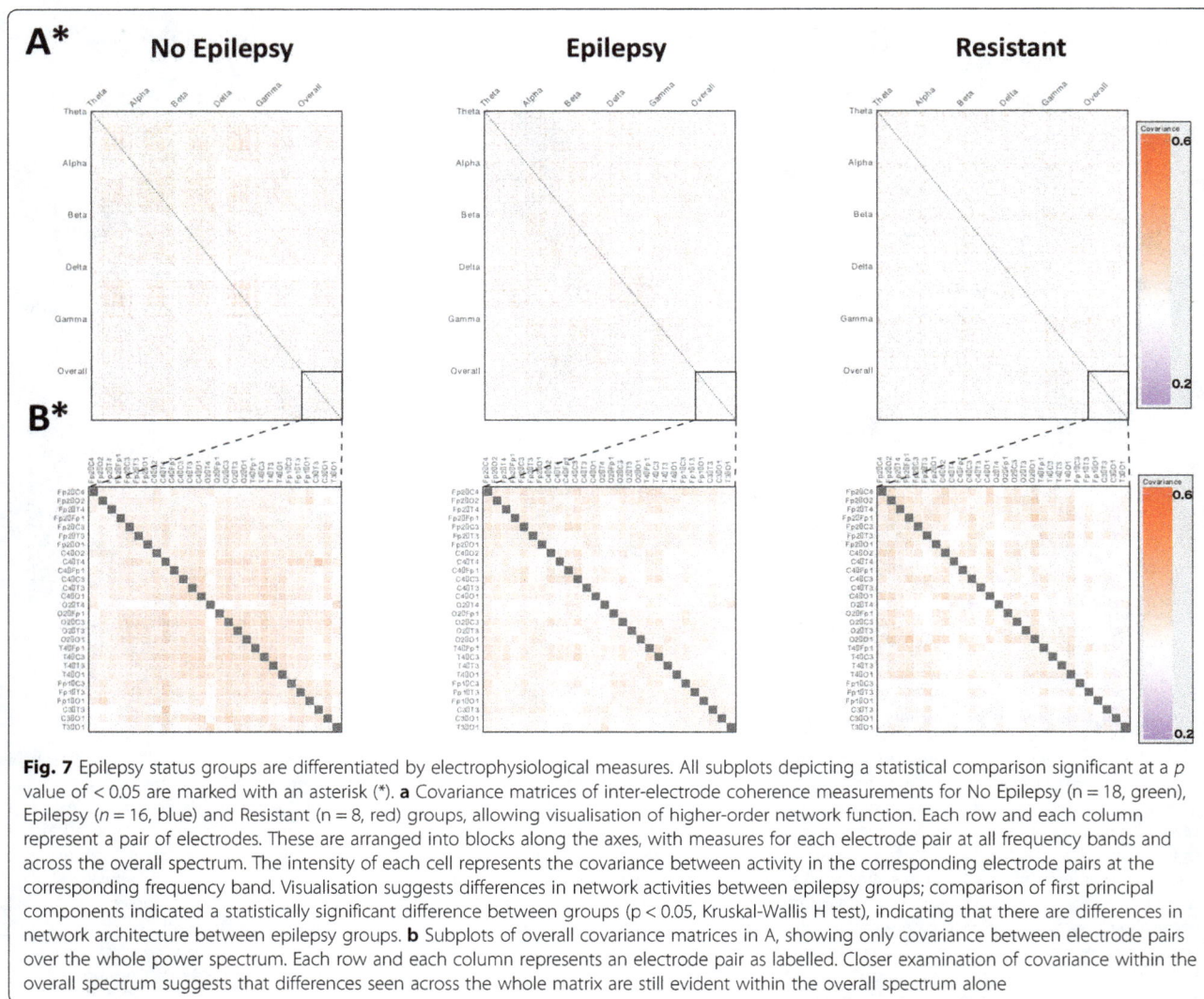

Fig. 7 Epilepsy status groups are differentiated by electrophysiological measures. All subplots depicting a statistical comparison significant at a *p* value of < 0.05 are marked with an asterisk (*). **a** Covariance matrices of inter-electrode coherence measurements for No Epilepsy (n = 18, green), Epilepsy (*n* = 16, blue) and Resistant (n = 8, red) groups, allowing visualisation of higher-order network function. Each row and each column represent a pair of electrodes. These are arranged into blocks along the axes, with measures for each electrode pair at all frequency bands and across the overall spectrum. The intensity of each cell represents the covariance between activity in the corresponding electrode pairs at the corresponding frequency band. Visualisation suggests differences in network activities between epilepsy groups; comparison of first principal components indicated a statistically significant difference between groups (p < 0.05, Kruskal-Wallis H test), indicating that there are differences in network architecture between epilepsy groups. **b** Subplots of overall covariance matrices in A, showing only covariance between electrode pairs over the whole power spectrum. Each row and each column represents an electrode pair as labelled. Closer examination of covariance within the overall spectrum suggests that differences seen across the whole matrix are still evident within the overall spectrum alone

Resistant groups were combined into one overall group of patients with epilepsy, irrespective of treatment resistance, and compared to the No Epilepsy group in order to assess whether specific features drive the electrophysiologic profile evident in epilepsy in an effort to identify markers that may aid the prediction of epilepsy status in a patient whose epilepsy status is otherwise unknown.

Analysis of the features that had emerged as differing between groups demonstrated no difference in overall network architecture as assessed by principal component analysis of inter-electrode coherence measures (*p* = 0.970, Mann-Whitney U test), and a strong pattern of difference in overall occipital asymmetry (No Epilepsy: − 2.50 +/− 5.81, Epilepsy: 1.66 +/− 5.14; *p* = 0.019, Mann-Whitney U test), as well as differences in all individual frequency bands, indicating that asymmetry in the occipital regions is the primary driver of differences in electrophysiological profile evident in

patients with epilepsy (see Additional file 1: Table S20, for results of all asymmetry comparisons).

The Epilepsy and Resistant groups were then directly compared in order to assess whether, in a population with epilepsy, treatment resistance was associated with specific abnormalities. Analysis of the features that had been identified on Kruskal-Wallis testing demonstrated strong differentiation based on overall network architecture (*p* = 0.029, Mann-Whitney U test), while differences in occipital asymmetry measures did not emerge as statistically significant (Epilepsy: 0.78 +/− 4.60, Resistant: 3.41 +/− 6.01; *p* = 0.444, Mann-Whitney U test) between groups, indicating that asymmetry measures differentiated less clearly between the treatment responsive and resistant groups (see Additional file 1: Table S21, for results of all asymmetry comparisons).

These results indicate that the presence of epilepsy is predominantly marked by differences in occipital asymmetry, while treatment resistance is indicated by network-level abnormalities.

Discussion

We present the first quantitative electrophysiological characterization of Rett Syndrome variants, demonstrating that these variants are characterized by specific electrophysiological patterns, that these features are stable over time, and that these network-level abnormalities may contribute to the determination of epilepsy status and treatment responsiveness.

These findings provide insight into the specific abnormalities underlying different variants and presentations of RTT, and may have valuable applications in the clinical evaluation of RTT.

Genetic and phenotypic groups are characterized by specific patterns of network activity

Both genetic and clinical variants of RTT were associated with distinct patterns of inter-electrode coherence measures, indicating differences in network architecture between these subgroups.

These results reveal a role for network dysfunction in mediating the clinical heterogeneity observed in RTT, providing a mechanism through which genetic abnormalities altering synaptic regulation produce varying clinical syndromes. This framework of RTT as a disorder of neural connectivity is consistent with the underlying molecular biology, with previous evidence of electrophysiological abnormalities, and with other related neurodevelopmental disorders such as ASD, where the role of aberrant network function is well established (Murias et al. [21]).

Notably, there were no statistically significant differences in measures of spectral power either in the overall spectrum or within specific bands both overall and between specific electrode locations, between genetic or clinical subgroups. This suggests that the observed differences are not simply due to a gross focal abnormality in neural functioning, but rather a more subtle, systemic alteration at the network level.

Network architecture provides a stable endophenotype in RTT

Remarkably, longitudinal analysis of a subgroup of patients demonstrates that network measures are stable across time. This further supports a potential role for network-level dysfunction in mediating the phenotypic expression of specific genetic abnormalities, as the observed differences between subgroups appear to be conserved over time, rather than simply a transitory phenomenon at the time of testing.

This stable nature of the electrophysiologic characteristics of RTT variants suggests that they may prove useful as biomarkers for the classification and prognostication of RTT patients. Furthermore, greater characterisation of the electrophysiologic profiles of RTT subtypes may be able to provide an objective, electrophysiologic framework for the classification of this heterogeneous neurodevelopmental disorder, rather than the currently used clinical methods.

Interestingly, despite stability of network level features over time, we observed a widespread reduction in power at follow-up (Fig. 5). Although this analysis is limited by the relatively small numbers available for longitudinal analysis, the results suggest that the progression of RTT is marked by gradual reduction in global spectral power, a feature typically observed in advanced ageing and neurodegeneration, potentially offering insight into the neuropathological course of RTT. Greater characterization with a larger prospective cohort in a design more suited to evaluating such longitudinal changes may be warranted to further investigate the precise nature of these power abnormalities with disease progression.

Occipito-temporal dysfunction drives differences in RTT subgroups

While the existence of stable neurophysiological correlates of genetic and phenotypic subtypes is interesting in itself, analysis of the nature of the between-groups differences offer insight into the nature of the dysfunctions responsible for the observed differences at the clinical level.

Notably, differences in global connectivity of occipital and temporal networks appear to be tightly linked to the clinical severity of RTT. Loss of these functioning within these networks is consistent with a loss of normal sensory integration, providing a logical neurologic correlate to the severity of neurodevelopmental deficit produced. Furthermore, preservation of speech in the PSV variant appears to be particularly related to increased integration of parietal networks, which may offer a mechanistic insight into the reasons for the language loss observed in the typical Rett phenotype.

Additionally, more clinically "severe" syndromes such as those produced by *CDKL5* mutations tend to be associated with marked abnormalities in within- and cross-frequency network function in delta band. Given typical associations of such slow-wave activity with unconsciousness, neurodegenerative conditions and temporal lobe epilepsy, abnormalities in delta network in these severe syndromes may play a role in the observed rapid regression, lack of responsiveness and treatment-refractory epilepsy.

Epilepsy status is associated with specific network features in RTT

Both the presence of epilepsy and its response to treatment are also associated with specific electrophysiological features. Notably, the presence of epilepsy is largely driven by measures of occipital asymmetry across all bands. This is suggestive of an abnormal distribution of activity in occipital regions in patients with epilepsy, consistent with the proposed role of dysfunction in occipital networks in determining clinical severity. Given that epilepsy is classically attributed to abnormal synchronous neuronal discharges, this may suggest the presence of excessively active networks in the occipital regions acting as a focus for seizure onset in these patients, further underlining the particular role played by abnormalities of occipital network formation in the clinical phenotype of RTT.

Within those with clinically evident epilepsy, treatment resistance was marked by specific network-level abnormalities; in particular, a pattern of low global integration of frontotemporal networks was observed in those refractory to treatment, a pattern not observed as particularly characteristic of any genetic or clinical subtype. This suggests that reduced response to treatment is associated with increasingly disordered network architecture, beyond that observed in non-epileptic or treatment-responsive patients. This particularly disordered network function may increase seizure predisposition to such an extent that it is not overcome by medical therapies to the same extent as in those with less disordered architecture. Such an explanation also ties into the association of epilepsy with particular mutations and particularly severe clinical pictures, in that more "severe" network-level abnormalities may further increase the predisposition to epilepsy, and the likelihood that the epilepsy will be treatment-refractory.

Interestingly, as both coherence measures and asymmetry were demonstrated to remain stable over time, these features may serve as predictive markers of epilepsy and treatment responsiveness in RTT. This would provide a very valuable biomarker for the prediction of patient outcomes. A prospective analysis of the ability of occipital asymmetry and global measures of network integration to predict onset of epilepsy in new cases of RTT would be valuable in validating these features as clinically useful biomarkers in RTT.

Despite being the first report on the electrophysiological characterization of Rett Syndrome variants, the current study was limited by a relatively small number of the rare subtypes of RTT. This may have limited the ability to detect differences in some measures, particularly those marked by a large degree of variance. Several features showed interesting trends, such as a marked pattern of asymmetry observed in the *CDKL5* group, which may have reached statistical significance if greater statistical power were available, potentially offering even greater insight into the differences between these subtypes. However, for a disorder with a population prevalence of 1 per 10,000 live female births, and where the

known variants are rare, our sample is very large and presents the first report on electrophysiological differences between these variants.

Additionally, the use of small numbers of electrodes limited the amount of electrophysiological data collected. Greater data availability may allow further characterisation of the specific features of each of these subtypes. This limitation was largely due to the need to use small caps with limited montages with the young children with behavioural disorders included in the study. Notably, marked differences at the network level were still distinguished despite these limitations, suggesting strong differences in these measures.

Conclusion

This study represents the first electrophysiological characterisation of RTT subtypes. We demonstrate the role of dysfunctional network architecture as an important intermediary between genetic dysregulation of synapse formation and clinical phenotype. We further provide evidence for a specific role of occipito-temporal networks in the pathogenesis of RTT, and demonstrate that electrophysiological features are strongly associated with co-morbid epilepsy status. We show that network features appear to be stable over time, outlining potential value as a biomarker for diagnosis, classification and prognostication of RTT subtypes. Further work using a longitudinal analysis of a prospective cohort will allow greater elucidation of the prognostic value of electrophysiologic measures in this rare disorder.

Abbreviations
CDLK5: Cyclin dependent kinase-like 5; EEG: Electroencephalogram; MeCP2: Methyl CpG binding protein 2; PSV: Preserved speech variant; RTT: Rett syndrome

Acknowledgements
We sincerely thanks the patients (and their families) who participated in the present study.

Funding
No funding was received to carry out the work in this paper. However, the International Rett Syndrome Foundation (IRSF) contributed towards the publication fees for the manuscript.

Authors' contributions
We adhere to the International Committee of Medical Journal Editors (ICMJE) for authorship. CK was responsible for study conceptualisation, analysis of all

patient EEG, clinical and genetic data, preparation of the original manuscript. DT & GP designed and conceptualised the present study and were responsible for critical appraisal of the manuscript. AHD was responsible for preliminary EEG and clinical data analysis, manuscript drafting and editing. IG, PdM, SB were responsible for patient assessment and acquiring patient data. RR gave substantial advise on EEG data analysis and interpretation. He also contributed to the preparation of the manuscript. All authors read and approved the final manuscript.

Competing interests
The authors declare that they have no competing interests.

Author details
[1]School of Medicine, Trinity College Dublin, 152-160 Pearse Street, Dublin 2, Ireland. [2]Tuscany Rett Center, Ospedale Versilia, 55043 Lido di Camaiore, Italy. [3]Medical Genetic Unit, Ferrara University Hospital, Ferrara, Italy. [4]Trinity Centre for Bioengineering, Trinity College Dublin, Dublin 2, Ireland. [5]Neuropsychiatric Genetics, Trinity Centre for Health Sciences, St. James's Hospital, D8 Dublin, Ireland. [6]Trinity College Institute of Neuroscience (TCIN), Lloyd Building, Trinity College Dublin, Dublin 2, Ireland.

References
1. Cahrour M, Zoghbi HY. The story of Rett syndrome: from clinic to neurobiology. Neuron. 2007;56:422–37. https://doi.org/10.1016/j.neuron.2007.10.001.
2. Neul JL, Zoghbi HY. Rett syndrome: a prototypical neurodevelopmental disorder. Nueroscientist. 2004;10:118–28.
3. Kozinetz CA, Skender ML, MacNaughton N, Almes MJ, Schultz RJ, Percy AK, et al. Epidemiology of Rett syndrome: a population based registry. Pediatrics. 1993;91(2):445–50.
4. Pini G, Bigoni S, Congiu L, Romanelli AM, Scusa MF, Di Marco P, et al. Rett syndrome: a wide clinical and autonomic picture. Orphanet J Rare Dis. 2016; 11:132. https://doi.org/10.1186/s13023-016-0499-7.
5. Cheng TL, Qiu Z. MeCP2: multifaceted roles in gene regulation and neural development. Neurosci Bull. 2014;30(4):601–9.
6. Kaufman WE, Johnston MV, Blue ME. MeCP2 expression and function during brain development: implications for Rett syndrome's pathogenesis and clinical evolution. Brain Dev. 2005;27(1):77–87.
7. Amir RE, Van den Veyver IB, Wan M, Tran CQ, Francke U, Zoghbi HY. Rett syndrome is caused by mutations in X-linked MECP2, encoding methyl-CpG-binding protein 2. Nat Genet. 1999;23(2):185–8.
8. Chen Q, Zhu YC, Yu J, Miao S, Zheng J, Xu L, et al. CDKL5, a protein associated with Rett syndrome, regulates neuronal morphogenesis via Rac1 signalling. J Neurosci. 2010;30:12777–86.
9. Pini G, Bigoni S, Engerstrom IW, Calabrese O, Felloni B, Scusa MF, et al. Variant of Rett syndrome and CDLK 5 gene: clinical and autonomic description of 10 cases. Neuropaediatrics. 2012;43(1):37–43.
10. Kalscheuer VM, Tao J, Donnelly A, Hollway G, Schwinger E, Kubary S, et al. Disruption of the serine/threonine kinase 9 gene causes severe X-linked infantile spasms and mental retardation. Am J Hum Genet. 2003;72:1401–11.
11. Zapella M, Meloni I, Longo I, Hayek G, Renieri A. Preserved speech variants of the Rett syndrome: molecular and clinical analysis. Am J Med Genet. 2001;104:14–22.
12. Renieri A, Mari F, Mencarelli MA, Scala E, Ariani F, Longo I, et al. Diagnostic criteria for the Zapella variant of Rett Snydrome (the preserved speech variant). Brain and Development. 2009;31:208–16.
13. LeBlanc JJ, DeGregoria G, Centofante E, Vogel-Farley VK, Barnes K, Kaufman WE, Fagiolini M, Nelson CA. Visual evoked potentials detect cortical processing deficits in Rett syndrome. Ann Neurol. 2015;78:775–86.
14. Stauder JE, Smeets EE, van Mil SG, Curfs LG. The development of visual and auditory processing in Rett syndrome: an ERP study. Brain and Development. 2006;28(8):487–94.
15. Peters SU, Katzenstein A, Jones D, Key AP. Distinguishing Response to Names in Rett and MECP2 Duplication Syndrome: An ERP Study of Auditory Social Information Processing. 2017 1675: 71–77. https://doi.org/10.1016/j.brainres.2017.08.028.
16. Ammanuel S, Chan WC, Adler DA, Lakshamanan BM, Gupta SS, Ewen JB. Heightened Delta power during slow wave sleep in patients with Rett syndrome associated with poor sleep efficacy. PLoS One. 2015;10(10): e0138113. https://doi.org/10.1271/jurnal/pone.0138113.
17. Glaze DG. Neurophysiology of Rett syndrome. J Child Neurol. 2005;20(9): 740–6.
18. Wang J, Barstein J, Ethridge LE, Mosconi MW, Takarae Y, Sweeney JA. Resting state EEG abnormalities in autism Spectrum disorders. J Neurodev Disord. 2013;5:24.
19. Heunis TM, Aldrich D, de Vries PJ. Recent advances in resting-state electroencephalography biomarkers for autism Spectrum disorder – a review of methodological and clinical challenges. Pediatr Neurol. 2016; 61:28–37.
20. Billeci L, Sicca F, Maharana K, Apicella F, Narzisi A, Campatelli G, et al. On the application of quantitative EEG for Characterising autistic brain: a systematic review. Front Hum Neurosci. 2013;7:442. https://doi.org/10.3389/fnhum.2013.00442.
21. Murias M, Webb SJ, Greenson J, Dawson G. Resting state cortical connectivity reflected in EEG coherence in individuals with autism. Biol Psychiatry. 2007;62:270–3.
22. Coben R, Mohammad-Rezazadeh I, Cannon RL. Using quantitative and analytic EEG methods in the understanding of connectivity in autism Spectrum disorders: a theory of mixed over and under connectivity. Front Hum Neurosci. 2014. https://doi.org/10.3389/fnhum.2014.00045.
23. De Rubeis S, He X, Goldberg AP, Poultney CS, Samocha K, Cicek AE, et al. Synaptic, transcriptional and chromatin genes disrupted in autism. Nature. 2014;515(7526):209–15.
24. Nunez P & Srinivasan R. Electric fields of the brain: Oxford University press, 2006.
25. Bullmore E, Sporns O. Complex brain networks: graph theoretical analysis of structural and functional systems. Nat. Rev. Neurosci. 2009;10:186–98.

22

How often parents make decisions with their children is associated with obesity

Adrita Rahman[1], Kimberly G. Fulda[2,3]*(iD), Susan F. Franks[2,3], Shane I. Fernando[2,4], Nusrath Habiba[4] and Omair Muzaffar[2,3]

Abstract

Background: Evidence supports that better parental involvement and communication are related to reduced obesity in children. Parent-child collaborative decision-making is associated with lower BMI among children; while child-unilateral and parent-unilateral decision-making are associated with overweight children. However, little is known about associations between joint decision-making and obesity among Hispanic youth. The purpose of this analysis was to determine the relationship between parent-child decision making and obesity in a sample of predominantly Hispanic adolescents.

Methods: Data from two studies focused on risk for type II diabetes were analyzed. A total of 298 adolescents 10–14 years of age and their parent/legal guardian were included. Parents completed questionnaires related to psychosocial, family functioning, and environmental factors. Multiple logistic regression was used to determine the association between obesity ($\geq$ 95th percentile for age and gender), the dependent variable, and how often the parent felt they made decisions together with their child (rarely/never, sometimes, usually, always), the primary independent variable. Covariates included gender, age, ethnicity, total family income, and days participated in a physical activity for at least 20 min. ORs and 95% CIs were calculated.

Results: Adolescent participants were predominantly Hispanic $n = 233$ (78.2%), and approximately half $n = 150$ (50.3%) were female. In multivariate analyses, adolescents who rarely/never made decisions together with their family had significantly higher odds (OR = 3.50; 95% CI [1.25–9.83]) of being obese than those who always did. No association was observed between either those who sometimes make decisions together or those who usually did and those that always did.

Conclusions: Parents and children not making decisions together, an essential aspect of parent-child communication, is associated with increased childhood obesity. The results of our study contribute to evidence of parental involvement in decision-making as an important determinant of adolescent health. Further studies should explore temporal relationships between parenting or communication style and obesity.

Keywords: Obesity, Adolescent – Parent communication, Decision making between parents and adolescents

* Correspondence: kimberly.fulda@unthsc.edu
[2]North Texas Primary Care Practice-Based Research Network (NorTex),
University of North Texas Health Science Center at Fort Worth, 3500 Camp
Bowie Blvd, Fort Worth, TX 76107, USA
[3]Department of Family Medicine, Texas College of Osteopathic Medicine,
University of North Texas Health Science Center at Fort Worth, 3500 Camp
Bowie Blvd, Fort Worth, TX 76107, USA
Full list of author information is available at the end of the article

Background

Disparities between Hispanic and non-Hispanic populations in the area of childhood and adolescent obesity are critically important to understand, as these may predict related health disparities that can continue throughout life [1–4]. In 2015-2016, 25.8% of Hispanic youth were obese, compared to 22.0% of non-Hispanic black youth and 14.1% of non-Hispanc white youth [5]. Studies have shown that, similar to other ethnic groups [6], the rise in obesity among Hispanic youth is multifactorial involving a combination of genetic factors [7] and environmental factors [1], which include parental influence [8].

Lack of parental involvement and communication have consistently been highly related to obesity in children and adolescents [9–14]. Healthy family functioning, which consists of good communication, problem solving, roles, affective responsiveness, affective involvement, and behavioral control, is associated with more frequent family meals, greater daily vegetable and fruit consumption, more frequent breakfast consumption, fewer hours of sedentary behavior, lower BMI and lower percent overweight in adolescent girls [9]. Greater communication between parents and children also promotes healthier nutritional habits, lower weight and greater physical activity [10–12]. Furthermore, shared parent-child activities have been associated with less overweight and obesity [13]. One study found that children who made more decisions themselves, especially regarding nutrition, were more likely to be obese [14]. Parent-child collaborative decision-making is associated with better health behaviors, including healthy eating behaviors [15].

Unhealthy nutritional habits, physical inactivity, and being overweight or obese are all well-established modifiable risk factors for type II diabetes [16]. Also, having the perception of insufficient parental care and inadequate parental communication has been linked to higher risk for mental and behavioral problems, including unhealthy weight control habits among adolescents [17]. Lower maternal sensitivity is associated with adolescent obesity [18], and poor maternal-child relationships at the ages of 15, 24 and 36 months of age is associated with higher adolescent obesity [19]. Having good communication with parents, therefore, may be a protective factor for obesity and type II diabetes among adolescents.

Children whose parents talk to them about weight loss and restrict their eating practices are more likely to engage in unhealthy and disordered eating habits and gain weight, while those whose parents discuss healthy eating are less likely to eat unhealthy [20–23]. Parents using more lax and coercive disciplinary strategies, fewer health promoting techniques, and possessing less confidence in child lifestyle behavior management are more likely to have obese children [24]. In summation, an authoritative parenting style, where decision-making is collaborative, is associated with lower BMI among children and adolescents [25, 26], while more permissive/indulgent and rejecting/uninvolved parenting styles, where decision-making is child-unilateral, and authoritarian parenting and feeding styles, where decision-making is parent-unilateral, are associated with overweight children [8, 27–30].

Restriction of dietary intake is more common among parents who are racial or ethnic minorities, have low income, and have less than a high school education [31]. However, little is known about associations between parent-child communication and obesity among Hispanic youth. Studies have shown that Mexican-American adolescents have greater respect for parental authority and interdependence and less personal autonomy and independence, indicating less child-unilateral decision making, compared to white American adolescents [32–36]. For instance, Mexican mothers of young teenage daughters expect increases in parent-child mutual decision-making after their daughters turn 15 years old, a delayed age compared to other ethnic groups in the U.S. [36] Furthermore, Mexican-American mothers of very young children are the primary decision-makers when it comes to behaviors related to obesity, including sleep, physical activity and television screen time, although parents and children sometimes or often make decisions together regarding nutrition [37]. There is, however, a lack of a complete understanding of the determinants of the disparities in obesity. For example, participants in focus groups with low-income Hispanic mothers said their children liked fast food, and they placed no restrictions on the food their child wanted and decided to eat [38]. In another study, Hispanic parents said they allowed their child to decide what to eat as alternatives, and pressured them to eat more food [39]. We hypothesized that parent-child cooperative decision making as reported by the parent is associated with childhood obesity in Hispanic and non-Hispanic adolescents.

Methods

Study design

The association between parent-child decision making and obesity was explored using data from two cross-sectional studies focused on risk for type II diabetes and adolescence. These studies were titled "Factors Associated with Being at Risk for Type 2 Diabetes among Mexican and Mexican-American Children" (DMMX) and "Psychosocial and Physiological Predictors of Type 2 Diabetes Mellitus among Children Aged 10-14" (PedDM). Data were collected from 298 participants in Tarrant County, Texas between both study protocols. Subjects included adolescents (age 10 to 14 years, male or female, English or Spanish speaking) with a parent or legal guardian. The DMMX study only included Mexican (recruited at a partner institution in Mexico) or Mexican-American (recruited locally in the US) adolescents; whereas, the PedDM study included all race/ethnicities (recruited in the US). Only the Mexican American child participants from the DMMX study were included in the current analysis. The participants recruited in Mexico were not included in this analysis. Identical methods were used for both studies, and participants were recruited from the same geographical area, which allows for combining the data to have a larger sample size. Both studies included nondiabetic child participants. Exclusion criteria from the original studies consisted of having cystic fibrosis, diabetes mellitus, genetic syndromes, hypo- or hyperthyroidism, adrenal disease (Addison's or Cushing syndrome), taking oral corticosteroids (prednisone, prednisolone, orapred, decadron, dexamethasone) during the past year, or inability to provide consent. Parental consent and child assent were obtained since adolescent subjects were minors. Study procedures included one encounter at the University of North Texas Health Science Center (UNTHSC) that lasted about two hours. Parents completed surveys related to psychosocial, family functioning, and environmental factors. Survey questions were obtained from the National Survey of Children's Health 2012. Demographic information, such as gender, date of birth, race/ethnicity, socioeconomic status and household size were also obtained. Study materials were available in English and Spanish.

Study methodologies were approved by the Institutional Review Board of UNTHSC at Fort Worth, Texas.

Dependent variables

The primary dependent variable for this analysis is obesity, a categorical variable. Adolescent participants were classified as obese and non-obese. Body mass index (BMI) was calculated, and participants were categorized into BMI percentiles based on age and gender, according to CDC guidelines [40]. Those who were at the 95th percentile or above were classified as "obese", and those under the 95th percentile were classified as "non-obese" [41]. BMI was used instead of other measures of obesity since it is routinely collected in a clinic setting.

Primary independent variables

Parents/legal guardians were asked the question "How often do you feel that your child and you make decisions about his/her life together?" The responses were recorded in a Likert scale as "never," "rarely", "sometimes", "usually" and "always." The five categories were condensed into four categories; "rarely or never," "sometimes", "usually" and "always". "Rarely" and "never" were combined because there were very few people in the "never" category. This question is used by the Centers of Disease Control and Prevention in the National Survey of Children's Health, 2007 and the National Survey of Adoptive Parents to assess the subdomain Parent/Child Relationship under Family Functioning [42].

Covariates

Potential covariates in the current analysis included gender, age, ethnicity (Hispanic, non-Hispanic), total family income per year (less than $10,000, $10,000 to 19,999, $20,000 to $29,999, $30,000 to $39,999, $40,000 or more), and days participated in a physical activity for at least 20 min (less than 7 days, 7 days, I don't know). The category "I don't know" was included because the association between the lack of parent's knowledge regarding their child's physical activities and the child's BMI needed to be examined as well as lack of physical activity. It was perceived as representative of the parent's lack of involvement in the child's daily activities.

Statistical analysis

All analyses were conducted using SPSS software version 22 [43]. Descriptive statistics such as means and frequencies are provided for all variables and for levels of the dependent variable BMI (95th percentile or greater and less than the 95th percentile). Independent samples T-tests were used to assess differences between obese and non-obese participants for the continuous variable age, and chi-square tests were used to assess differences in categorical variables between levels of obesity. Simple and multiple logistic regression models were employed to examine associations between obesity and independent variables. Crude and adjusted odds ratios and 95% confidence intervals were estimated. Missing data were excluded from the analysis. Only 2% of cases had missing data. Multi-collinearity between independent variables was tested using Tolerance and Variation Inflation Factor (VIF). Results of the multicollinearity tests showed that collinearity between the variables was very low, with VIF values ranging from 1.005 to 1.023 and Tolerance values between 0.995 and 0.977.

Results

Table 1 presents the characteristics of the adolescent participants by presence of obesity (BMI equal to or greater than 95th percentile). A total of 298 adolescent participants were included. After missing data were excluded, 292 participants were included in the final multivariate analysis. The adolescent participants were predominantly Hispanic (78.2%) with an average age of 11.9 (SD = 1.4) years. Distribution of gender was essentially equivalent with 50.3% girls. Of participants, 80.5% of parents/guardians reported that they usually or always made decisions with their child. Only 14.9% of adolescents exercised for at least 20 min all seven days of the weeks. One hundred and forty (47.8%) reported a total household yearly income of less than $20,000. Total household income ($p = 0.04$) significantly differed between obese and non-obese adolescents. A majority of youth (52.8%) who live in households with an income of

Table 1 Characteristics of the Mexican and Mexican-American Children Study participants by BMI ≥ 95th percentile - Fort Worth, Texas, (N = 298)

Variable	Total number (%) of participants for category	BMI ≥ 95th percentile, n (%)	BMI <95th percentile, n (%)	p-value
How often parents make decisions together with child	n = 298			0.15
Rarely or never	20 (6.7)	12 (60.0)	8 (40.0)	
Sometimes	38 (12.8)	14 (36.8)	24 (63.2)	
Usually	117 (39.3)	51 (43.6)	66 (56.4)	
Always	123 (41.3)	41 (33.3)	82 (66.7)	
Age, mean (SD)	n = 298			0.57
	11.87 (1.405)	11.81 (1.5)	11.90 (1.4)	
Sex	n = 298			0.74
Male	148 (49.7)	60 (40.5)	88 (59.5)	
Female	150 (50.3)	58 (38.7)	92 (61.3)	
Ethnicity	n = 298			0.17
Hispanic	233 (78.2)	97 (41.6)	136 (58.4)	
Non-Hispanic	65 (21.8)	21 (32.3)	44 (67.7)	
Days of physical activity for at least 20 min	n = 296			0.16
7 days	44 (14.9)	12 (27.3)	32 (72.7)	
Less than 7 days	211 (71.3)	90 (42.7)	121 (57.3)	
I don't know	41 (13.9)	16 (39.0)	25 (61.0)	
Household income	n = 293			0.04
Less than $10,000	53 (18.1)	28 (52.8)	25 (47.2)	
$10,000 to $19,999	87 (29.7)	30 (34.5)	57 (65.5)	
$20,000 to $29,999	59 (20.1)	23 (39.0)	36 (61.0)	
$30,000 to $39,999	40 (13.7)	21 (52.5)	19 (47.5)	
$40,000 or more	54 (18.4)	16 (29.6)	38 (70.47)	

SD standard deviation

less than $10,000 were obese, compared to a small proportion of obese youth (29.6%) who lived in households with incomes of $40,000 and above.

Results of simple logistic regression are shown in Table 2. In bivariate analyses, parent-child decision-making and household income are both significant predictors of obesity. How often youth were reported to make decisions with their parents was significantly associated with obesity. Youth whose parents reported they rarely or never made decisions together were (OR = 3.000; 95% CI [1.137–7.914] more likely to be obese compared to youth whose parents reported they always made decisions together. Additionally, of the covariates, adolescents in households with a total income of less than $10,000 (OR = 2.660; 95% CI [1.201–5.890]) or with a total income of $30,000 to $39,999 (OR = 2.625; 95% CI [1.119–6.155]) were more likely to be obese than those in households with a total income of $40,000 or more.

Table 3 displays the results of a multiple logistic regression model with obesity as the dependent variable and all other variables as predictors. Adjusting for all other variables, youth whose parents report they rarely or never make decisions together with their parents had significantly higher odds (OR = 3.501; 95% CI [1.247–9.829]) of being obese than those who were reported as always making decisions with their parents. Of the covariates, age, gender, physical activity, and ethnicity had no association with obesity, while household income did. Adolescents living in very low-income households of less than $10,000 (OR = 3.329; 95% CI [1.439–7.703]) and from household incomes between $30,000 and $39,999 (OR = 2.698; 95% CI [1.117–6.515]) had a greater odds of being obese than those who came from families with a household income of $40,000 or greater income even though there were no significant differences between the middle income groups and the highest income group.

Discussion

Parents and children not making decisions together, an essential aspect of parent-child communication, is associated with increased childhood obesity. The results of the present study contribute to evidence of parental involvement in decision-making as an

Table 2 Simple logistic regression for BMI ≥ 95th percentile with crude odds ratios

Variable	Crude OR	95% CI
How often parents make decisions together with child		
Always	...	...
Rarely or never	3.000	(1.137–7.914)
Sometimes	1.167	(0.547–2.490)
Usually	1.545	(0.916–2.609)
Age	0.957	(0.811 - 1.129)
Sex		
Female	...	...
Male	1.082	(0.680–1.721)
Household Income		
$40,000 or more	...	...
Less than $10,000	2.660	(1.201–5.890)
$10,000 to $19,999	1.250	(0.601–2.600)
$20,000 to $29,999	1.517	(0.693–3.324)
$30,000 to $39,999"	2.625	(1.119–6.155)
Ethnicity		
Non-Hispanic	...	...
Hispanic	1.494	(0.836–2.673)
Days of physical activity for at least 20 min		
7 days	...	...
Less than 7 days vs 7 days	1.983	(0.968–4.064)
I don't know vs 7 days	1.707	(0.685–4.253)

... = reference group, *OR* odds ratio, *95% CI* 95% confidence interval

Table 3 Multiple logistic regression for BMI ≥ 95th percentile with adjusted odds ratios

Variable	Adjusted OR	95% CI
How often parents make decisions together with child		
Always	...	...
Rarely or never	3.501	(1.247–9.829)
Sometimes	1.136	(0.511–2.527)
Usually	1.639	(0.940–2.855)
Age	0.956	(0.800 - 1.144)
Sex		
Female	...	...
Male	1.095	(0.669–1.792)
Household Income		
$40,000 or more	...	...
Less than $10,000	3.329	(1.439–7.703)
$10,000 to $19,999	1.170	(0.551–2.486)
$20,000 to $29,999	1.537	(0.687–3.438)
$30,000 to $39,999	2.698	(1.117–6.515)
Ethnicity		
Non-Hispanic	...	...
Hispanic	1.636	(0.862–3.104)
Days of physical activity for at least 20 min		
7 days	...	...
less than 7 days vs 7 days	2.109	(0.981–4.536)
I don't know vs 7 days	2.266	(0.852–6.025)

... = reference group; *OR* odds ratio, *95% CI* 95% confidence interval

important determinant of adolescent health. In this study, youth whose parents reported they rarely or never made decisions with their parents were more likely to have a BMI in the 95th percentile or above compared to those who always made decisions with their parents. The results complement the findings of studies that support relationships between better parent-child communication and reduced child obesity [8, 28–30, 44].

The significant association found in this study between BMI and how often children are reported as making decisions together with their parents complements the literature. How often adolescents make their life decisions with their parents may be representative of how involved the parents are in their children's lives, and also how close the parent-child relationship is in terms of communication and trust. Greater parental involvement may lead to children making fewer negative choices, including those regarding their nutritional and lifestyle habits. Better nutritional and lifestyle choices may in turn make them less likely to be obese compared to peers who make unhealthy decisions. Unhealthy nutritional habits include eating disorders, which are associated with

perception of low parental caring, poor parent-child communication, and valuing peers' opinions over parents' [17]. Therefore, in accordance with previous findings on communication and obesity, adolescents whose parents report rarely make decisions with their families are more likely to be obese.

Interestingly, age does not appear to be a good predictor of obesity in this sample, even though in 2011–2014, there were disparities in obesity prevalence between the age groups of 2 to 5 years, 6 to 11 years and 12 to 19 years [5]. However, the range of our sample is only between the years of 10 and 14 years. Perhaps exploring these associations in a cohort consisting of a wider age range might show different results. Furthermore, the current study did not find gender to be a predictor of high BMI, and there was no statistically significant difference in obesity between Hispanics and non-Hispanics. Being physically active for at least 20 min every day of the week is not associated with decreased obesity in this population, although research shows that physical activity is associated with reduced overweight and obesity among youth [45]. The CDC, however, recommends 60 min of exercise every day for

7 days [46], so perhaps the children in this study were not getting sufficient exercise. A relationship between household annual income of less than $10,000 and presence of obesity is also consistent with the literature, as low socioeconomic status is associated with child obesity. The finding that families earning between $30,000 and $39,999 are more likely to have children with obesity needs further exploration. Results of one study showed that among Mexican-origin families, fathers reported more joint parent-child decision making when they were of high SES, and mothers reported less child-unilateral decision-making when they were of high SES [47]. Despite controlling for the effects of household income, however, a statistically significant association between parent-child decision-making and child obesity remained in our study.

Strengths

One of the strengths of this study is that weight and height were measured and not self-reported by the subjects. Some studies use self-reported weight and height as opposed to measured weight and height [44, 48]. Although overall self-reported height and weight are positively associated with measured height and weight, females and obese children are statistically more likely to under-report their weight, and children who are shorter than 150 cm are more likely to under-report their height [48]. The BMI percentiles are based on those objective measurements, and the study used the online CDC calculator with age and sex of the child.

Limitations

A limitation of this study is its cross-sectional nature. This prevents inferring causation between parent-child decision making and child obesity status. Another limitation is that only one component of parent-child decision making is assessed in this study. Additionally, parent-child decision making was measured using a single item. This item has been used by the CDC to measure family functioning in national surveys; however, future research should include a more robust measure. Information about parental obesity, which is positively associated with childhood obesity [49–54], is also not available for this study. The number of children above a BMI percentile of 95 who were reported to have rarely or never made decisions with their parents was also small, leading to wide confidence intervals in our model. Studies should explore this further by recruiting a larger sample of parents who rarely report joint decision-making with their children.

Conclusions

Future studies should explore temporal or dyadic relationships between parenting or communication style and obesity. Further investigations should explore these associations using causal inference. A longitudinal study would be able to examine these relationships temporally. Those that used self-reported BMI [46] were done in young children, were done in samples not representative of the US youth population [55], or only used maternal relationships [56]. Many cross-sectional studies have been done, but few have been done on how parent-child relationships predict obesity and other cardio-metabolic outcomes later in adulthood. Thus, longitudinal studies should also include cardio-metabolic biological markers in addition to weight and behavioral outcomes.

Additional studies should also include children from different ethnic and cultural backgrounds, as cultural backgrounds could influence relationships between parent-child decision making and obesity in children. For example, a study conducted on Chinese-American youth showed that authoritarian parenting style was associated with lower child obesity, contradictory to studies done on American populations, likely because of greater parental authority and child obedience in Chinese culture compared to American culture [57]. Therefore similar studies should also be conducted with other ethnic populations to see how decision-making is related to weight-related practices and weight status.

Evidence shows that eating behavior can be influenced by sibling behavior [58], and that having an obese sibling increases the likelihood of child obesity [51]. However, most studies investigating parent-child decision making and child weight do not look at sibling relationships, and many that do look at siblings are genetic studies. Therefore, future studies should include relationships between siblings as a potential confounder. One of the limitations was that only one aspect of parent-child communication was explored. Other aspects of communication in relation to obesity status need to be studied. Different developmental ages should be included, as adolescents give more value to their own opinions for making decisions and gradually spend less time with their parents as they grow older [59]. Increasing the age range may help determine when decision-making comes into play and how it affects weight and nutritional health in youth.

Abbreviations
95% CI: 95% confidence interval; OR: Odds ratio

Acknowledgements
We would like to acknowledge the research staff of the North Texas Primary Care Practice-Based Research Network (NorTex) for their help in processing research participants.

Funding
This research was funded through an intramural grant program at the UNT Health Science Center.

Authors' contributions

All authors give consent for publication and approved of the final manuscript. AR conducted the data analysis, drafted the initial manuscript, and approved the final manuscript. KF was PI on one study and co-I on the other study from which data were analyzed, oversaw the data analysis, drafted the initial manuscript, and approved the final manuscript. SFF provided input for the design and analysis of the study, edited the initial manuscript, and approved the final manuscript. SIF provided input for the design and analysis of the study, edited the initial manuscript, and approved the final manuscript. NH was PI on one study and co-I on the other study from which data were analyzed, edited the initial manuscript, and approved the final manuscript. OM edited the initial manuscript and approved the final manuscript.

Competing interests

The authors declare that they have no competing interests.

Author details

[1]Division of Epidemiology and Community Health, School of Public Health, University of Minnesota, 1300 S 2nd Street, Suite 300, Minneapolis, MN 55454, USA. [2]North Texas Primary Care Practice-Based Research Network (NorTex), University of North Texas Health Science Center at Fort Worth, 3500 Camp Bowie Blvd, Fort Worth, TX 76107, USA. [3]Department of Family Medicine, Texas College of Osteopathic Medicine, University of North Texas Health Science Center at Fort Worth, 3500 Camp Bowie Blvd, Fort Worth, TX 76107, USA. [4]Department of Pediatrics, Texas College of Osteopathic Medicine, University of North Texas Health Science Center at Fort Worth, 3500 Camp Bowie Blvd, Fort Worth, TX 76107, USA.

References

1. Butte NF, Cai G, Cole SA, Wilson TA, Fisher JO, Zakeri IF, Ellis KJ, Comuzzie AG. Metabolic and behavioral predictors of weight gain in Hispanic children: the viva la Familia study. Am J Clin Nutr. 2007;85(6):1478–85.
2. Pérez-Morales M, Bacardí-Gascón M, Jiménez-Cruz A. Childhood overweight and obesity prevention interventions among hispanic children in the United States: systematic review. Nutricion Hospitalria. 2012;27(5):1415–21.
3. Wiley J, Cloutier M, Wakefield D, et al. Acculturation determines BMI percentile and noncore food intake in Hispanic children. J Nutr. 2014;144(3):305–10.
4. Zoorob R, Buchowski M, Beech B, et al. Healthy families study: design of a childhood obesity prevention trial for Hispanic families. Contemporary Clinical Trials. 2013;35(2):108–21.
5. Centers for Disease Control and Prevention. Childhood obesity facts. https://www.cdc.gov/obesity/data/childhood.html. Accessed 09 Sept 2018.
6. Böttcher Y, Körner A, Kovacs P, Kiess W. Obesity genes: Implication in childhood obesity. Paediatrics Child Health. 2012;22(1):31–6. http://dx.doi.org.proxy.hsc.unt.edu/10.1016/j.paed.2011.08.009.
7. Butte N, Cai G, Cole S, Comuzzie A. Viva la Familia study: genetic and environmental contributions to childhood obesity and its comorbidities in the Hispanic population. Am J Clin Nutr. 2006;84(3):646–54.
8. Johnson R, Welk G, Saint-Maurice PF, Ihmels M. Parenting styles and home obesogenic environments. Int J Environ Res Public Health. 2012;9(4):1411–26. https://doi.org/10.3390/ijerph9041411.
9. Berge JM, Wall M, Larson N, Loth KA, Neumark-Sztainer D. Family functioning: Associations with weight status, eating behaviors, and physical activity in adolescents. J Adolesc Health. 2013;52(3):351–7. https://doi.org/10.1016/j.jadohealth.2012.07.006.
10. Borra ST, Kelly L, Shirreffs MB, Neville K, Geiger CJ. Developing health messages: qualitative studies with children, parents, and teachers help identify communications opportunities for healthful lifestyles and the prevention of obesity. J Am Diet Assoc. 2003;103(6):721–8.
11. Halliday JA, Palma CL, Mellor D, Green J, Renzaho AM. The relationship between family functioning and child and adolescent overweight and obesity: a systematic review. Int J Obes. 2014;38:480–93.
12. Pinquart M. Associations of general parenting and parent-child relationship with pediatric obesity: A meta-analysis. J Pediatr Psychol. 2014;39(4):381–93. https://doi.org/10.1093/jpepsy/jst144.
13. Benson L, Mokhtari M. Parental employment, shared parent–child activities and childhood obesity. J Fam Econ Iss. 2011;32(2):233–44.
14. Murphy E, Ice C, Mccartney K, Leary J, Cottrell L. Is parent and child weight status associated with decision making regarding nutrition and physical activity opportunities? Appetite. 2012;59(2):563–9.
15. Ndiaye K, Silk KJ, Anderson J, Horstman HK, Carpenter A, Hurley A, Proulx J. Using an ecological framework to understand parent-child communication about nutritional decision- making and behavior. J Appl Commun Res. 2013;41(3):253–74. https://doi.org/10.1080/00909882.2013.792434.
16. Centers for Disease Control and Prevention. Prediabetes: Your Chance to Prevent Type 2 Diabetes. https://www.cdc.gov/diabetes/basics/prevention.html. Updated 2016. Accessed 21 Dec 2016.
17. Ackard DM, Neumark-Sztainer D, Story M, Perry C. Parent–Child connectedness and behavioral and emotional health among adolescents. Am J Prev Med. 2006;30(1):59–66. https://doi.org/10.1016/j.amepre.2005.09.013.
18. Davis R, Ashba J, Appugliese D, et al. Adolescent obesity and maternal and paternal sensitivity and monitoring. Int J Pediatr Obes. 2011; 6(3): 457–463. doi: http://www.tandfonline.com/doi/abs/10.3109/17477166.2010.549490 [doi].
19. Anderson S, Gooze R, Lemeshow S, et al. Quality of Early Maternal – Child Relationship and Risk of Adolescent Obesity. American Academy of Pediatrics. 2011;129(1):132–40. http://pediatrics.aappublications.org/content/129/1/132.long.
20. Gubbels JS, Kremers SP, Stafleu A, et al. Association between parenting practices and children's dietary intake, activity behavior and development of body mass index: The KOALA birth cohort study. Int J Behav Nutr Phys Act. 2011;8:18–5868-8-18. doi: https://doi.org/10.1186/1479-5868-8-18 [doi].
21. Berge JM, Maclehose R, Loth KA, Eisenberg M, Bucchianeri MM, Neumark-Sztainer D. Parent conversations about healthful eating and weight: Associations with adolescent disordered eating behaviors. JAMA Pediatr. 2013;167(8):746–53. https://doi.org/10.1001/jamapediatrics.2013.78.
22. Clark HR, Goyder E, Bissell P, Blank L, Peters J. How do parents' child-feeding behaviours influence child weight? Implications for childhood obesity policy. J Public Health (Oxf). 2007;29(2):132–41. https://doi.org/10.1093/pubmed/fdm012.
23. Loth KA, MacLehose RF, Fulkerson JA, Crow S, Neumark-Sztainer D. Food-related parenting practices and adolescent weight status: A population-based study. Pediatrics. 2013;131(5):e1443–50. https://doi.org/10.1542/peds.2012-3073.
24. Morawska A, West F. Do parents of obese children use ineffective parenting strategies? J Child Health Care. 2013;17(4):375–86. https://doi.org/10.1177/1367493512462263.
25. Berge JM. A review of familial correlates of child and adolescent obesity: what has the 21st century taught us so far? Int J Adolesc Med Health. 2009; 21(4):457–83.
26. Kim MJ, McIntosh WA, Anding J, Kubena KS, Reed DB, Moon GS. Perceived parenting behaviours predict young adolescents' nutritional intake and body fatness. Matern Child Nutr. 2008;4(4):287–303. https://doi.org/10.1111/j.1740-8709.2008.00142.x.
27. Berge JM, Wall M, Bauer KW, Neumark-Sztainer D. Parenting characteristics in the home environment and adolescent overweight: A latent class analysis. Obesity (Silver Spring). 2010;18(4):818–25. https://doi.org/10.1038/oby.2009.324.
28. Hennessy E, Hughes SO, Goldberg JP, Hyatt RR, Economos CD. Parent-child interactions and objectively measured child physical activity: A cross-sectional study. Int J Behav Nutr Phys Act. 2010;7:71–5868-7-71. https://doi.org/10.1186/1479-5868-7-71.
29. Moens E, Braet C, Soetens B. Observation of family functioning at mealtime: A comparison between families of children with and without overweight. J Pediatr Psychol. 2007;32(1):52–63. https://doi.org/10.1093/jpepsy/js1011.
30. Rodenburg G, Kremers SP, Oenema A, van de Mheen D. Psychological control by parents is associated with a higher child weight. Int J Pediatr Obes. 2011;6(5–6):442–9. https://doi.org/10.3109/17477166.2011.590203.
31. Loth KA, MacLehose RF, Fulkerson JA, Crow S, Neumark-Sztainer D. Eat this, not that! parental demographic correlates of food-related parenting practices. Appetite. 2013;60(1):140–7. https://doi.org/10.1016/j.appet.2012.09.019.
32. Fuligni AJ. Authority, autonomy, and parent–adolescent conflict and cohesion: a study of adolescents from Mexican, Chinese, Filipino, and European backgrounds. Dev Psychol. 1998;34(4):782–92.
33. Love JA, Buriel R. Language brokering, autonomy, parent-child bonding, biculturalism, and depression- a study of Mexican American adolescents from immigrant families. Hisp J Behav Sci. 2007;29(4):472–91.

34. Nadeem E, Romo LF. Low-income Latina mothers' expectations for their pregnant daughters' autonomy and interdependence. J Res Adolesc. 2008; 18(2):215–38.

35. Roche K, Caughy M, Schuster M, Bogart L, Dittus P, Franzini L. Cultural orientations, parental beliefs and practices, and Latino adolescents' autonomy and independence. Journal of Youth and Adolescence. 2014; 43(8):1389–403.

36. Romo LF, Mireles-Rios R, Lopez-Tello G. Latina mothers' and daughters' expectations for autonomy at age 15 (La Quinceanera). J Adolesc Res. 2014; 29(2):271–94.

37. Davis RE, Cole SM, Blake CE, McKenney-Shubert SJ, Peterson KE. Eat, play, view, sleep: exploring Mexican American mothers' perceptions of decision making for four behaviors associated with childhood obesity risk. Appetite. 2016;101:104–13.

38. O'dougherty M, Story M, Lytle L. Food choices of young African-American and Latino adolescents- where do parents fit in? J Am Diet Assoc. 2006; 106(11):1846–50.

39. Sherry B, Mcdivitt J, Birch LL, Cook FH, Sanders S, Prish JL, Francis LA, Scanlon KS. Attitudes, practices, and concerns about child feeding and child weight status among socioeconomically diverse white, Hispanic, and African-American mothers. J Am Diet Assoc. 2004;104(2):215–21.

40. Centers for Disease Control and Prevention. BMI Percentile Calculator for Child and Teen English Version. https://www.cdc.gov/healthyweight/bmi/calculator.html. Accessed 07 July 2017.

41. Centers for Disease Control and Prevention. Defining childhood obesity. https://www.cdc.gov/obesity/childhood/defining.html. Updated 2017. Accessed 07 July 2017.

42. Centers for Disease Control and Prevention. National Survey of Children's Health. http://www.cdc.gov/nchs/slaits/nsch.htm. Updated 2013. Accessed 06 Oct 2015.

43. IBM Corporation. IBM SPSS statistics for Macintosh. 2013.

44. Berge JM, Wall M, Loth K, Neumark-Sztainer D. Parenting style as a predictor of adolescent weight and weight-related behaviors. J Adolesc Health. 2010; 46(4):331–8. https://doi.org/10.1016/j.jadohealth.2009.08.004.

45. Center for Disease Control and Prevention. Physical activity and health. https://www.cdc.gov/physicalactivity/basics/pa-health/index.htm. Updated 2015. Accessed 21 Dec 16.

46. Centers for Disease Control and Prevention. How much physical activity do children need? http://www.cdc.gov/physicalactivity/everyone/guidelines/children.html. Updated 2011. Accessed 05 Jan 2014.

47. Perez-Brena NJ, Updegraff KA, Umaña-Taylor AJ. Father- and mother-adolescent decision-making in Mexican-origin families. Journal of Youth and Adolescence. 2012;41(4):460–73.

48. Strauss RS. Comparison of measured and self-reported weight and height in a cross-sectional sample of young adolescents. Int J Obes Relat Metab Disord. 1999;23(8):904–8.

49. Gibson L, Byrne S, Davis E, et al. The role of family and maternal factors in childhood obesity. Med J Aust. 2007;186(11):591–5.

50. Maffeis C, Talamini G, Tato L. Influence of diet, physical activity and parents' obesity on children's adiposity: a four-year longitudinal study. Int J Obes Relat Metab Disord. 1998;22(8):758–64.

51. Pachuki M, Lovenheim M, Harding M. Within-family obesity associations: evaluation of parent, child, and sibling relationships. American Journal of Preventive Medicine. 2014;47(4):382–91. https://doi.org/10.1016/j.amepre.2014.05.018.

52. Schaefer-Graf UM, Pawliczak J, Passow D, et al. Birth weight and parental BMI predict overweight in children from mothers with gestational diabetes. Diabetes Care. 2005;28(7):1745–50.

53. Wang Z, Patterson CM, Hills AP. Association between overweight or obesity and household income and parental body mass index in Australian youth: analysis of the Australian National Nutrition Survey, 1995. Asia Pac J Clin Nutr. 2002;11(3):200–5.

54. Whitaker RC, Wright JA, Pepe MS, Seidel KD, Dietz WH. Predicting obesity in young adulthood from childhood and parental obesity. N Engl J Med. 1997; 337(13):869–73.

55. Lehto R, Ray C, Roos E. Longitudinal associations between family characteristics and measures of childhood obesity. Int J Public Health. 2012; 57:495–503.

56. Rhee KE, Lumeng JC, Appugliese DP, Kaciroti N, Bradley RH. Parenting styles and overweight status in first grade. Pediatrics. 2006;117:2047.

57. Vollmer RL, Mobley AR. Parenting styles, feeding styles, and their influence on child obesogenic behaviors and body weight. A review. Appetite. 2013; 71:232–41. https://doi.org/10.1016/j.appet.2013.08.015.

58. de RNH L, Snoek HM, van JFJ L, van Strien T, Engels RCME. Similarities and reciprocal influences in eating behavior within sibling pairs: a longitudinal study. Eat Behav. 2007;8:464–73.

59. Fuligni AJ, Eccles JS. Perceived parent-child relationships and early adolescents' orientation toward peers. Dev Psychol. 1993;29(4):622–32. https://doi.org/10.1037/0012-1649.29.4.622.

Growth patterns from birth to 24 months in Chinese children: a birth cohorts study across China

Fengxiu Ouyang[1*], Fan Jiang[1,2], Fangbiao Tao[3], Shunqing Xu[4], Yankai Xia[5], Xiu Qiu[6] and Jun Zhang[1*]

Abstract

Background: Assessment of child growth is important in detecting under- and over-growth. We aimed to examine the growth patterns of healthy Chinese infants from birth to 24 months.

Methods: This study was based on six recent birth cohorts across China, which provided data (from 2015) on 4251 children (2174 boys, 2077 girls) who were born at term to mothers without gestational or preexisting diabetes, chronic hypertension, preeclampsia, or eclampsia. Analyses were performed using 28,298 longitudinal anthropometric measures in 4251 children and the LMS method to generate smoothed Z-score growth curves, which were compared to the WHO growth standards (which are based on data from 2003) and current Chinese growth references (which are based on data from 2005).

Results: Most (80.3%) of mother had college education or more, and maternal smoking was rare (0.4%). Compared to the WHO longitudinal growth standards for children aged 0 to 2 years, the growth references from this longitudinal study (length-, weight-, head circumference-, BMI-for-age, and weight-for-length) were significantly higher, for boys and girls; Specifically, the median length-, weight-, head circumference-, BMI-for-age, and weight-for-length was on average 0.9 (range 0.2–1.3) cm, 0.51 (range 0.09–0.74) kg, 0.17 (range − 0.24 to 0.37) cm, 0.70 (range 0.01 to 0.92) kg/m^2, and 0.43 (range 0.01 to 1.07) kg higher in Chinese boys, and 1.3 (range 0.5–1.9) cm, 0.73 (range 0.10–0.91) kg, 0.45 (range 0.15–0.62) cm, 0.7 (range 0.0 to 1.0) kg/m^2, and 0.42 (range 0.00 to 0.64) kg greater in Chinese girls, respectively. Compared to the current China cross-sectional growth references (based on data from a decade ago), growth references from this study were also higher, but the difference was less than that between growth references of this study and WHO growth standards.

Conclusions: This recent multicenter prospective birth cohort study examined early growth patterns in China. The new growth curves represent the growth patterns of healthy Chinese infants evaluated longitudinally from 0 to 24 months of age, and provide references for monitoring growth in early life in modern China that are more recent than WHO longitudinal growth standards from other countries and previous cross-sectional growth references for China.

Keywords: Growth standards, Chinese children, Infancy

* Correspondence: ouyangfengxiu@xinhuamed.com.cn;
ouyangfengxiu@126.com; junjimzhang@sina.com
[1]Ministry of Education and Shanghai Key Laboratory of Children's
Environmental Health, Xinhua Hospital, Shanghai Jiao Tong University School
of Medicine, 1665 Kong Jiang Road, Shanghai 200092, China
Full list of author information is available at the end of the article

Background

The assessment of child growth is important in detecting under- and over-growth, which can provide information for timely intervention. The first 1000 days of life (from conception to 2 years of age) is a period of rapid growth and development, and vulnerable to nutritional and environmental influences [1]. Identifying normal child growth patterns is of fundamental importance in growth assessment.

Both the World Health Organization (WHO) growth standards [2] and the China growth references [3] are being applied in China. The WHO growth standards for children aged 0 to 24 months were constructed based on longitudinal data of children (n = 882) by using selection criteria of having socioeconomic conditions favorable to growth and having access to breastfeeding support (for qualifying as "standard") from the WHO Multicenter Growth Reference Study (MGRS) conducted in six countries from 1997 to 2003 (without a site in China). The China growth charts were constructed from a large (n = 44,250) cross-sectional study based on stratified random sampling of children in nine cities of China, which was conducted from May to October in 2005 [3]. Comparison of the growth curves over the restricted range of ages from 0 to 2 years indicated the reference for China was significant higher for BMI for boys and girls. However, the comparisons were complicated by differences in inclusion/exclusion criteria (for the WHO sample, strict criteria about known constraints on growth and cooperation with feeding recommendations, which led to over 80% of mother-infant pairs being ineligible; for the China sample, multistage stratified cluster sampling was used based on urban/suburban areas, districts, and community, with several exclusion criteria), as well as by differences in the design of the studies (longitudinal for the WHO study and cross-sectional for the study in China). The difference between China growth references and WHO growth standards could have been an artifact, so confirmation study is warranted.

Historically, in some circumstances, secular trends of height have occurred from one generation to the next generation [4]. China has a diverse population, environment, dietary habits and tradition, and it is going through rapid modernization and urbanization. Early child growth has drawn much attention since these factors may affect growth. China started the 1st National Survey on the Physical Growth and Development of Children (NSPGDC) in the nine cities of China in 1975, and conducted the survey every 10 years from 1975 to 2005 to address possible secular trends, with the most recent data (from 2005) providing the current references for growth in China [3] (but in need of a 10-year update in 2015). Longitudinal data from a sample with stricter inclusion/exclusion criteria would provide a better comparison to the WHO standards. A small cohort [5]

recruited in 2007 (n = 1531 retained up to 1 year of age) with strict WHO criteria applied showed significant differences (heavier in weight, longer in length, and bigger in head circumference) compared to WHO standards, as well as compared to the current cross-sectional references, which showed similar differences (except for the 97th percentiles that were lower rather than higher).

Long-term follow-up data has enormous value in evaluating the optimal individual growth trajectory, which may not be captured by cross-sectional data [3, 6]. Between 2012 and 2014, six longitudinal birth cohort studies were launched in China. A number of common exposures shared by all cohorts were collected and common outcomes were observed, which formed the foundation of China Birth Cohort Consortium (CBCC). This collaboration provided, for the first time in China, longitudinal growth data from birth cohorts from various regions of the country, but it still is a convenience sample from an efficient combination of cohorts.

This report examines growth patterns from birth to 24 months in Chinese children by pooling the individual level anthropometric follow-up measures from CBCC. The growth references from the 2015 CBCC will be used for comparison to the 2006 WHO longitudinal growth standards and the 2005 China cross-sectional growth references to provide an update on how healthy infants are growing in modern China.

Methods

Study population and data collection

This study used data from six birth cohorts of CBCC which were located at Shanghai (2 cohorts), Anhui, Guangdong, Hubei, and Jiangsu Provinces and were initiated between 2012 and 2014 (Additional file 1: Table S1_1 and S1_2). Additional file 1: Table S1_2 presents the study objective of each of the 6 cohorts. The original aims of these prospective cohorts were to study the environmental, genetic and behavioral factors during pregnancy and in early childhood, and their effects on pregnancy outcomes, fetal and child growth and development, and risks of diseases. Pregnant women were recruited at hospitals when they came for their routine prenatal care visits.

Weight, length, head circumference, and gestational age at birth were obtained from obstetrical medical records. Child anthropometric measurements including weight, length, and head circumference were conducted by trained study staff or trained pediatric nurses in maternal and child health care centers according to the WHO protocol at 7 targeted ages (42 days, 3, 6, 9, 12, 18 and 24 months; http://www.who.int/childgrowth/training/en/). Recumbent length on infants was measured with infant head position in the Frankfort Vertical Plane, and the soles of the feet flat on the moveable footboard. The cohort staffs were trained by group-watching WHO training video course on weight, length, and head circumference. The pediatric nurse measurements were made as routine care was provided. Infant age was calculated by date at measurement minus date of birth. Feeding type in the first 6 months was classified into three types: exclusive breastfeeding, mixed feeding (i.e., combination of breastfeeding and formula feeding), and exclusive/only formula feeding [7]. Infant passive smoking exposure was defined by the mother or father smoking, or for anyone else living in the home smoking. The diagnosis of gestational diabetes mellitus (GDM) in pregnant women was based on the recommendations of International Association of Diabetes and Pregnancy Study Groups (IADPSG) [8].

For this project, we requested each of the six birth cohort studies to contribute longitudinal child growth data of 1000 singleton children from birth to 2 years of age, or maximum number available at the time of our data request in July, 2016. Two cohorts contributed child follow-up measurements up to 12 months due to later starting date (2014) or child follow-up schedule (Additional file 1: Table S1). The inclusion criteria included singleton live births. The exclusion criteria included: (1) infants born with congenital malformations; (2) pregnancy conceived by assisted reproductive technologies (ART); (3) women with medical complication of sexually transmitted diseases (syphilis, HIV infection, and AIDS); (4) women with pre-existed diabetes. There were 5152 mother-child pairs, which provided a sample almost 6 times greater than the WHO longitudinal cohort from 2003 and over 3 times greater than the previous China longitudinal cohort from 2007. While birth cohort studies used better trained personnel for the growth assessments, more observations can also offset "imprecise observations".

Among the 5152 mothers, 672 had GDM, 213 had preterm deliveries (gestational age < 37 weeks), and 71 had hypertensive disorders in pregnancy. Among the remaining 4258, 7 had missing data on infant sex. To generate the growth references, we used data from 4251 normal term-born children and excluded children of mothers with GDM, hypertensive disorders in pregnancy (e.g., chronic hypertension, gestational hypertension, preeclampsia and eclampsia),children born preterm to avoid the potential influences of known prenatal risk factors [10–12],and children with missing data on sex.

Statistical analysis

We used the LMS method to fit smooth z-score curves for length, weight, head circumference and BMI according to age, and for weight according to length respectively in normal term-born healthy children, stratified by infant sex. [13] The three curves of median (M), coefficient of variation (S) and skewness (L, which is expressed as a Box-Cox power) across age/or length

were fitted as cubic splines by using maximum penalized likelihood [13]. The z-score of child growth measures y (length, weight, head circumference and BMI) at time t (or length t, for weight-for-length) was calculated from the smooth curve L(t), M(t), and S(t) by the formula:

$$z = \frac{[y/M(t)]^{L(t)}-1}{L(t)S(t)}, \text{if } L(t) \neq 0; \; z$$
$$= \frac{\log[y/M(t)]}{S(t)}, \text{if } L(t) = 0$$

By using the maximum penalized likelihood and LMS method, all available data of infants from birth to 27 months, including those followed up to 12 months were able to be used to estimate the smoothing parameters and generate the smoothed curves [9, 13]. The age-based references were truncated at 24 completed months to avoid the right-edge effect [14]. We compared z-scores of 0, ±2, and ± 3 for the growth measures in this study with the WHO standards (http://www.who.int/childgrowth/standards/en/), and the China 2005 references for children aged 0 to 2 years [3], both of which were constructed using similar LMS methods for smoothing procedures [3, 14]. The two-sided t-test was used to test statistical significance of the difference at a $p < 0.05$. The growth curves were constructed by using LMSchartmaker Pro version 2.54 software (Medical Research Council, UK).

We also calculated the 3rd, 10th, 50th, 90th and 97th percentiles of all growth measures in both boys and girls by age with subgroup sample size > 100 observations to summarize our data (without using smoothing technique), and compared these percentiles with WHO standards to show the differences. The analyses were conducted by using SAS 9.4 software (SAS Institute, Cary, North Carolina).

Results

This report presented the z-score curves of 4251 children who were born at term to mothers without gestational or preexisting diabetes, chronic hypertension, preeclampsia, or eclampsia. A total of 28,298 anthropometric measures were obtained from ages 0 to 27 months (Additional file 1: Tables S2 and S3). All were urban children. 51.1% were boys and 54.0% were delivered via C-section. The mean maternal and paternal height was 161.4 (SD 4.9) cm and 174.4 (SD 5.3) cm, respectively. Mean (pre-pregnancy) BMI was 20.6 (SD 2.8) kg/m^2 for mothers and 23.9 (SD 3.3) kg/m^2 for fathers. As expected, boy infants had greater birthweight, length and head circumference than girl infants (Table 1). Most (80.3%) of mother had college education or more and 98.3% of mother were Han ethnicity. During the first 6 months, most (77.6%) of infants were mixed fed, and 13.4% had exclusive breast-feeding. In the first 2 years,

Table 1 Characteristics of 4251 mothers, fathers and children by child sex

	Infant sex		p value
	Boy	Girl	
Sample size	2174	2077	
Maternal factors			
Maternal age (years)	28.7 ± 3.4	28.6 ± 3.5	0.51
Pre-pregnancy weight (kg)	53.8 ± 7.8	53.7 ± 8.1	0.92
Maternal height (cm)	161.3 ± 4.9	161.4 ± 5.0	0.33
Prepregnancy BMI (kg/m²)	20.7 ± 2.8	20.6 ± 2.8	0.46
Mother Education			
Junior high school or lower	136(6.3)	135(6.6)	0.90
High school	287(13.4)	266(13.0)	
College or above	1725(80.3)	1641(80.4)	
Mother smoke during pregnancy			
Yes	10(0.5)	7(0.3)	0.53
No	2148(99.5)	2047(99.7)	
Parity			
Primiparous	1958(90.2)	1885(90.9)	0.44
parous	212(9.8)	188(9.1)	
Mode of Delivery			
Vaginal delivery	994(45.8)	957(46.2)	0.79
C-section	1177(54.2)	1115(53.8)	
Paternal factors			
Father age (years)	30.6 ± 4.4	30.6 ± 4.6	0.69
Father height (cm)	174.2 ± 5.2	174.6 ± 5.3	0.04
Father weight (kg)	72.5 ± 11.2	73.1 ± 11.7	0.14
Father BMI (kg/m²)	23.9 ± 3.2	23.9 ± 3.3	0.56
Father smoke during mother pregnancy			
Yes	568(32.1)	567(34.0)	0.25
No	1199(67.9)	1101(66.0)	
Infant factors			
Birth weight (g)	3399 ± 404	3309 ± 392	< 0.001
Birth length (cm)	50.2 ± 1.4	49.8 ± 1.3	< 0.001
Birth head circumference (cm)	34.1 ± 1.1	34.0 ± 1.0	0.01
Gestational age (weeks)	39.1 ± 1.0	39.3 ± 1.0	< 0.001
Breastfeeding Type (0–6 months)			
Formula feeding	168(8.7)	172(9.4)	0.36
Exclusive Breastfeeding	252(13.0)	252(13.7)	
Mixed feeding	1518(78.3)	1412(76.9)	
Children passive smoking			
No	1187(72.7)	1125(71.5)	0.44
Yes	445(27.3)	448(28.5)	

Data were presented as mean ± SD, and n (%)
χ^2 test for categorical variables and t-test for continuous variables

27.9% of children were exposed to passive-smoking. There was no sex difference for these factors (Table 1). Over the follow-up assessments (see Fig. 1), the children aged 0 to 2 years in this cohort were taller, heavier, and had greater head circumference than the children in the WHO cohort.

Length-for-age

Table 2 presents the growth references of length-for-age at 0, ±1, ±2, and ± 3 SD in our study. In comparison with the corresponding WHO growth standard from 0 to 24 months of age, the median length-for-age was on average 0.9 cm (range 0.2–1.3 cm) higher in Chinese boys, and 1.3 cm (range 0.5–1.9 cm) higher in Chinese girls (Fig. 1). Similarly, for z-score of − 2 (i.e. the cutoffs for defining stunting), child length was on average 1.1 cm taller (range 0.8–1.8 cm) in Chinese boys and 1.6 (range 1.1–2.0) cm taller in Chinese girls than the corresponding sex-specific WHO curves. Likewise, for z-score of − 3 was higher in Chinese boys and girls across age.

Compared to the China growth reference (2005 data), the median length-for-age in our study (2015 data) was on average 0.3 cm higher in boys, and 0.5 cm higher in girls across age (Fig. 2). This might be evidence of a small secular trend. The comparisons to the 2005 China references were more similar than that for the comparisons to the WHO standards (Figs. 1 and 2).

Weight-for-age

Table 3 presents the growth reference of weight-for-age at 0, ±1, ±2, and ± 3 SD in our study. For weight-for-age z-score of − 2 (cutoff point for defining underweight), weight was on average 0.60 (range 0.13–0.94) kg heavier in Chinese boys and 0.80 (range 0.19–1.10) kg heavier in Chinese girls than those of WHO standards across age (Fig. 1).

Compared to China reference from 2005 data, the weight-for-age median in our study (China 2015 data) was on average 0.25 kg higher (range 0.07–0.33 kg) in boys, and 0.34 kg higher (range 0.09–0.42 kg) in girls across age (Fig. 2).

Head circumference-for-age

Table 4 presents the growth reference of head circumference-for-age at 0, ±1, ±2, and ± 3 SD in our study. At the z-score of − 2, head circumference was 0.36 cm greater (range 0.08 to 0.86 cm) in Chinese boys, and 0.76 cm greater (range 0.54 to 1.04 cm) in Chinese girls, than the corresponding WHO standards (Fig. 1).

Compared to cross-sectional 2005 norms for China, the median head circumference-for-age in our study was similar in boys, but on average 0.3 cm greater (range 0.1–0.7 cm) in girls across age (Fig. 2).

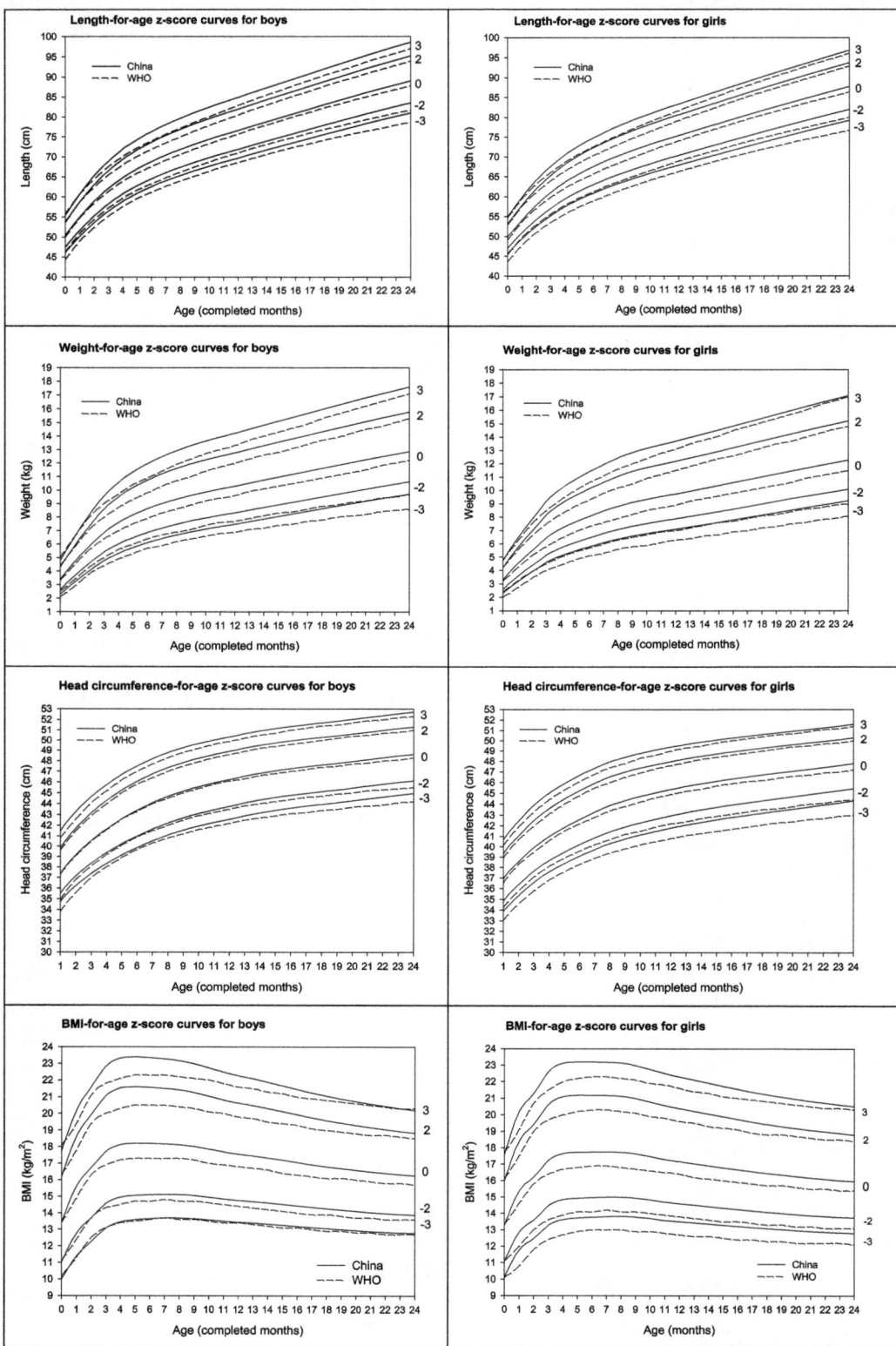

Fig. 1 Comparison of growth-for-age z-score curves with WHO standards in boys and girls

Table 2 Length (cm)-for-age z-score curves at 0, ±1, ±2, and ± 3 SD for Chinese boys and girls from birth to 24 months

Age (month)	Boys										Girls									
	L	M	S	-3SD	-2SD	-1SD	0SD	1SD	2SD	3SD	L	M	S	-3SD	-2SD	-1SD	0SD	1SD	2SD	3SD
0	−0.7996	50.3	0.0306	46.0	47.4	48.8	50.3	51.9	53.6	55.3	−1.0973	49.9	0.0305	45.7	47.0	48.4	49.9	51.5	53.2	55.0
1	−0.7996	54.9	0.0318	50.1	51.6	53.2	54.9	56.7	58.6	60.6	−0.9519	54.2	0.0320	49.4	50.9	52.5	54.2	55.9	57.9	59.9
2	−0.7996	58.9	0.0326	53.6	55.3	57.1	58.9	60.9	63.0	65.3	−0.6922	57.9	0.0331	52.6	54.3	56.0	57.9	59.9	62.0	64.2
3	−0.7996	62.2	0.0330	56.6	58.3	60.2	62.2	64.3	66.6	69.0	−0.3981	61.0	0.0338	55.3	57.1	59.0	61.0	63.2	65.4	67.7
4	− 0.7996	64.8	0.0331	58.9	60.8	62.8	64.8	67.1	69.4	71.9	−0.1356	63.6	0.0342	57.4	59.4	61.4	63.6	65.8	68.1	70.5
5	−0.7996	67.0	0.0332	60.9	62.8	64.8	67.0	69.3	71.7	74.3	0.0640	65.7	0.0343	59.2	61.3	63.5	65.7	68.0	70.3	72.8
6	−0.7996	68.8	0.0331	62.6	64.5	66.6	68.8	71.2	73.7	76.3	0.2052	67.5	0.0344	60.8	63.0	65.2	67.5	69.9	72.3	74.8
7	−0.7996	70.5	0.0330	64.0	66.1	68.2	70.5	72.9	75.4	78.1	0.2974	69.1	0.0344	62.2	64.5	66.8	69.1	71.5	74.0	76.5
8	−0.7996	71.9	0.0330	65.4	67.4	69.6	71.9	74.4	76.9	79.7	0.3533	70.6	0.0344	63.5	65.8	68.2	70.6	73.0	75.6	78.1
9	−0.7996	73.2	0.0329	66.6	68.7	70.9	73.2	75.7	78.3	81.1	0.3867	71.9	0.0344	64.7	67.1	69.5	71.9	74.4	77.0	79.6
10	−0.7996	74.4	0.0329	67.7	69.8	72.0	74.4	76.9	79.6	82.5	0.4064	73.1	0.0343	65.8	68.2	70.7	73.1	75.7	78.3	80.9
11	−0.7996	75.5	0.0328	68.7	70.8	73.1	75.5	78.1	80.8	83.7	0.4167	74.3	0.0342	66.9	69.3	71.8	74.3	76.9	79.5	82.1
12	−0.7996	76.6	0.0328	69.7	71.9	74.2	76.6	79.2	82.0	84.9	0.4203	75.4	0.0342	67.9	70.3	72.8	75.4	78.0	80.6	83.3
13	−0.7996	77.7	0.0328	70.7	72.9	75.2	77.7	80.3	83.1	86.1	0.4205	76.5	0.0341	68.9	71.4	73.9	76.5	79.1	81.8	84.5
14	− 0.7996	78.8	0.0328	71.7	73.9	76.3	78.8	81.5	84.3	87.3	0.4189	77.6	0.0341	69.9	72.4	74.9	77.6	80.2	82.9	85.7
15	−0.7996	79.9	0.0327	72.7	74.9	77.3	79.9	82.6	85.4	88.5	0.4166	78.6	0.0340	70.9	73.4	76.0	78.6	81.3	84.1	86.9
16	−0.7996	81.0	0.0327	73.7	76.0	78.4	81.0	83.7	86.6	89.7	0.4142	79.7	0.0339	71.8	74.4	77.0	79.7	82.5	85.2	88.1
17	−0.7996	82.1	0.0327	74.7	77.0	79.4	82.1	84.8	87.8	90.9	0.4125	80.8	0.0339	72.8	75.4	78.1	80.8	83.6	86.4	89.2
18	−0.7996	83.1	0.0327	75.6	78.0	80.5	83.1	85.9	88.9	92.1	0.4121	81.8	0.0338	73.8	76.4	79.1	81.8	84.6	87.5	90.4
19	−0.7996	84.1	0.0327	76.6	78.9	81.5	84.1	87.0	90.0	93.2	0.4134	82.9	0.0337	74.7	77.4	80.1	82.9	85.7	88.6	91.5
20	−0.7996	85.2	0.0327	77.5	79.9	82.4	85.2	88.0	91.1	94.3	0.4154	83.9	0.0336	75.7	78.3	81.1	83.9	86.7	89.6	92.6
21	−0.7996	86.1	0.0327	78.4	80.8	83.4	86.1	89.0	92.1	95.4	0.4169	84.9	0.0336	76.6	79.3	82.0	84.9	87.7	90.7	93.7
22	−0.7996	87.1	0.0327	79.3	81.7	84.3	87.1	90.0	93.2	96.5	0.4172	85.8	0.0335	77.5	80.2	83.0	85.8	88.8	91.7	94.7
23	−0.7996	88.1	0.0327	80.1	82.6	85.3	88.1	91.0	94.2	97.5	0.4164	86.8	0.0335	78.4	81.1	83.9	86.8	89.8	92.7	95.8
24	−0.7996	89.0	0.0327	81.0	83.5	86.2	89.0	92.0	95.2	98.6	0.4146	87.8	0.0334	79.2	82.0	84.9	87.8	90.7	93.8	96.8

BMI-for-age

Table 5 presents the growth reference of BMI-for-age at 0, ±1, ±2, and ± 3 SD in our study. As shown in Fig. 1, median BMI-for-age was on average 0.70 kg/m^2 (range 0.01 to 0.92 kg/m^2) higher in Chinese boys, and 0.7 (range 0.0 to 1.0) kg/m^2 higher in Chinese girls than the corresponding WHO standards across the age of 0–24 months. For z-score of 2, BMI on average ~ 0.70 kg/m^2 higher in Chinese boys and girls than the WHO standards.

Compared to the China corresponding growth references from 2005 data, the median BMI-for-age in our study was on average 0.3 kg/m^2 higher in boys and 0.4 kg/m^2 higher in girls across age (Fig. 2).

Weight-for-length

Table 6 presents the growth references of weight-for-length at 0, ±1, ±2, and ± 3 SD in our study. Median weight-for-length was on average 0.43 kg greater (range 0.01 to 1.07 kg) than WHO standards in boys, and 0.42 kg greater (range 0.00 to 0.64 kg) in Chinese girls from body length ≥ 50 cm (Fig. 3), but lighter weight at the very short length in Chinese girls (< 52 cm).

For z-score of – 2 (cutoff for wasting definition) in boys, weight was ~ 0.29 kg higher (range 0.003–0.94 kg) than the WHO standard at length ≥ 64 cm; between length 45–63 cm, it was 0.08 kg lower (ranged 0.02 to – 0.17) (Fig. 3). In Chinese girls, the weight-for-length values at z-score of – 2 were on average 0.44 kg heavier (ranging 0.001 to 0.85 kg) than the WHO standards for length ≥ 49 cm. For z-score of 2 (cutoff for overweight definition), compared to the WHO standards, weight was on average 0.39 kg higher (range 0.04 to 0.75 kg) in Chinese boys, and 0.34 kg higher (range 0.06 to 0.64 kg) in Chinese girls for the length ≥ 50 cm. Similarly, for z-score of 3, weight-for-length was on average 0.16 kg higher (range – 0.11to 0.36 kg) in Chinese boys, and was 0.30 kg higher (range 0.00 to 0.64 kg) at most length (49 cm to 95 cm) in Chinese girls than the WHO standards.

Compared to cross-sectional 2005 growth references for China, the median weight-for-length was on average

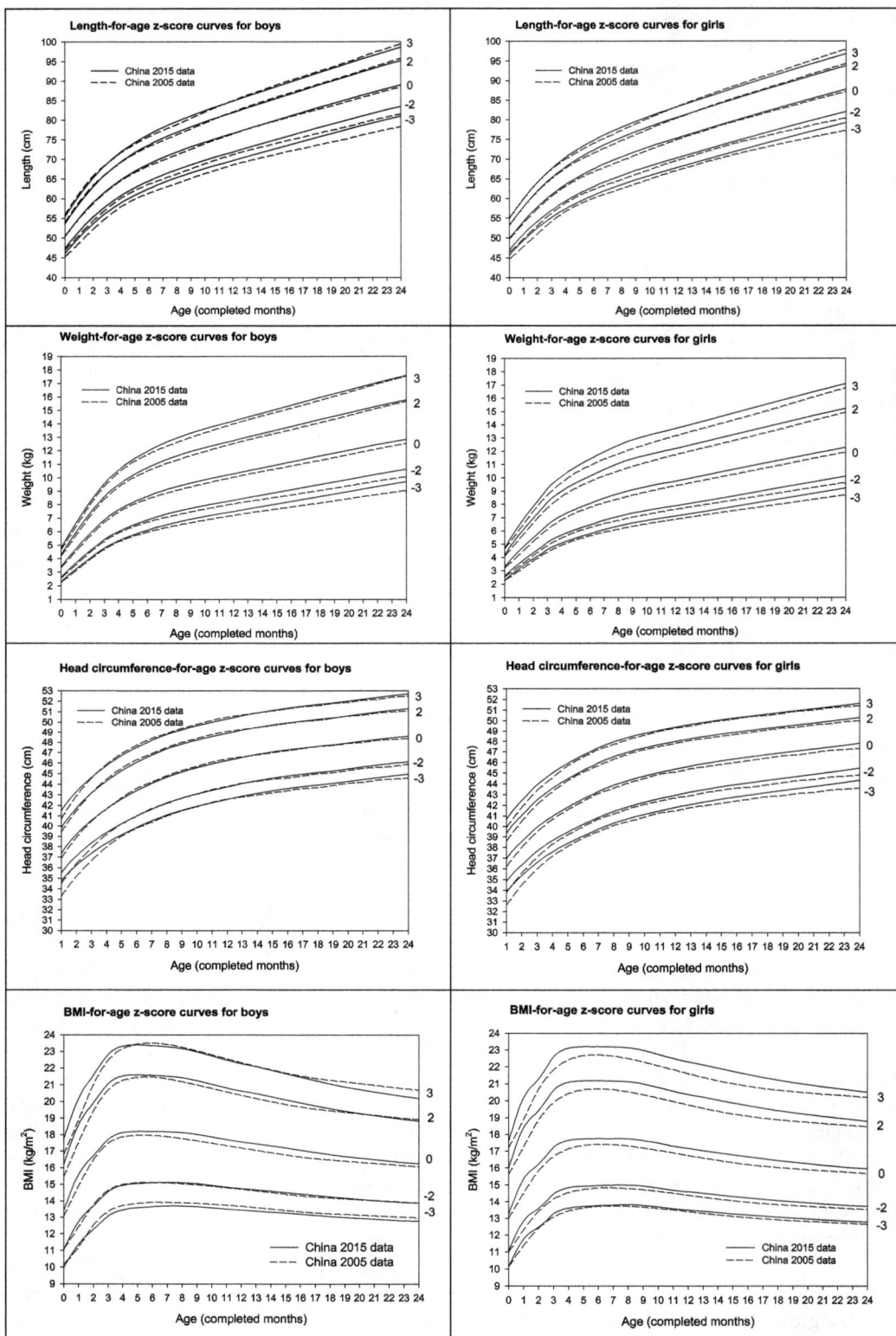

Fig. 2 Comparison of growth-for-age z-score curves from China 2015 data (the present study) with those from China 2005 data in boys and girls

Table 3 Weight (kg)-for-age z-score curves at 0, ±1, ±2, and ± 3 SD for Chinese boys and girls from birth to 24 months

Age (months)	Boys										Girls									
	L	M	S	-3SD	-2SD	-1SD	0SD	1SD	2SD	3SD	L	M	S	-3SD	-2SD	-1SD	0SD	1SD	2SD	3SD
0	0.3325	3.39	0.1213	2.30	2.63	2.99	3.39	3.82	4.28	4.78	0.0359	3.30	0.1196	2.30	2.59	2.92	3.30	3.71	4.18	4.71
1	0.3465	4.70	0.1196	3.21	3.66	4.16	4.70	5.29	5.92	6.60	-0.0184	4.51	0.1182	3.17	3.56	4.01	4.51	5.08	5.71	6.44
2	0.3315	5.87	0.1178	4.03	4.59	5.20	5.87	6.59	7.36	8.20	-0.0550	5.48	0.1168	3.88	4.35	4.88	5.48	6.17	6.94	7.81
3	0.2872	6.87	0.1159	4.76	5.41	6.11	6.87	7.70	8.60	9.57	-0.0886	6.46	0.1155	4.60	5.14	5.76	6.46	7.26	8.16	9.19
4	0.2373	7.61	0.1143	5.32	6.01	6.78	7.61	8.52	9.51	10.58	-0.1129	7.13	0.1145	5.09	5.69	6.37	7.13	8.01	9.00	10.13
5	0.1874	8.16	0.1130	5.75	6.48	7.28	8.16	9.13	10.18	11.33	-0.1331	7.63	0.1137	5.47	6.10	6.82	7.63	8.56	9.62	10.82
6	0.1414	8.61	0.1118	6.11	6.86	7.69	8.61	9.62	10.73	11.95	-0.1515	8.06	0.1130	5.79	6.45	7.20	8.06	9.03	10.14	11.41
7	0.1005	9.00	0.1107	6.42	7.19	8.05	9.00	10.05	11.20	12.48	-0.1690	8.45	0.1122	6.09	6.78	7.56	8.45	9.46	10.62	11.95
8	0.0648	9.34	0.1098	6.69	7.48	8.36	9.34	10.42	11.61	12.93	-0.1858	8.81	0.1115	6.37	7.08	7.89	8.81	9.86	11.07	12.45
9	0.0344	9.62	0.1089	6.92	7.73	8.62	9.62	10.72	11.95	13.31	-0.2003	9.11	0.1109	6.60	7.33	8.16	9.11	10.19	11.43	12.85
10	0.0082	9.86	0.1082	7.12	7.94	8.85	9.86	10.99	12.24	13.64	-0.2125	9.34	0.1103	6.78	7.53	8.38	9.34	10.44	11.71	13.17
11	-0.0159	10.08	0.1076	7.30	8.13	9.05	10.08	11.22	12.50	13.93	-0.2238	9.54	0.1098	6.94	7.70	8.56	9.54	10.67	11.95	13.44
12	-0.0398	10.29	0.1069	7.48	8.32	9.25	10.29	11.45	12.75	14.21	-0.2356	9.74	0.1093	7.10	7.87	8.74	9.74	10.88	12.19	13.70
13	-0.0650	10.51	0.1062	7.67	8.51	9.45	10.51	11.69	13.01	14.50	-0.2487	9.94	0.1088	7.26	8.04	8.93	9.94	11.10	12.43	13.97
14	-0.0919	10.73	0.1055	7.86	8.71	9.66	10.73	11.93	13.28	14.79	-0.2635	10.15	0.1082	7.44	8.23	9.13	10.15	11.33	12.69	14.26
15	-0.1199	10.95	0.1048	8.05	8.91	9.87	10.95	12.17	13.54	15.09	-0.2798	10.37	0.1076	7.61	8.41	9.33	10.37	11.57	12.95	14.55
16	-0.1485	11.18	0.1040	8.24	9.11	10.08	11.18	12.41	13.81	15.39	-0.2974	10.59	0.1070	7.80	8.61	9.53	10.59	11.81	13.21	14.84
17	-0.1776	11.40	0.1033	8.43	9.30	10.29	11.40	12.65	14.07	15.68	-0.3161	10.81	0.1063	7.98	8.80	9.74	10.81	12.05	13.47	15.13
18	-0.2070	11.62	0.1026	8.62	9.50	10.49	11.62	12.88	14.32	15.96	-0.3357	11.03	0.1057	8.16	8.99	9.94	11.03	12.28	13.73	15.42
19	-0.2365	11.83	0.1019	8.80	9.69	10.70	11.83	13.11	14.58	16.25	-0.3558	11.24	0.1051	8.34	9.18	10.14	11.24	12.51	13.98	15.70
20	-0.2659	12.04	0.1012	8.99	9.88	10.89	12.04	13.34	14.82	16.52	-0.3766	11.45	0.1045	8.51	9.36	10.33	11.45	12.73	14.23	15.98
21	-0.2953	12.24	0.1006	9.17	10.07	11.09	12.24	13.56	15.06	16.79	-0.3981	11.65	0.1039	8.69	9.54	10.53	11.65	12.96	14.48	16.25
22	-0.3246	12.45	0.0999	9.35	10.26	11.28	12.45	13.78	15.30	17.06	-0.4204	11.86	0.1033	8.86	9.73	10.72	11.86	13.18	14.72	16.53
23	-0.3539	12.65	0.0993	9.53	10.44	11.47	12.65	13.99	15.54	17.33	-0.4432	12.07	0.1027	9.04	9.91	10.92	12.07	13.41	14.97	16.81
24	-0.3832	12.85	0.0986	9.71	10.62	11.66	12.85	14.21	15.77	17.59	-0.4665	12.28	0.1021	9.22	10.10	11.11	12.28	13.63	15.21	17.08

Table 4 Head circumference (cm)-for-age z-score curves at 0, ±1, ±2, and ± 3 SD for Chinese boys and girls from birth to 24 months

Age (months)	Boys										Girls									
	L	M	S	-3SD	-2SD	-1SD	0SD	1SD	2SD	3SD	L	M	S	-3SD	-2SD	-1SD	0SD	1SD	2SD	3SD
0	−7.0263	34.3	0.0262	32.2	32.8	33.4	34.3	35.3	36.6	38.4	−1.4337	34.1	0.0300	31.3	32.1	33.1	34.1	35.1	36.3	37.5
1	−4.4686	37.3	0.0280	34.8	35.5	36.4	37.3	38.5	39.8	41.5	−1.2431	36.9	0.0304	33.9	34.8	35.8	36.9	38.1	39.3	40.7
2	−2.7515	39.2	0.0291	36.3	37.1	38.1	39.2	40.4	41.8	43.3	−1.0791	38.6	0.0304	35.4	36.4	37.4	38.6	39.8	41.1	42.5
3	−1.7763	40.6	0.0294	37.4	38.4	39.5	40.6	41.8	43.2	44.7	−0.9472	40.0	0.0303	36.6	37.7	38.8	40.0	41.2	42.5	43.9
4	−1.2600	41.7	0.0295	38.3	39.4	40.5	41.7	43.0	44.3	45.8	−0.8444	41.0	0.0301	37.6	38.6	39.8	41.0	42.2	43.6	45.0
5	−0.9752	42.6	0.0293	39.2	40.2	41.4	42.6	43.9	45.3	46.7	−0.7629	41.8	0.0298	38.4	39.5	40.6	41.8	43.1	44.5	45.9
6	−0.7968	43.4	0.0291	39.9	41.0	42.1	43.4	44.7	46.0	47.5	−0.6960	42.6	0.0295	39.1	40.2	41.4	42.6	43.9	45.2	46.7
7	−0.6658	44.1	0.0289	40.5	41.6	42.8	44.1	45.4	46.7	48.2	−0.6377	43.3	0.0292	39.7	40.9	42.0	43.3	44.6	45.9	47.4
8	−0.5616	44.7	0.0286	41.1	42.2	43.4	44.7	46.0	47.4	48.8	−0.5863	43.9	0.0289	40.3	41.5	42.6	43.9	45.2	46.5	48.0
9	−0.4796	45.2	0.0284	41.6	42.7	43.9	45.2	46.5	47.9	49.3	−0.5444	44.3	0.0286	40.8	41.9	43.1	44.3	45.6	47.0	48.4
10	−0.4171	45.6	0.0282	41.9	43.1	44.3	45.6	46.9	48.2	49.7	−0.5097	44.7	0.0283	41.2	42.3	43.5	44.7	46.0	47.4	48.8
11	−0.3699	45.9	0.0280	42.3	43.4	44.7	45.9	47.2	48.6	50.0	−0.4793	45.1	0.0280	41.5	42.6	43.8	45.1	46.3	47.7	49.1
12	−0.3349	46.2	0.0278	42.6	43.8	45.0	46.2	47.5	48.9	50.3	−0.4516	45.4	0.0278	41.8	42.9	44.1	45.4	46.6	48.0	49.4
13	−0.3116	46.5	0.0277	42.9	44.1	45.3	46.5	47.8	49.2	50.6	−0.4262	45.6	0.0275	42.1	43.2	44.4	45.6	46.9	48.3	49.6
14	−0.3002	46.8	0.0275	43.2	44.3	45.6	46.8	48.1	49.5	50.9	−0.4029	45.9	0.0273	42.3	43.5	44.7	45.9	47.2	48.5	49.9
15	−0.2977	47.1	0.0274	43.4	44.6	45.8	47.1	48.4	49.7	51.1	−0.3819	46.1	0.0271	42.6	43.7	44.9	46.1	47.4	48.7	50.1
16	−0.2997	47.3	0.0273	43.6	44.8	46.0	47.3	48.6	49.9	51.4	−0.3629	46.3	0.0269	42.8	43.9	45.1	46.3	47.6	48.9	50.3
17	−0.3039	47.4	0.0272	43.8	45.0	46.2	47.4	48.8	50.1	51.5	−0.3456	46.5	0.0267	43.0	44.1	45.3	46.5	47.8	49.1	50.5
18	−0.3091	47.6	0.0271	43.9	45.1	46.3	47.6	48.9	50.3	51.7	−0.3293	46.7	0.0265	43.2	44.3	45.5	46.7	48.0	49.3	50.6
19	−0.3155	47.8	0.0270	44.1	45.3	46.5	47.8	49.1	50.4	51.9	−0.3135	46.9	0.0263	43.4	44.5	45.7	46.9	48.1	49.4	50.8
20	− 0.3232	47.9	0.0269	44.3	45.5	46.7	47.9	49.3	50.6	52.0	−0.2976	47.1	0.0261	43.6	44.7	45.9	47.1	48.3	49.6	50.9
21	−0.3320	48.1	0.0268	44.5	45.6	46.9	48.1	49.4	50.8	52.2	−0.2811	47.2	0.0260	43.7	44.9	46.0	47.2	48.5	49.8	51.1
22	−0.3414	48.3	0.0267	44.6	45.8	47.0	48.3	49.6	51.0	52.4	−0.2641	47.4	0.0258	43.9	45.1	46.2	47.4	48.7	50.0	51.3
23	−0.3506	48.5	0.0266	44.8	46.0	47.2	48.5	49.8	51.1	52.6	−0.2473	47.6	0.0256	44.1	45.3	46.4	47.6	48.9	50.1	51.5
24	−0.3592	48.6	0.0265	45.0	46.1	47.4	48.6	49.9	51.3	52.7	−0.2313	47.8	0.0254	44.3	45.4	46.6	47.8	49.0	50.3	51.6

0.31 kg-cm higher (range 0.03–1.00 kg-cm) in boys and 0.28 (range 0.02–0.56) kg-cm higher in girls across length in this study (Fig. 3).

The difference between our raw data and WHO standards
The numbers of anthropometric measurements used for generating smoothed growth curves was shown in Additional file 1: Tables S2 and S3. This study measured the children at 7 targeted ages (42 days, 3, 6, 9, 12, 18 and 24 months), but in fact provided adequate monthly numbers in the first 12 months (Additional file 1: Tables S2 and S3). In addition to above comparison of the LMS-method-fitted smoothing curves, we also presented the 3rd, 10th, 50th, 90th and 97th percentiles of growth measures by age in both boys (Additional file 1: Table S4) and girls (Additional file 1: Table S5). Compared to the corresponding 2006 WHO percentile standards, the 3rd, 10th, 50th, 90th and 97th percentiles (across the ages evaluated in this study from 0 to 2 years) for length, weight, and BMI (Additional file 1: Table S4 for boys and

Additional file 1: Table S5 for girls) were consistently higher in healthy Chinese boys (Additional file 1: Table S6) and girls (Additional file 1: Table S7) in 2015. For example, the median lengths from 0 to 2 years were 50.0–89.5 cm in boys (Additional file 1: Table S4), which were 0.1–3.1 cm taller than the WHO percentile standards (Additional file 1: Table S6). The differences compared to WHO standards also were present for weight by length in both boys and girls (Additional file 1: Tables S8 and S9). This indicates the robust of our results.

Discussion
This report of growth measures is based on a large cohort of children (n = 4251) from six recent birth cohorts from China. Growth references from this study represent normal growth of today's Chinese children from birth to 24 months by using the multicenter data collected recently (from 2012 to 2015). Compared with the WHO standards (collected more than 10 years ago from mid-1997 to end of 2003) and the current China

Table 5 BMI-for-age z-score at 0, ±1, ±2, and ± 3 SD for Chinese boys and girls from birth to 24 months

Age (month)	Boys										Girls									
	L	M	S	-3SD	-2SD	-1SD	0SD	1SD	2SD	3SD	L	M	S	-3SD	-2SD	-1SD	0SD	1SD	2SD	3SD
0	0.1590	13.4	0.0958	10.0	11.0	12.2	13.4	14.7	16.2	17.8	−0.1727	13.3	0.0920	10.1	11.1	12.1	13.3	14.5	16.0	17.6
1	0.7178	15.6	0.0943	11.4	12.8	14.2	15.6	17.1	18.6	20.2	−0.0900	15.4	0.0898	11.8	12.9	14.1	15.4	16.8	18.4	20.2
2	0.6937	16.7	0.0930	12.3	13.7	15.2	16.7	18.3	19.9	21.6	−0.1078	16.2	0.0891	12.5	13.6	14.8	16.2	17.7	19.4	21.3
3	0.6483	17.7	0.0920	13.1	14.6	16.1	17.7	19.4	21.1	22.8	−0.1322	17.2	0.0886	13.3	14.5	15.8	17.2	18.8	20.6	22.6
4	0.6054	18.1	0.0909	13.5	14.9	16.5	18.1	19.8	21.5	23.3	−0.1567	17.7	0.0880	13.6	14.8	16.2	17.7	19.3	21.1	23.1
5	0.5683	18.2	0.0899	13.6	15.1	16.6	18.2	19.9	21.6	23.4	−0.1810	17.7	0.0875	13.7	14.9	16.3	17.7	19.4	21.2	23.2
6	0.5384	18.2	0.0890	13.6	15.1	16.6	18.2	19.8	21.6	23.4	−0.2055	17.7	0.0869	13.8	15.0	16.3	17.7	19.4	21.2	23.2
7	0.5161	18.2	0.0880	13.7	15.1	16.6	18.2	19.8	21.5	23.3	−0.2298	17.8	0.0863	13.8	15.0	16.3	17.8	19.4	21.2	23.2
8	0.5000	18.1	0.0871	13.7	15.1	16.6	18.1	19.7	21.4	23.2	−0.2535	17.7	0.0857	13.8	15.0	16.3	17.7	19.3	21.1	23.1
9	0.4888	18.0	0.0862	13.7	15.0	16.5	18.0	19.6	21.3	23.0	−0.2763	17.6	0.0851	13.8	14.9	16.2	17.6	19.2	21.0	23.0
10	0.4814	17.9	0.0854	13.6	14.9	16.4	17.9	19.4	21.0	22.7	−0.2981	17.5	0.0845	13.7	14.8	16.1	17.5	19.0	20.8	22.7
11	0.4767	17.7	0.0846	13.5	14.8	16.2	17.7	19.2	20.8	22.5	−0.3192	17.3	0.0839	13.6	14.7	15.9	17.3	18.8	20.6	22.5
12	0.4735	17.6	0.0838	13.4	14.7	16.1	17.6	19.1	20.6	22.3	−0.3398	17.2	0.0834	13.5	14.6	15.8	17.2	18.7	20.4	22.3
13	0.4713	17.4	0.0830	13.4	14.7	16.0	17.4	18.9	20.5	22.1	−0.3598	17.0	0.0828	13.4	14.5	15.7	17.0	18.5	20.2	22.1
14	0.4693	17.3	0.0823	13.3	14.6	15.9	17.3	18.8	20.3	21.9	−0.3794	16.9	0.0823	13.4	14.4	15.6	16.9	18.4	20.0	21.9
15	0.4673	17.2	0.0816	13.3	14.5	15.8	17.2	18.6	20.1	21.7	−0.3984	16.8	0.0818	13.3	14.3	15.5	16.8	18.2	19.9	21.7
16	0.4654	17.1	0.0809	13.2	14.4	15.7	17.1	18.5	19.9	21.5	−0.4169	16.7	0.0814	13.2	14.2	15.4	16.7	18.1	19.7	21.5
17	0.4635	16.9	0.0802	13.1	14.3	15.6	16.9	18.3	19.7	21.3	−0.4349	16.5	0.0809	13.1	14.1	15.3	16.5	18.0	19.6	21.4
18	0.4616	16.8	0.0795	13.0	14.2	15.5	16.8	18.2	19.6	21.1	−0.4524	16.4	0.0805	13.1	14.1	15.2	16.4	17.8	19.4	21.2
19	0.4598	16.7	0.0789	13.0	14.2	15.4	16.7	18.0	19.4	20.9	−0.4695	16.3	0.0801	13.0	14.0	15.1	16.3	17.7	19.3	21.1
20	0.4581	16.6	0.0783	12.9	14.1	15.3	16.6	17.9	19.3	20.7	−0.4862	16.2	0.0797	13.0	13.9	15.0	16.2	17.6	19.2	20.9
21	0.4564	16.5	0.0777	12.9	14.0	15.2	16.5	17.8	19.2	20.6	−0.5024	16.2	0.0793	12.9	13.9	15.0	16.2	17.5	19.1	20.8
22	0.4547	16.4	0.0772	12.8	14.0	15.2	16.4	17.7	19.0	20.4	−0.5181	16.1	0.0789	12.9	13.8	14.9	16.1	17.4	19.0	20.7
23	0.4531	16.3	0.0766	12.8	13.9	15.1	16.3	17.6	18.9	20.3	−0.5334	16.0	0.0786	12.8	13.8	14.8	16.0	17.4	18.9	20.6
24	0.4516	16.2	0.0761	12.8	13.9	15.0	16.2	17.5	18.8	20.2	−0.5482	16.0	0.0782	12.8	13.7	14.8	16.0	17.3	18.8	20.5

references (collected 10-years ago in late 2005), the median values of length-, weight-, and BMI-for-age reported here were all higher across the ages from 0 to 2 years, and also for median head circumference-for-age except for boys in our study compared to the 2005 references for China. The weight-for-length in our study was also slightly higher at most times in both boys and girls. The magnitude of differences between the WHO standards and the current large cohort (assessed in 2015) was larger than the magnitude of differences previously reported compared to the outdated 2005 references for China. Our report provides improved references for evaluating growth of children aged 0–24 months in modern China.

The height- and weight-for-age values were higher in our longitudinal cohort assessed in five cities of China (Shanghai, Ma'anshan Anhui, Wuhan, Jiangsu, and Guangzhou) than in the cohort based on a cross-sectional study in nine cities of China (Beijing, Shanghai, Harbin, Xi'an, Nanjing, Wuhan, Guangzhou, Fuzhou, and

Kunming) [3]. This could be a secular trend. The CBCC cohorts recruited pregnant women in provincial or large tertiary maternity and child hospitals. Most mothers had high education (college or higher), maternal smoking was rare, and the living standard were relatively high. Thus, the growth data in this study may reflect infant growth patterns under near-optimal circumstances. Since our data were acquired recently (10 years since 2005), the higher length and weight may also reflect an ongoing secular trend [4]. The WHO data suggest that secular trend may depend on where the cohort was acquired: the predicted adult height from the child's length at 2 years suggested there would be no parent-offspring difference in Norway and the United States (i.e., no increase due to a secular trend), but the predicted adult height was much larger than mid-parental height for the other four countries (Brazil, Ghana, India and Oman). [15] Based on the taller height reported here for ages 0 to 24 months than the 2005 China data, we expect a secular trend (i.e., we predict that average adulthood the height of the children in China

Table 6 Weight (kg)- for-length (cm) z-score curves at 0, ±1, ±2, and ± 3 SD for Chinese boys and girls from birth to 24 months

Length (cm)	Boys										Girls									
	L	M	S	-3SD	-2SD	-1SD	0SD	1SD	2SD	3SD	L	M	S	-3SD	-2SD	-1SD	0SD	1SD	2SD	3SD
45	1.0000	2.54	0.1032	1.76	2.02	2.28	2.54	2.80	3.07	3.33	-0.5434	2.37	0.0928	1.83	1.99	2.17	2.37	2.61	2.89	3.21
46	1.0000	2.67	0.1028	1.85	2.12	2.40	2.67	2.95	3.22	3.50	-0.5303	2.56	0.0927	1.97	2.14	2.34	2.56	2.81	3.11	3.46
47	1.0000	2.81	0.1025	1.95	2.24	2.53	2.81	3.10	3.39	3.68	-0.5173	2.74	0.0927	2.12	2.30	2.51	2.74	3.02	3.33	3.70
48	1.0000	2.97	0.1021	2.06	2.36	2.66	2.97	3.27	3.57	3.88	-0.5041	2.93	0.0926	2.26	2.45	2.68	2.93	3.22	3.56	3.95
49	1.0000	3.15	0.1017	2.19	2.51	2.83	3.15	3.47	3.79	4.11	-0.4904	3.12	0.0926	2.41	2.62	2.85	3.12	3.44	3.79	4.21
50	1.0000	3.36	0.1012	2.34	2.68	3.02	3.36	3.70	4.04	4.38	-0.4757	3.34	0.0925	2.58	2.80	3.06	3.34	3.68	4.06	4.50
51	1.0000	3.61	0.1007	2.52	2.88	3.25	3.61	3.97	4.34	4.70	-0.4597	3.60	0.0924	2.77	3.02	3.29	3.60	3.96	4.37	4.84
52	1.0000	3.89	0.1001	2.72	3.11	3.50	3.89	4.28	4.67	5.06	-0.4434	3.88	0.0923	2.99	3.25	3.55	3.88	4.26	4.71	5.22
53	1.0000	4.18	0.0995	2.93	3.35	3.76	4.18	4.59	5.01	5.42	-0.4276	4.16	0.0922	3.20	3.48	3.80	4.16	4.57	5.04	5.58
54	1.0000	4.45	0.0990	3.13	3.57	4.01	4.45	4.89	5.33	5.77	-0.4126	4.42	0.0921	3.40	3.70	4.03	4.42	4.85	5.35	5.92
55	1.0000	4.71	0.0984	3.32	3.78	4.25	4.71	5.17	5.64	6.10	-0.3983	4.66	0.0920	3.58	3.90	4.26	4.66	5.12	5.64	6.24
56	1.0000	4.95	0.0978	3.50	3.99	4.47	4.95	5.44	5.92	6.41	-0.3841	4.90	0.0918	3.77	4.10	4.48	4.90	5.38	5.93	6.56
57	1.0000	5.21	0.0972	3.69	4.20	4.70	5.21	5.72	6.22	6.73	-0.3702	5.16	0.0917	3.98	4.33	4.72	5.16	5.67	6.24	6.90
58	1.0000	5.49	0.0966	3.90	4.43	4.96	5.49	6.02	6.55	7.08	-0.3572	5.46	0.0915	4.21	4.58	4.99	5.46	6.00	6.60	7.29
59	1.0000	5.81	0.0959	4.14	4.69	5.25	5.81	6.36	6.92	7.48	-0.3463	5.79	0.0912	4.46	4.85	5.29	5.79	6.35	6.99	7.72
60	1.0000	6.14	0.0952	4.39	4.97	5.56	6.14	6.73	7.31	7.90	-0.3376	6.11	0.0910	4.71	5.12	5.59	6.11	6.70	7.38	8.14
61	1.0000	6.48	0.0945	4.64	5.25	5.87	6.48	7.09	7.70	8.32	-0.3307	6.41	0.0907	4.94	5.38	5.86	6.41	7.03	7.73	8.53
62	1.0000	6.79	0.0938	4.88	5.52	6.16	6.79	7.43	8.07	8.71	-0.3252	6.69	0.0904	5.16	5.61	6.12	6.69	7.33	8.06	8.88
63	1.0000	7.09	0.0931	5.11	5.77	6.43	7.09	7.75	8.41	9.07	-0.3212	6.94	0.0901	5.35	5.82	6.35	6.94	7.60	8.35	9.21
64	1.0000	7.36	0.0925	5.32	6.00	6.68	7.36	8.05	8.73	9.41	-0.3184	7.19	0.0898	5.55	6.04	6.58	7.19	7.87	8.65	9.52
65	1.0000	7.63	0.0918	5.53	6.23	6.93	7.63	8.33	9.03	9.73	-0.3169	7.44	0.0894	5.75	6.25	6.81	7.44	8.14	8.94	9.84
66	1.0000	7.89	0.0912	5.73	6.45	7.17	7.89	8.61	9.33	10.05	-0.3170	7.69	0.0891	5.95	6.47	7.04	7.69	8.42	9.24	10.17
67	1.0000	8.14	0.0906	5.93	6.67	7.40	8.14	8.88	9.62	10.36	-0.3188	7.94	0.0887	6.15	6.68	7.27	7.94	8.68	9.53	10.48
68	1.0000	8.39	0.0900	6.13	6.88	7.64	8.39	9.15	9.90	10.66	-0.3223	8.18	0.0883	6.34	6.89	7.49	8.18	8.94	9.81	10.78
69	1.0000	8.64	0.0894	6.32	7.10	7.87	8.64	9.42	10.19	10.96	-0.3270	8.41	0.0879	6.53	7.09	7.71	8.41	9.19	10.08	11.08
70	1.0000	8.89	0.0889	6.52	7.31	8.10	8.89	9.68	10.47	11.26	-0.3328	8.63	0.0875	6.71	7.28	7.92	8.63	9.43	10.34	11.36
71	1.0000	9.13	0.0883	6.71	7.52	8.33	9.13	9.94	10.74	11.55	-0.3391	8.85	0.0871	6.89	7.47	8.12	8.85	9.67	10.59	11.63
72	1.0000	9.36	0.0878	6.90	7.72	8.54	9.36	10.19	11.01	11.83	-0.3458	9.06	0.0867	7.07	7.66	8.32	9.06	9.90	10.84	11.90
73	1.0000	9.59	0.0872	7.08	7.92	8.76	9.59	10.43	11.27	12.10	-0.3527	9.28	0.0863	7.25	7.85	8.53	9.28	10.13	11.09	12.18
74	1.0000	9.82	0.0867	7.26	8.12	8.97	9.82	10.67	11.52	12.37	-0.3597	9.50	0.0858	7.43	8.04	8.73	9.50	10.37	11.34	12.45
75	1.0000	10.04	0.0861	7.44	8.31	9.17	10.04	10.90	11.77	12.63	-0.3667	9.72	0.0854	7.61	8.23	8.93	9.72	10.60	11.59	12.72
76	1.0000	10.26	0.0856	7.62	8.50	9.38	10.26	11.13	12.01	12.89	-0.3737	9.93	0.0850	7.78	8.42	9.13	9.93	10.83	11.84	12.98

Table 6 Weight (kg)- for-length (cm) z-score curves at 0, ±1, ±2, and ± 3 SD for Chinese boys and girls from birth to 24 months (*Continued*)

Length (cm)	Boys										Girls									
	L	M	S	-3SD	-2SD	-1SD	0SD	1SD	2SD	3SD	L	M	S	-3SD	-2SD	-1SD	0SD	1SD	2SD	3SD
77	1.0000	10.47	0.0851	7.80	8.69	9.58	10.47	11.36	12.25	13.14	-0.3806	10.14	0.0846	7.96	8.60	9.33	10.14	11.05	12.07	13.24
78	1.0000	10.68	0.0846	7.97	8.87	9.78	10.68	11.58	12.49	13.39	-0.3872	10.34	0.0842	8.13	8.78	9.52	10.34	11.26	12.30	13.48
79	1.0000	10.88	0.0841	8.14	9.05	9.97	10.88	11.80	12.71	13.63	-0.3933	10.53	0.0837	8.29	8.96	9.70	10.53	11.47	12.53	13.72
80	1.0000	11.07	0.0836	8.30	9.22	10.15	11.07	12.00	12.93	13.85	-0.3988	10.72	0.0834	8.45	9.12	9.88	10.72	11.67	12.74	13.95
81	1.0000	11.26	0.0832	8.45	9.39	10.32	11.26	12.20	13.13	14.07	-0.4036	10.91	0.0830	8.60	9.29	10.05	10.91	11.87	12.95	14.18
82	1.0000	11.44	0.0828	8.60	9.55	10.49	11.44	12.39	13.33	14.28	-0.4076	11.09	0.0826	8.76	9.45	10.22	11.09	12.06	13.16	14.40
83	1.0000	11.62	0.0823	8.75	9.71	10.67	11.62	12.58	13.54	14.49	-0.4109	11.28	0.0822	8.92	9.62	10.40	11.28	12.26	13.37	14.63
84	1.0000	11.81	0.0819	8.91	9.87	10.84	11.81	12.78	13.74	14.71	-0.4134	11.47	0.0819	9.08	9.79	10.58	11.47	12.47	13.59	14.86
85	1.0000	12.00	0.0815	9.07	10.05	11.03	12.00	12.98	13.96	14.94	-0.4149	11.68	0.0815	9.25	9.98	10.78	11.68	12.69	13.83	15.11
86	1.0000	12.21	0.0810	9.24	10.23	11.22	12.21	13.20	14.19	15.18	-0.4151	11.90	0.0811	9.44	10.17	10.99	11.90	12.92	14.08	15.38
87	1.0000	12.43	0.0806	9.42	10.42	11.42	12.43	13.43	14.43	15.43	-0.4137	12.13	0.0807	9.63	10.38	11.21	12.13	13.17	14.34	15.66
88	1.0000	12.66	0.0801	9.62	10.63	11.64	12.66	13.67	14.69	15.70	-0.4105	12.38	0.0803	9.84	10.60	11.44	12.38	13.44	14.62	15.96
89	1.0000	12.91	0.0797	9.82	10.85	11.88	12.91	13.94	14.96	15.99	-0.4056	12.65	0.0799	10.06	10.83	11.69	12.65	13.72	14.92	16.28
90	1.0000	13.17	0.0792	10.04	11.09	12.13	13.17	14.22	15.26	16.30	-0.3987	12.92	0.0796	10.28	11.07	11.94	12.92	14.01	15.23	16.60
91	1.0000	13.46	0.0787	10.28	11.34	12.40	13.46	14.52	15.58	16.64	-0.3901	13.19	0.0792	10.51	11.31	12.20	13.19	14.30	15.54	16.93
92	1.0000	13.75	0.0782	10.53	11.60	12.68	13.75	14.83	15.91	16.98	-0.3797	13.47	0.0789	10.74	11.56	12.47	13.47	14.60	15.86	17.27
93	1.0000	14.06	0.0778	10.78	11.87	12.97	14.06	15.15	16.25	17.34	-0.3677	13.75	0.0786	10.97	11.80	12.73	13.75	14.89	16.17	17.60
94	1.0000	14.37	0.0773	11.04	12.15	13.26	14.37	15.48	16.59	17.71	-0.3543	14.03	0.0783	11.20	12.05	12.99	14.03	15.19	16.48	17.93
95	1.0000	14.68	0.0769	11.30	12.43	13.56	14.68	15.81	16.94	18.07	-0.3398	14.30	0.0780	11.42	12.29	13.24	14.30	15.48	16.79	18.25
96	1.0000	15.00	0.0764	11.56	12.71	13.85	15.00	16.15	17.29	18.44	-0.3243	14.57	0.0777	11.64	12.52	13.50	14.57	15.77	17.10	18.57
97	1.0000	15.32	0.0760	11.82	12.99	14.15	15.32	16.48	17.65	18.81	-0.3081	14.84	0.0775	11.86	12.76	13.75	14.84	16.05	17.39	18.89
98	1.0000	15.63	0.0756	12.09	13.27	14.45	15.63	16.82	18.00	19.18	-0.2914	15.10	0.0772	12.07	12.99	13.99	15.10	16.33	17.69	19.20
99	1.0000	15.95	0.0751	12.36	13.56	14.75	15.95	17.15	18.35	19.55	-0.2744	15.37	0.0769	12.29	13.22	14.24	15.37	16.61	17.98	19.51
100	1.0000	16.27	0.0747	12.62	13.84	15.06	16.27	17.49	18.70	19.92	-0.2575	15.63	0.0767	12.50	13.45	14.49	15.63	16.89	18.28	19.81

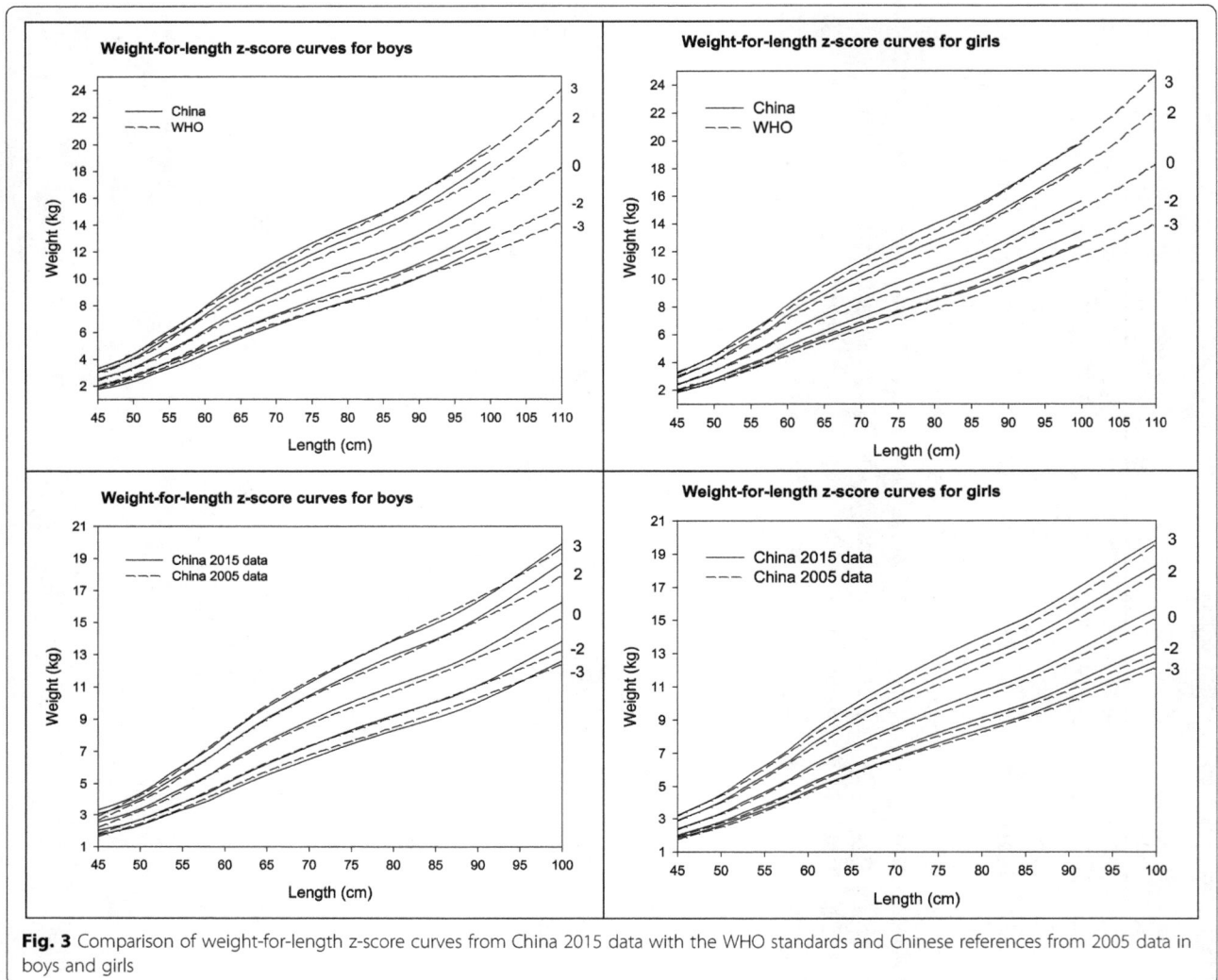

Fig. 3 Comparison of weight-for-length z-score curves from China 2015 data with the WHO standards and Chinese references from 2005 data in boys and girls

will exceed the average height of their parents). While China has undergone dramatic progress in economic and social development, the differences still exist between urban and rural areas, different ethnics, and different social economic. The growth pattern observed in this study may reflect infant growth patterns under more optimal circumstances.

Some studies have found that some child population might have their own growth pattern [16], and our study confirmed that Chinese children may be one of them [3, 17, 18]. The difference in values for height-, weight- and BMI-for-age, weight-for-length, and head circumference in this report in comparison to the WHO standards suggests an interesting country difference, and adds to previous comparison that have been summarized in a recent review [19]. Based on studies from both longitudinal and cross-sectional designs, this review concluded that the WHO standards for height and weight "... endorsed slenderness in the

midst of an obesity epidemic" and for head circumference were underestimates (and "... would put many children at risk for misdiagnosis of macrocephaly and microcephaly"). Healthy children in some countries are classified (perhaps inappropriately) as "stunted" [16]. In opposite of findings from some countries (overestimating stunting) [16], overall, our study confirmed that the values of growth measures were higher for the key z-score cutoffs in Chinese children in comparison with WHO growth standards [3, 5].

Our references provide the potential cutoffs for evaluating child growth in a population (like in modern China), where children are the center of attention in the family and are growing under favorable environments. Length has been widely used in early detection of stunting, while weight is commonly used as a measure responsive to short-term influences [20]. Head circumference is then the next most-used measure in clinical settings. To reflect the growth centile (position) of a Chinese child in local population, conditioned on age and sex, the Chinese growth standards need to be considered. It may help identify the infants who suffer from poor and modifiable conditions, and thus target those who may benefit most from intervention. In this study, while another term was considered ("growth pattern"), the term "growth reference" was used to maintain consistency with the term used in other publications about Chinese cohorts and to contrast to the term "growth standard" used for the WHO cohort.

One characteristic of this study (the large-scale multi-center prospective birth cohort design) allows us to obtain data on pre- and perinatal risk factors including GDM, chronic hypertension, pre-eclampsia and preterm status. Based on this strength, we could exclude affected mother-infant pairs cases at risk for abnormal patterns of child growth. In this study, the difference of mean paternal age among the three groups of children (mothers with GDM, born preterm, and healthy children) is interesting. Older fathers have more de novo mutations in DNA, and this probably contributes to growth in some cases [21]. Another strength of this study is the longitudinal rather than cross-sectional design. Additional longitudinal analysis [22, 23] of these longitudinal data could better capture and describe the tempo of growth, but due to space limitations will be presented elsewhere. Also, in this sample the educational level of mothers was high, and few of the mothers smoked, so the children lived in advantaged condition, and approach the criteria used for establishing the WHO standards (reflecting how children should grow). Therefore, the data here may reflect growth in near-optimal conditions in China, and provide a growth pattern for contemporary Chinese children.

On the other hand, one limitation of this study is that in some cases head circumference at birth was not measured, and some of children were just followed up to 12 months, which reduced the sample size for this measurement. However, our sample size is still larger than the sample sizes in similar longitudinal birth cohort studies conducted in other countries. We have also performed sensitivity analysis to summary the 3rd, 10th, 50th, 90th and 97th percentiles of all growth measures in infant who had all observations up to 24 months (i.e., without missing observations) and the results were similar to those from all observations (data not shown). Thus, the missing data should be "at random" [9] Also, the birth measures obtained from medical records may not be ideal despite of the high number of the participating hospitals (which were all provincial or large tertiary maternity and child hospitals). Thirdly, this was a convenience sample without specific entry criteria as in the WHO study.

Conclusions

The growth curves in this study represent the growth pattern of today's normal Chinese children, and may provide references for evaluation of the individual growth status of children growing up in modern China.

Abbreviations
ART: Assisted reproductive technologies; CBCC: China Birth Cohort Consortium; GDM: Gestational diabetes mellitus; IADPSG: International Association of Diabetes and Pregnancy Study Groups; MGRS: Multicenter Growth Reference Study; WHO: World Health Organization

Acknowledgements
We thank Dr. James Swanson, Dr. Michael Hermanussen and Dr. Zhong-Cheng Luo for their intensive reviews and insightful comments on this manuscript.

Funding
This work was funded by the Gates Foundation Healthy Birth, Growth & Development knowledge integration (HBGDki) project (No. OPP1153191). Dr. F. Ouyang was also supported by grants from National Natural Science Foundation of China (grant numbers 81673178; 81372954) and Coordinated Research Project E43032 from International Atomic Energy Agency (IAEA). The funders were not involved in the study design, data collection, analysis, and interpretation, or manuscript preparation.

Authors' contributions
FO conceptualized, designed and conducted this study, performed the statistical analysis, and drafted the manuscript. JZ conceptualized this study, and critically reviewed the manuscript. All authors (JZ, FO, FJ, FT, SX, YX, and XQ) took responsibility for one cohort, and critically reviewed the manuscript. All authors read and approved the final manuscript as submitted.

Competing interests
The authors declare that they have no competing interests.

Author details
[1]Ministry of Education and Shanghai Key Laboratory of Children's Environmental Health, Xinhua Hospital, Shanghai Jiao Tong University School of Medicine, 1665 Kong Jiang Road, Shanghai 200092, China. [2]Department of Developmental and Behavioral Pediatrics, Shanghai Pediatric Transitional Institution, Shanghai Children's Medical Center affiliated with Shanghai Jiao Tong University School of Medicine, Shanghai 200127, China. [3]School of Public Health, Anhui Medical University, Hefei 230032, China. [4]Key Laboratory of Environment and Health (HUST), Ministry of Education & Ministry of Environmental Protection, and State Key Laboratory of Environmental Health (Incubation), School of Public Health, Tongji Medical College, Huazhong University of Science and Technology, Wuhan 430074, Hubei, China. [5]School of Public Health, Nanjing Medical University, Nanjing 211166, China. [6]Division of Birth Cohort Study, Guangzhou Women and Children's Medical Center, Guangzhou Medical University, Guangzhou 510000, China.

References
1. Blake-Lamb TL, Locks LM, Perkins ME, Woo Baidal JA, Cheng ER, Taveras EM. Interventions for childhood obesity in the first 1,000 days a systematic review. Am J Prev Med. 2016;50(6):780–9.
2. de Onis M, Onyango A, Borghi E, Siyam A, Blossner M, Lutter C, Group WHOMGRS. Worldwide implementation of the WHO child growth standards. Public Health Nutr. 2012;15(9):1603–10.
3. Zong XN, Li H. Construction of a new growth references for China based on urban Chinese children: comparison with the WHO growth standards. PLoS One. 2013;8(3):e59569.
4. Cole TJ. The secular trend in human physical growth: a biological view. Econ Hum Biol. 2003;1(2):161–8.
5. Huang X, Chang J, Feng W, Xu Y, Xu T, Tang H, Wang H, Pan X. Development of a new growth standard for breastfed Chinese infants: what is the difference from the WHO growth standards? PLoS One. 2016;11(12):e0167816.
6. Tanner JM, Whitehouse RH, Takaishi M. Standards from birth to maturity for height, weight, height velocity, and weight velocity: British children, 1965. II. Arch Dis Child. 1966;41(220):613–35.

7.   Xu F, Qiu L, Binns CW, Liu X. Breastfeeding in China: a review. Int Breastfeed J. 2009;4:6.

8.   American Diabetes A. Diagnosis and classification of diabetes mellitus. Diabetes Care. 2013;36(Suppl 1):S67–74.

9.   Croy CD, Novins DK. Methods for addressing missing data in psychiatric and developmental research. J Am Acad Child Adolesc Psychiatry. 2005;44(12):1230–40.

10. Gillman MW, Rifas-Shiman S, Berkey CS, Field AE, Colditz GA. Maternal gestational diabetes, birth weight, and adolescent obesity. Pediatrics. 2003; 111(3):e221–6.

11. Paauw ND, van Rijn BB, Lely AT, Joles JA. Pregnancy as a critical window for blood pressure regulation in mother and child: programming and reprogramming. Acta Physiol (Oxf). 2016.

12. Ogland B, Vatten LJ, Romundstad PR, Nilsen ST, Forman MR. Pubertal anthropometry in sons and daughters of women with preeclamptic or normotensive pregnancies. Arch Dis Child. 2009;94(11):855–9.

13. Cole TJ, Green PJ. Smoothing reference centile curves: the LMS method and penalized likelihood. Stat Med. 1992;11(10):1305–19.

14. Borghi E, de Onis M, Garza C, Van den Broeck J, Frongillo EA, Grummer-Strawn L, Van Buuren S, Pan H, Molinari L, Martorell R, et al. Construction of the World Health Organization child growth standards: selection of methods for attained growth curves. Stat Med. 2006;25(2):247–65.

15. Garza C, Borghi E, Onyango AW, de Onis M, Group WHOMGRS. Parental height and child growth from birth to 2 years in the WHO multicentre growth reference study. Matern Child Nutr. 2013;9(Suppl 2):58–68.

16. Aman B, Pulungan MJ, Batubara JRL, Hermanussen M. Indonesian national synthetic growth charts. Acta Scientific Paediatrics. 2018;1(1):15.

17. Dang S, Yan H, Wang D. Implication of World Health Organization growth standards on estimation of malnutrition in young Chinese children: two examples from rural western China and the Tibet region. J Child Health Care. 2014;18(4):358–68.

18. Hui LL, Schooling CM, Cowling BJ, Leung SS, Lam TH, Leung GM. Are universal standards for optimal infant growth appropriate? Evidence from a Hong Kong Chinese birth cohort. Arch Dis Child. 2008;93(7):561–5.

19. Natale V, Rajagopalan A. Worldwide variation in human growth and the World Health Organization growth standards: a systematic review. BMJ Open. 2014;4(1):e003735.

20. Tanner JM, Whitehouse RH, Takaishi M. Standards from birth to maturity for height, weight, height velocity, and weight velocity: British children, 1965. I. Arch Dis Child. 1966;41(219):454–71.

21. Acuna-Hidalgo R, Veltman JA, Hoischen A. New insights into the generation and role of de novo mutations in health and disease. Genome Biol. 2016;17(1):241.

22. Tanner JM, Whitehouse RH. Clinical longitudinal standards for height, weight, height velocity, weight velocity, and stages of puberty. Arch Dis Child. 1976;51(3):170–9.

23. Wachholder A, Hauspie RC. Clinical standards for growth in height of Belgian boys and girls, aged 2 to 18. International Journal of Anthropology. 1986;1(4):327–38.

Permissions

List of Contributors

M. G. Sathiadas, Arunath Viswalingam and Karunya Vijayaratnam
Department of Paediatrics, University of Jaffna, Adiyapatham Raod, Jaffna, Sri Lanka

Michelle Jackman
School of Child and Adolescent Medicine, The University of Sydney, Sydney, Australia
Occupational Therapy Department, John Hunter Children's Hospital, Newcastle, Australia

Iona Novak
School of Child and Adolescent Medicine, The University of Sydney, Sydney, Australia
Cerebral Palsy Alliance Research Institute, The University of Sydney, Sydney, Australia

Claire Galea
Cerebral Palsy Alliance Research Institute, The University of Sydney, Sydney, Australia

Natasha Lannin
Alfred Health, La Trobe University, Melbourne, Australia

Elspeth Froude
School of Health Science, Australian Catholic University, Sydney, Australia

Laura Miller
School of Health Science, Australian Catholic University, Brisbane, Australia

Seung Jun Choi
Department of Pediatrics, Asan Medical Center Children's Hospital, University of Ulsan College of Medicine, Seoul, Republic of Korea
Graduate School of Medicine, The Catholic University of Korea, College of Medicine, Seoul, Republic of Korea

Sena Moon, Ui Yoon Choi, Yoon Hong Chun, Jung Hyun Lee and Jung Woo Rhim
Department of Pediatrics, College of Medicine, The Catholic University of Korea, 222, Banpodaero, Seocho-gu, Seoul 06591, Republic of Korea

Dae Chul Jeong
Department of Pediatrics, College of Medicine, The Catholic University of Korea, 222, Banpodaero, Seocho-gu, Seoul 06591, Republic of Korea

Vaccine Bio-research Institute, College of Medicine, The Catholic University of Korea, Seoul, Republic of Korea

Jin Lee
Department of Pediatrics, Hanjin General Hospital, Seoul, Republic of Korea

Hwang Min Kim
Department of Pediatrics, Yonsei Christian Hospital, Wonju, Republic of Korea

Y. Amare
Consultancy for Social Development, Addis Ababa, Ethiopia

S. Paul
Nell Hodgson Woodruff School of Nursing, Emory University, 1520 Clifton Road NE, 30322 Atlanta, Georgia

L. M. Sibley
Nell Hodgson Woodruff School of Nursing and Rollins School of Public Health, Emory University, 1520 Clifton Road NE, 30322 Atlanta, Georgia

Katherine M. Morrison and Lehana Thabane
Department of Pediatrics, McMaster University, Hamilton, ON, Canada
Population Health Research Institute, McMaster University, Hamilton, ON, Canada

Pam Mackie
Population Health Research Institute, McMaster University, Hamilton, ON, Canada

Geoff D. C. Ball
Department of Pediatrics, University of Alberta, Edmonton, AB, Canada

Josephine Ho
Department of Pediatrics, University of Calgary, Calgary, AB, Canada

Annick Buchholz and Mark Tremblay
Children's Hospital of Eastern Ontario, Ottawa, ON, Canada

Jean-Pierre Chanoine
Department of Pediatrics, University of British Columbia, Vancouver, BC, Canada

Jill Hamilton
The Hospital for Sick Children, Toronto, ON, Canada

Anne-Marie Laberge
Department of Pediatrics, CHU Ste Justine, Montreal, QC, Canada

Laurent Legault
Department of Pediatrics, McGill University, Montreal, QC, Canada

Ian Zenlea
Credit Valley Hospital, Mississauga, ON, Canada

Mahama Saaka, Fusena Ali and Felicia Vuu
University for Development Studies, School of Allied Health Sciences, 1883 Tamale, Ghana

Maryam Barzin, Shayan Aryannezhad, Sara Serahati, Akram Beikyazdi, Majid Valizadeh, Maryam Ziadlou and Farhad Hosseinpanah
Obesity Research Center, Research Institute for Endocrine Sciences, Shahid Beheshti University of Medical Sciences, Tehran, Iran

Fereidoun Azizi
Endocrine Research Center, Research Institute for Endocrine Sciences, Shahid Beheshti University of Medical Sciences, Tehran, Iran

Tao Zhou, Tianli Zheng, Chunping Jiang and Xiaofang Pei
Department of Public Health Laboratory Sciences, West China School of Public Health (No.4 West China Teaching Hospital), Sichuan University, 16#, Section 3, Renmin Road South, Chengdu 610041, Sichuan, People's Republic of China

Jiayi Chen
Department of Public Health Laboratory Sciences, West China School of Public Health (No.4 West China Teaching Hospital), Sichuan University, 16#, Section 3, Renmin Road South, Chengdu 610041, Sichuan, People's Republic of China
Research Center for Occupational Respiratory Diseases, West China School of Public Health (No.4 West China Teaching Hospital), Sichuan University, 16#, Section 3, Renmin Road South, Chengdu 610041, Sichuan, China

Pengwei Hu
Department of Public Health Laboratory Sciences, West China School of Public Health (No.4 West China Teaching Hospital), Sichuan University, 16#, Section 3, Renmin Road South, Chengdu 610041, Sichuan, People's Republic of China
Shenzhen Nanshan Center for Disease Control and Prevention, 95#, Nanshang Road, Shenzhen 518054, Guangdong, China

Lingxu Zhou
Department of Public Health Laboratory Sciences, West China School of Public Health (No.4 West China Teaching Hospital), Sichuan University, 16#, Section 3, Renmin Road South, Chengdu 610041, Sichuan, People's Republic of China
Chongqing Yuzhong District Center for Disease Control and Prevention, 254#, Heping Road, Yuzhong District, Chongqing 400010, China

Lara Nasreddine
Department of Nutrition and Food Science, Faculty of Agricultural and Food Sciences, American University of Beirut, Riad El Solh, Beirut, Lebanon

Hani Tamim and Aurelie Mailhac
Clinical Research Institute, Biostatistics Unit, American University of Beirut Medical Center, Riad El Solh, Beirut, Lebanon

Fadia S. AlBuhairan
Department of Pediatrics and Adolescent Medicine, AlDara Hospital and Medical Center, Riyadh 11431, Saudi Arabia
Department of Population, Family, and Reproductive Health, Bloomberg School of Public Health, Johns Hopkins University, Baltimore, MD, USA

Zhenjiang Bai, Zhong Xu and Jiao Chen
Pediatric Intensive Care Unit, Children's Hospital of Soochow University, Suzhou, JiangSu province, China

Fang Fang, Jian Pan and Jian Wang
Institute of Pediatric Research, Children's Hospital of Soochow University, Suzhou, JiangSu province, China

Yanhong Li
Institute of Pediatric Research, Children's Hospital of Soochow University, Suzhou, JiangSu province, China

Department of nephrology, Institute of pediatric research, Children's Hospital of Soochow University, Suzhou, JiangSu province, China

Chunjiu Lu and Xueqin Wang
Department of nephrology, Institute of pediatric research, Children's Hospital of Soochow University, Suzhou, JiangSu province, China

Hartono Gunardi, Soedjatmiko, Rini Sekartini, Hindra Irawan Satari, Bernie Endyarni Medise and Sri Rezeki S. Hadinegoro
Department of Child Health, Faculty of Medicine, Universitas Indonesia/Dr. Cipto Mangunkusumo Hospital, Jl. Diponegoro No 71, Jakarta 10430, Indonesia

Kusnandi Rusmil, Eddy Fadlyana, Meita Dhamayanti, Rodman Tarigan, Cissy B. Kartasasmita
Department of Child Health, Faculty of Medicine, Padjadjaran University/Dr. Hasan Sadikin Hospital, Jl. Pasteur No 38, Bandung 40161, Indonesia

Rini Mulia Sari and Novilia Sjafri Bachtiar
PT Bio Farma, Jl. Pasteur No 28, Bandung, Jawa Barat, Indonesia

Agnieszka Guzik, Mariusz Drużbicki, Andrzej Kwolek, Grzegorz Przysada, Katarzyna Bazarnik-Mucha, Magdalena Szczepanik and Andżelina Wolan-Nieroda
Institute of Physiotherapy, University of Rzeszów, Warszawska 26 a, 35-205 Rzeszów, Poland

Marek Sobolewski
Rzeszów University of Technology, Rzeszów, Poland

João Valente-dos-Santos
CIDAF (UID/DTP/04213/2016), University of Coimbra, Coimbra, Portugal
Portuguese Foundation for Science and Technology (SFRH/BPD/100470/2014), Lisbon, Portugal
Institute for Biomedical Imaging and Life Sciences (IBILI), Faculty of Medicine, University of Coimbra, Coimbra, Portugal
Faculty of Physical Education and Sport, Lusófona University of Humanities and Technologies, Lisbon, Portugal

Paulo M. Sousa-e-Silva, Luís M. Rama and Manuel J. Coelho-e-Silva
CIDAF (UID/DTP/04213/2016), University of Coimbra, Coimbra, Portugal

Faculty of Sports Sciences and Physical Education, University of Coimbra, Coimbra, Portugal

João P. Duarte
CIDAF (UID/DTP/04213/2016), University of Coimbra, Coimbra, Portugal
Faculty of Sports Sciences and Physical Education, University of Coimbra, Coimbra, Portugal
Portuguese Foundation for Science and Technology (SFRH/BD/101083/2014), Lisbon, Portugal

Óscar M. Tavares
Department of Medical Imaging and Radiation Therapy, School of Health and Technology, Polytechnical Institute of Coimbra, Coimbra, Portugal

José M. Casanova
Faculty of Medicine, University of Coimbra, Coimbra, Portugal

Carlos A. Fontes-Ribeiro
Laboratory of Pharmacology and Experimental Therapeutics, Institute for Biomedical Imaging and Life Sciences (IBILI), Faculty of Medicine, University of Coimbra, Coimbra, Portugal
Center for Neuroscience and Cell Biology (CNC), Institute for Biomedical Imaging and Life Sciences (IBILI), Faculty of Medicine, University of Coimbra, Coimbra, Portugal

Elisa A. Marques
Research Center in Sports Sciences, Health Sciences and Human Development (CIDESD), University Institute of Maia (ISMAI), Maia, Portugal

Daniel Courteix
Laboratory of Metabolic Adaptations to Exercise in Physiological and Pathological conditions (AME2P), Université Clermont Auvergne, Clermont-Ferrand, France
School of Exercise Science, Faculty of Health, Australian Catholic University, East Melbourne, Victoria, Australia

Enio R. V. Ronque and Edilson S. Cyrino
Metabolism, Nutrition, and Exercise Laboratory (GEPEMENE), State University of Londrina (UEL), Londrina, Brazil

Jorge Conde
School of Health and Technology, Polytechnical Institute of Coimbra, Coimbra, Portugal

Katherine Moreau
University of Ottawa, 451 Smyth Road, Ottawa, ON K1H 8M5, Canada

Elizabeth Esselmont and Catherine M. Pound
University of Ottawa, 451 Smyth Road, Ottawa, ON K1H 8M5, Canada
Children's Hospital of Eastern Ontario, 401 Smyth Road, Ottawa, ON K1H 8L1, Canada

Mary Aglipay
Children's Hospital of Eastern Ontario Research Institute, 401 Smyth Road, Ottawa, ON K1H 5B2, Canada

Nanlesta A. Pilgrim and Samuel Kalibala
Population Council, 4301 Connecticut Avenue NW, Suite 280, Washington, DC 20008, USA

Jerry Okal and James Matheka
Population Council, Nairobi, Kenya

Irene Mukui
National AIDS and STI Control Programme, Nairobi, Kenya

Mandy M. Archibald
College of Nursing and Health Sciences, Flinders University, Sturt Road, Bedford Park, Adelaide, SA 5042, Australia

Lisa Hartling and Samina Ali
Department of Pediatrics, Faculty of Medicine and Dentistry, University of Alberta, Edmonton Clinic Health Academy, 11405-87 Avenue, Alberta T6G 1C9, Canada

Vera Caine and Shannon D. Scott
Faculty of Nursing, University of Alberta, Level 3, Edmonton Clinic Health Academy, 11405-87 Avenue, Alberta T6G 1C9, Canada

Rogers Awoh Ajeh
R4D International Foundation, Yaounde, Cameroon

Habakkuk Azinyui Yumo
R4D International Foundation, Yaounde, Cameroon
Center for International Health (CIH), Ludwig-Maximilians-Universität, München, Germany

Akindeh Mbuh Nji
R4D International Foundation, Yaounde, Cameroon
University of Yaounde I, Yaounde, Cameroon

Marcus Beissner and Thomas Loescher
Center for International Health (CIH), Ludwig-Maximilians-Universität, München, Germany

Christopher Kuaban
Faculty of Health Sciences, University of Bamenda, Bamenda, Cameroon

Denis Nash
CUNY Graduate School of Public Health and Health Policy, New York, USA

Anastos Kathryn
Department of Epidemiology and Population Health, Albert Einstein College of Medicine, New York, USA
Montefiore Medical Center, New York, USA

Hailemariam Mekonnen Workie, Abdilahi Sharifnur Sharifabdilahi and Esubalew Muchie Addis
School of Nursing and Midwifery, College of Health and Medical Science, Haramaya University, Harar, Ethiopia

Silvia Maya-Enero, Francesc Botet-Mussons and Josep Figueras-Aloy
Neonatology Service, Hospital Clínic, seu Maternitat, ICGON (Institut Clínic de Ginecologia, Obstetrícia i Neonatologia), Barcelona University, Sabino de Arana, 1, 08028 Barcelona, Spain

Montserrat Izquierdo-Renau, Marta Thió and Martin Iriondo-Sanz
Neonatology Service, Hospital Sant Joan de Déu, BCNatal (Centre de Medicina Maternofetal i Neonatal de Barcelona, Hospital Sant Joan de Déu, Hospital Clínic), Barcelona University, Passeig de Sant Joan de Déu, 2, 08950 Esplugues de Llobregat, Barcelona, Spain

Zeray Baraki, Lidiya Tsegay, Hadgu Gerensea and Awoke Kebede
Department of Neonatal Nursing, School of Nursing, College of Health Sciences, Aksum University, Aksum, Ethiopia

Mebrahtu Abay
Department of Epidemiology and Biostatistics, School of Public Health, College of Health Sciences, Aksum University, Aksum, Ethiopia

Hafte Teklay
Department of Biomedical Sciences, School of Medicine, College of Health Sciences, Aksum University, Aksum, Ethiopia

Conor Keogh and Adam H. Dyer
School of Medicine, Trinity College Dublin, 152-160 Pearse Street, Dublin 2, Ireland

Giorgio Pini, Pietro DiMarco and Ilaria Gemo
Tuscany Rett Center, Ospedale Versilia, 55043 Lido di Camaiore, Italy

Stefania Bigoni
Medical Genetic Unit, Ferrara University Hospital, Ferrara, Italy

Richard Reilly
Trinity Centre for Bioengineering, Trinity College Dublin, Dublin 2, Ireland

Daniela Tropea
Neuropsychiatric Genetics, Trinity Centre for Health Sciences, St. James's Hospital, D8 Dublin, Ireland
Trinity College Institute of Neuroscience (TCIN),Lloyd Building, Trinity College Dublin, Dublin 2, Ireland

Adrita Rahman
Division of Epidemiology and Community Health, School of Public Health,University of Minnesota, 1300 S 2nd Street, Suite 300, Minneapolis, MN55454, USA

Kimberly G. Fulda, Susan F. Franks and Omair Muzaffar
North Texas Primary Care Practice-Based Research Network (NorTex), University of North Texas Health Science Center at Fort Worth, 3500 Camp Bowie Blvd, Fort Worth, TX 76107, USA
Department of Family Medicine, Texas College of Osteopathic Medicine, University of North Texas Health Science Center at Fort Worth, 3500 Camp Bowie Blvd, Fort Worth, TX 76107, USA

Shane I. Fernando
North Texas Primary Care Practice-Based Research Network (NorTex), University of North Texas Health Science Center at Fort Worth, 3500 Camp Bowie Blvd, Fort Worth, TX 76107, USA
Department of Pediatrics, Texas College of Osteopathic Medicine, University of North Texas Health Science Center at Fort Worth, 3500 Camp Bowie Blvd, Fort Worth, TX 76107, USA

Nusrath Habiba
Department of Pediatrics, Texas College of Osteopathic Medicine, University of North Texas Health Science Center at Fort Worth, 3500 Camp Bowie Blvd, Fort Worth, TX 76107, USA

Fengxiu Ouyang and Jun Zhang
Ministry of Education and Shanghai Key Laboratory of Children's Environmental Health, Xinhua Hospital, Shanghai Jiao Tong University School of Medicine, 1665 Kong Jiang Road, Shanghai 200092, China

Fan Jiang
Ministry of Education and Shanghai Key Laboratory of Children's Environmental Health, Xinhua Hospital, Shanghai Jiao Tong University School of Medicine, 1665 Kong Jiang Road, Shanghai 200092, China
Department of Developmental and Behavioral Pediatrics, Shanghai Pediatric Transitional Institution, Shanghai Children's Medical Center affiliated with Shanghai Jiao Tong University School of Medicine, Shanghai 200127, China

Fangbiao Tao
School of Public Health, Anhui Medical University, Hefei 230032, China

Shunqing Xu
Key Laboratory of Environment and Health (HUST), Ministry of Education and Ministry of Environmental Protection, and State Key Laboratory of Environmental Health (Incubation), School of Public Health, Tongji Medical College, Huazhong University of Science and Technology, Wuhan 430074, Hubei, China

Yankai Xia
School of Public Health, Nanjing Medical University, Nanjing 211166, China

Xiu Qiu
Division of Birth Cohort Study, Guangzhou Women and Children's Medical Center, Guangzhou Medical University, Guangzhou 510000, China

Index

www.ingramcontent.com/pod-product-compliance
Lightning Source LLC
Chambersburg PA
CBHW061258190326
41458CB00011B/3702